BLOOD PRESSURE MONITORING
IN CARDIOVASCULAR MEDICINE AND THERAPEUTICS

CONTEMPORARY CARDIOLOGY

CHRISTOPHER P. CANNON
SERIES EDITOR

BLOOD PRESSURE MONITORING IN CARDIOVASCULAR MEDICINE AND THERAPEUTICS

Edited by

WILLIAM B. WHITE, MD

University of Connecticut Health Center
Farmington, CT

Foreword by

Norman M. Kaplan, MD

University of Texas Southwestern Medical School
Dallas, TX

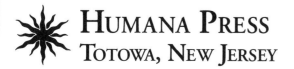
✳ HUMANA PRESS
TOTOWA, NEW JERSEY

Library of Congress Cataloging-in-Publication Data

Blood pressure monitoring in cardiovascular medicine and therapeutics / edited by William B. White
    p.   cm.—(Contemporary cardiology)
  Includes index.
    ISBN 0-89603-840-8 (alk. paper)
    1. Hemodynamic monitoring. 2. Blood pressure. 3. Circadian rhythms. 4. Cardiovascular system--Diseases--Diagnosis. 5. Hypertension. 6. Ambulatory blood pressure monitoring. I. White, William B., 1953- II. Contemporary cardiology (Totowa, N.J.: unnumbered)
    [DNLM: 1. Hypertension--diagnosis. 2. Blood Pressure--physiology. 3. Blood Pressure Monitoring, Ambulatory. 4. Cardiovascular Diseases--physiopathology. 5. Chronobiology. 6. Circadian Rhythm--physiology. 7. Heart Rate. 8. Hypertension--therapy. WG 340 B660 2001]
  RC670.5.H45 B56 2001
  616.1'32075--dc21

00-033588

To B. E. M.

FOREWORD

Blood Pressure Monitoring in Cardiovascular Medicine and Therapeutics provides information that will be especially useful to all who care for hypertensive patients. The various chapters provide a full account of the mounting scientific evidence that blood pressure recordings need to be obtained for proper diagnosis, prognosis, and therapy for these patients. The contributors are each directly involved in clinical studies of home and ambulatory blood pressure monitoring, as well as of the relationship of circadian variations in heart rate and blood pressure to cardiovascular events.

As a longtime observer of the multiple facets of clinical hypertension, I have been greatly impressed with the rapid advances in this area over the last two decades. Out-of-office blood pressure monitoring has grown from a curiosity to a necessity. In order to improve the currently inadequate control of hypertension throughout the world, such monitoring should become routine in the diagnosis and treatment of every patient.

The evidence for the role of out-of-office monitoring that is so well described in *Blood Pressure Monitoring in Cardiovascular Medicine and Therapeutics* should serve as a stimulus for the more widespread adoption of the procedure. Once this is understood, the constraints on the broader clinical use of ambulatory monitoring that now exist in the United States will be lifted as the value of such information becomes more generally recognized. In the meantime, self-recorded home measurements should be more widely utilized. Therapies that ensure 24-hour coverage of hypertension—in particular the early morning surge that is involved in the largest proportion of cardiovascular catastrophies—should surely be more widely prescribed.

In short, it is greatly to be hoped that the information provided in *Blood Pressure Monitoring in Cardiovascular Medicine and Therapeutics* will be rapidly translated into better care of millions of hypertensives, thereby helping to achieve the true goods of medicine: relief of suffering and prolongation of life.

Norman M. Kaplan, MD
Clinical Professor of Medicine
University of Texas
    Southwestern Medical School
Dallas, TX

PREFACE

Blood Pressure Monitoring in Cardiovascular Medicine and Therapeutics is devoted exclusively to the topic of circadian variation in cardiovascular disease, with a special emphasis on hypertension. New research findings on the self and ambulatory monitoring of blood pressure and heart rate have led to marked improvements in our ability to detect various clinical entities in patients with hypertension and vascular diseases. This research is important not only because hypertension is such a common problem among adults in industrialized countries, but also because the cardiovascular morbidity and mortality associated with the hypertensive disease process is so great.

Research efforts in basic and clinical hypertension have continued to accelerate during the past decade. Work devoted to the measurement of blood pressure and blood pressure variability has also been quite productive and a number of major outcome studies were completed during the latter half of the 1990s. In fact, several seminal papers in the field of ambulatory blood pressure monitoring and a number of international consensus conferences have been held in this field during the past three years. Furthermore, the field of cardiovascular chronobiology has also advanced during the 1990s and several therapeutic entities have been developed to provide improved pharmacologic coverage of the circadian rhythms of blood pressure elevations and myocardial ischemia. Thus, it is my premise that a book devoted to research and education involving blood pressure monitoring and cardiovascular chronobiology is needed at this time.

The four chapters in Part I describe the methodology of self and ambulatory blood pressure monitoring in research and clinical practice. Dr. Pickering first presents a comprehensive assessment of the utility of self blood pressure measurement for clinical practice by evaluating the validity of the devices, reviewing the epidemiologic data that are available, and discussing the potential for this technique in clinical trials and for the general management of patients. Drs. James and Mansoor describe the importance of diaries and physical activity recordings in cardiovascular disease. These techniques are crucial for obtaining meaningful data during ambulatory blood pressure recordings in clinical trials. Advances in actigraphy research have allowed investigators to pinpoint changes in physical activity that may directly impact on blood pressure variability. Dr. Anis Anwar and I have written an overview of ambulatory monitoring of the blood pressure, including descriptions of device validation, patterns of blood pressure variation discovered with the advent of this technique, and usefulness of the methodology in clinical hypertension.

The seven chapters in Part II describe a number of advances in our understanding of the pathophysiology of the circadian biology of cardiovascular disorders. Drs. Portaluppi and Smolensky begin with an overview of the chronobiology of blood pressure regulation in humans. This chapter lays the groundwork for the rest of the book with its comprehensive discussion of the progress that has been made in research involving the chronophysiology of human disease with major emphases on hypertension, coronary artery disease, and stroke. Drs. Celis, Staessen, Palatini, and Verdecchia present a number of epidemiologic and prognostic studies that examine the importance of blood pressure and heart rate ability as determinants of cardiovascular morbidity and mortality. During the past five years, the field of ambulatory blood pressure monitoring has advanced dramatically owing to the completion and publication of major prospective studies that relate circadian blood pressure to cardiovascular outcomes. These studies all show that ambulatory blood pressure values are independent predictors of cardiovascular morbidity and mortality. Drs. Sica and Wilson have examined the available data on the role of neurohormonal activity, salt sensitivity, and the renin–angiotensin system on blood pressure variability, especially as it relates to the blunting of the nocturnal decline in pressure.

Drs. Chasen and Muller have reported on the circadian variation of myocardial infarction and cardiovascular death. These authors remind us of the need to identify acute causes of sudden death and myocardial infarction since coronary disease remains the leading cause of death in so many countries around the globe. Drs. Vagaonescu, Phillips, and Tuhrim conclude this section by providing a review of the data on the relationship between blood pressure variability and stroke, as well as discussing the seasonal and daily variations in the incidence of stroke.

The two chapters in Part III focus on the effects of antihypertensive drug therapy on the circadian variation of blood pressure, heart rate, and myocardial ischemia. Dr. Lemmer has reviewed most of the available data on the effects of altering the timing of dosing of drugs (chronopharmacology) on circadian blood pressure variation; he provides data from the perspective of both the chronobiologist and the clinical hypertension specialist. In the final chapter, I have provided an extensive review of the usefulness of ambulatory blood pressure monitoring during antihypertensive drug development. In addition to the obvious benefits of ambulatory blood pressure measurement from a quantitative and statistical point-of-view, ambulatory monitoring elucidates the efficacy of new antihypertensive therapies versus placebo. It also is an important tool to compare antihypertensive agents after registration of the drug has occurred.

The authorities contributing to this text have provided us with a comprehensive up-to-date view of a rapidly advancing field in hypertension and vascular disease. The progress that has been made since Drs. Perloff, Sokolow, and Cowans' seminal study on awake ambulatory blood pressure and cardiovascular outcome 17 years ago is truly remarkable. Just 15–20 years ago, most research in the field of ambulatory monitoring of the blood pressure was descriptive and did not correlate the data to target organ disease. Thus, practicing physicians were not provided with enough useful information to have an impact on the day-to-day management of their patients. As the reader will note, this certainly is no longer the case and ambulatory blood pressure monitoring has matured into an important methodology for clinical hypertension research as well as an important aid in the management of patients with hypertension and vascular disease.

I am truly grateful for all of the outstanding manuscripts provided by my contributors, which greatly simplified the editorial process. I am especially fortunate to have supportive colleagues in the Section of Hypertension and Clinical Pharmacology at the University of Connecticut School of Medicine who helped in the practice and research program so diligently during the production of this book. Diane Webster from the Editorial office of *Blood Pressure Monitoring* at the University of Connecticut Health Center was extremely helpful in helping me to prepare and organize the manuscripts during the course of their production. Paul Dolgert at Humana Press in New Jersey provided his broad expertise and invaluable guidance during the publishing process. Finally, I would like to extend my appreciation to those organizations who provided unrestricted research and educational support during this project.

William B. White, MD

CONTENTS

CONTRIBUTORS

YUSRA ANIS ANWAR, MD • *Assistant Professor, Division of Hypertension and Clinical Pharmacology, Department of Medicine, University of Connecticut School of Medicine, Farmington, CT*

HILDE CELIS, MD • *Hypertension and Cardiovascular Rehabilitation Unit, Department of Molecular and Cardiovascular Research, University of Leuven, Belgium*

CRAIG A. CHASEN, MD • *Assistant Professor of Medicine, University of Kentucky School of Medicine , Lexington, KY*

GARY D. JAMES, PHD • *Research Professor of Nursing, State University of New York, Binghamton, NY*

BJÖRN LEMMER, MD • *Professor of Pharmacology and Toxicology, Ruprecht-Karls-Universität Heidelberg, Germany*

GEORGE A. MANSOOR, MD, MRCP • *Assistant Professor of Medicine, Section of Hypertension and Clinical Pharmacology, University of Connecticut School of Medicine, Farmington, CT*

JAMES E. MULLER, MD • *Professor of Medicine, Harvard Medical School; Chief of Cardiovascular Clinical Research, Massachusetts General Hospital, Boston, MA*

PAOLO PALATINI, MD • *Professor of Medicine, Deparment of Clinical and Experimental Medicine, University of Padova, Padova, Italy*

ROBERT A. PHILLIPS, MD, PHD, FACC • *Hypertension Section and Cardiac Health Program, Cardiovascular Institute and the Department of Neurology, Mt. Sinai Medical Center, New York, NY*

THOMAS G. PICKERING, MD, DPHIL • *Professor of Medicine, Cornell University Medical College, New York, NY*

FRANCESCO PORTALUPPI, MD • *Hypertension Unit, University of Ferrara, Ferrara, Italy*

GIUSEPPE SCHILLACI, MD • *Department of Clinical and Experimental Medicine, University of Perugia Medical School, Perugia, Italy*

DOMENIC A. SICA, MD • *Professor of Medicine and Pharmacology, Medical College of Virginia of Virginia Commonwealth University, Richmond, VA*

MICHAEL H. SMOLENSKY, PHD • *Professor of Physiology, Hermann Center for Chronobiology and Chronotherapeutics, School of Public Health, University of Texas-Houston, TX*

JAN A. STAESSEN, MD, PHD • *Academisch Consulent, Hypertension and Cardiovascular Rehabilitation Unit, Department of Molecular and Cardiovascular Research, Catholic University of Leuven, Belgium*

STANLEY TUHRIM, MD • *Hypertension Section and Cardiac Health Program, Cardiovascular Institute and the Department of Neurology, Mt. Sinai Medical Center, New York, NY*

TUDOR D. VAGAONESCU, MD, PHD • *Hypertension Section and Cardiac Health Program, Cardiovascular Institute and the Department of Neurology, Mt. Sinai Medical Center, New York, NY*

PAOLO VERDECCHIA, MD • *Hypertension and Echocardiography Laboratory, Department of Cardiology, "R. Silvestrini" Hospital, Perugia, Italy*

MICHAEL A. WIENER • *Cardiovascular Institute and the Department of Neurology, Mt. Sinai Medical Center, New York, NY*

WILLIAM B. WHITE, MD • *Professor of Medicine, Section of Hypertension and Clinical Pharmacology, University of Connecticut School of Medicine, Farmington, CT*

DAWN K. WILSON, PHD • *Associate Professor of Medicine, Medical College of Virginia Commonwealth University, Richmond, VA*

I

TECHNIQUES FOR OUT-OF-OFFICE BLOOD PRESSURE MONITORING

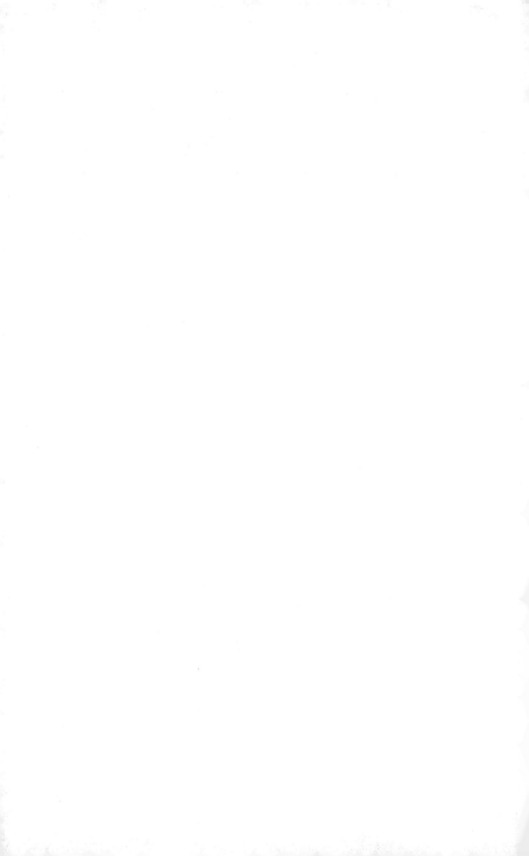

1

Self-Monitoring of Blood Pressure

Thomas G. Pickering, MD, DPHIL

CONTENTS

From: *Contemporary Cardiology:*
Blood Pressure Monitoring in Cardiovascular Medicine and Therapeutics
Edited by: W. B. White © Humana Press Inc., Totowa, NJ

Although the monitoring of antihypertensive treatment is usually performed using blood pressure readings made in the physician's office and having a blood pressure check is by far the commonest reason for visiting a physician, it is neither a reliable nor an efficient process. Thus, physician's measurements are often inaccurate as a result of poor technique, often unrepresentative because of the "white coat" effect, and rarely include more than three readings made at any one visit. It is often not appreciated how great the variations of blood pressure when measured in the clinic can be. In a study conducted by Armitage and Rose in 10 normotensive subjects, two readings were taken on 20 occasions over a 6-wk period by a single trained observer *(1)*. The authors concluded that "the clinician should recognize that the patient whose diastolic pressure has fallen 25 mm from the last occasion has not necessarily changed in health at all; or, if he is receiving hypotensive therapy, that there has not necessarily been any response to treatment." There is also a practical limitation to the number or frequency of clinic visits that can be made by the patient, who may have to take time off work to make the visit.

ADVANTAGES AND LIMITATIONS OF SELF-MONITORING

The potential utility of hypertensive patients having their blood pressures measured at home, either by using self-monitoring or by having a family member make the measurements was first demonstrated in 1940 by Ayman and Goldshine *(2)*. They demonstrated that home blood pressures could be 30 or 40 mmHg lower than the physicians' readings and that these differences might persist over a period of 6 mo. Self-monitoring has the theoretical advantage of being able to overcome the two main limitations of clinic readings: the small number of readings that can be taken and the "white coat" effect. It provides a simple and cost-effective means for obtaining a large number of readings, which are at least representative of the natural environment in which patients spend a major part of their day. Self-monitoring has four practical advantages: It is helpful for distinguishing sustained from "white coat" hypertension; it can assess the response to antihypertensive medication; it may improve patient compliance; and it may reduce costs (Table 1).

The limitations of self-monitoring also need to be specified. First, readings tend to be taken in a relatively relaxed setting, so that they may not reflect the blood pressure occurring during stress; second, patients may misrepresent their readings; and third, occasional patients may become more anxious as a result of self-monitoring.

Although the technique has been readily available for many years, it took a surprisingly long time to find its way into general clinical practice. There has been a recent explosion in the sale of devices for self-monitoring, few of which have been properly validated. Physicians are also endorsing the more widespread use of home monitoring and national guidelines, such as produced by the American Society of Hypertension, are beginning to appear.

Table 1
Advantages and Disadvantages of Self-Monitoring

Advantages	Disadvantages
Elimination of "white coat" effect	Limited prognostic data
Increased number of readings	May underestimate daytime pressure
Assess response to antihypertensive treatment	Patients may misreport readings
Reduced costs	
Improved compliance	

CHOICE OF MONITORS FOR HOME USE

There are three general types of monitor that could be used for self-monitoring: mercury sphygmomanometers, aneroid devices, and a variety of electronic ones. The mercury and aneroid devices require a good degree of manual dexterity and intact hearing, however, which makes them less suitable for elderly patients.

Mercury Sphygmomanometers

These monitors continue to be the gold standard against which all other devices are compared, although this situation is rapidly changing, and many countries have banned the use of mercury, or are about to do so. Although mercury sphygmomanometers can be used for self-monitoring, they are not usually recommended because of the potential dangers of spilled mercury (not a major problem in reality) and because they are relatively expensive and cumbersome.

Aneroid Devices

These devices have been traditionally recommended in the past. They are the least expensive, and there is relatively little to go wrong with them. However, they are subject to the same sources of observer error that beset clinic measurements, and the accuracy of the gage commonly deteriorates over time. In one survey of University Hospital clinics, 80% of aneroid devices were found to be out of calibration (3). They have largely been superseded by electronic devices. They can almost always be managed without problems by younger patients, but they may cause problems in the elderly. The zero setting on the dial should be checked, and also the accuracy of the gage by connecting it to a mercury column with a Y-piece and inflating the cuff to 100 and 200 mmHg.

Electronic Devices

These are available in a bewildering number and are rapidly gaining in popularity. They can take blood pressure from the arm, wrist, or finger, and they may use manual or automatic inflation. Some monitors have memories and printers. They typically operate on the oscillometric method, which requires no microphone, but work by detecting the oscillations of pressure in the cuff as it is gradually deflated. The maximum oscillation occurs at the mean arterial pressure, and systolic and diastolic pressure are derived from the increase and decrease of the pressure waveforms. The method is, in principle, about as accurate as the Korotkoff sound technique. However, the overriding issue with them is the accuracy, which varies greatly from one device to another. Unfortunately, few have been subjected to proper validation (*see* Table 2).

Arm Monitors

Monitors that measure the blood pressure in the brachial artery with a cuff placed on the upper arm continue to be the most reliable and have the additional advantage that the brachial artery pressure is the measure that has been used in all the epidemiological studies of high blood pressure and its consequences.

Wrist Monitors

Wrist monitors are the most recent type to be introduced and have the advantage of being the most convenient to use. They are also very compact. They have the potential advantage that the circumference of the wrist increases relatively little in obese individuals, so that there is less concern about cuff size. The smaller diameter of the wrist in comparison with the upper arm means that less battery power is needed to inflate and also that they cause less discomfort for the patient. A potential disadvantage is that the wrist must be held at the level of the heart when a reading is being taken, which increases the possibility of erroneous readings. Experience with wrist monitors is relatively limited at present, and properly carried out validation studies are few (Table 2).

Finger Monitors

These monitors, which work by a cuff encircling the finger, are easy to use and compact. To control for the hydrostatic effect of the difference between the level of the finger and the heart, it is recommended that the readings be taken with the finger held on the chest over the heart; even so, they are not very accurate *(4)*. Their use should be discouraged.

TESTING AND VALIDATION OF MONITORS

Ideally, the only monitors that should be recommended for use are those that have been tested according to the American (Association for the Advancement of Medical Instrumentation [AAMI]) *(5)* or British (British Hypertension Society [BHS]) *(6,7)* protocols by independent and unaffiliated investigators and that have received a passing grade according to findings published in a peer-reviewed medical journal. Both protocols require the monitor to be compared against readings taken with a mercury sphygmomanometer by trained observers on 85 subjects with varying ages and blood pressures. The two main criteria by which

Table 2
Self-Monitoring Devices Tested by the AAMI and BHS Protocols

Device	Mode	AAMI	BHS
Omron HEM-400C	Oscillometric	Fail	Fail
Philips HP5308	Auscultatory	Fail	Fail
Healthcheck CX-5 060020	Oscillometric	Fail	Fail
Nissei Analog Monitor	Auscultatory	Fail	Fail
Philips HP5306/B	Oscillometric	Fail	Fail
Systema Dr MI-100	Oscillometric	Fail	Fail
Fortec Dr MI-100	Oscillometric	Fail	Fail
Philips HP5332	Oscillometric	Fail	C/A
Nissei DS-175	Oscillometric	Fail	D/A
Omron HEM 705CP	Oscillometric	Pass	B/A
Omron HEM 706	Oscillometric	Pass	B/C
Omron HEM 403C	Oscillometric	Pass	NA
Omron HEM-703-CP	Oscillometric	Pass	NA
Omron R3	Wrist	Pass	NA
Omron M4	Oscillometric	Pass	A/A
Omron MX2	Oscillometric	Pass	A/A
DynaPulse 200m	Oscillometric	Pass	NA

their accuracy is judged are the offset (i.e., the average deviation between the monitor and the observers) and the consistency, measured as the standard deviation (SD) of the differences between the observers' and the devices' readings. So far, relatively few monitors have been tested according to the full BHS and AAMI protocols. Some that have are shown in Table 2. To be considered satisfactory, a device should obtain at least a B grading for both systolic and diastolic pressure from the BHS protocol and a Pass grade from the AAMI.

CHECKING MONITORS FOR ACCURACY

When a patient gets a new monitor, it is a good idea to check it for accuracy, even if it is a model that has passed the above-described AAMI or BHS criteria. With aneroid devices, all that is required is to check the accuracy of the dial. This can be done by connecting the monitor to a mercury column with a Y-tube. If the offset error is more than 5 mmHg the device should be returned. With the electronic monitors, the ideal way to test them is to insert a Y-connector in the tubing between the cuff and the device and to connect a mercury column to the third arm of the Y. Auscultatory readings can then be taken simultaneously with the device's readings, by listening for Korotkoff sounds with a stethoscope placed just below the cuff. If, as is commonly the case, a Y-piece cannot be inserted without cutting the tube, the alternatives are either to take sequential readings with the device and the mercury sphygmomanometer on the same arm or to take

Table 3
Schema for Evaluating
a Home Blood Pressure Monitor in Clinical Practice

Measurement	BP (mmHg)	Device error
1. Mercury	144/88	
2. Monitor	150/96	0/2
3. Mercury	152/94	
4. Monitor	153/91	1/0
5. Monitor	138/86	

readings at approximately the same time as the device on the opposite arm. Although easier to do, the problem with comparing readings from opposite arms is that an ideal monitor would give only 70% of readings within 5 mmHg. This is because differences between the two arms of up to 5 mmHg with any noninvasive technique are quite common.

A practical schema for checking monitors by the sequential–same arm technique is shown in Table 3. A sequence of five readings is taken, starting and ending with a mercury reading, and sandwiching two device readings in between. If the device's reading is between the two adjacent mercury readings, the offset of the device can be considered to be zero, and the device acceptable. If the device's reading is outside the mercury values, it can be subtracted from the closest one to give the offset. With this procedure, an ideal monitor would give about 90% of readings within 5 mmHg. It is recommended that all monitors be rechecked annually.

TECHNIQUE AND ACCURACY
OF HOME BLOOD PRESSURE MONITORING

Until recently, the recommended techniques for self-monitoring were to use either mercury or aneroid devices. For the majority of patients, one of the approved electronic devices is preferable. It is certainly true that patients can be taught to record home blood pressures with reasonable accuracy, but it is important that they receive proper instruction in the technique. This should include cuff placement, body position, when to take readings, and how many. If an aneroid device is used, patients will also need to be taught the auscultatory technique. Training videos are helpful here.

It is often not appreciated that the physical act of inflating one's own sphygmomanometer cuff produces a transient elevation of blood pressure of around 12 mmHg, which lasts about 10 s. As shown in Fig. 1, this increase of blood pressure is the result of the muscular activity involved in cuff inflation rather than to the compressing effects of the cuff on the arm. If the cuff is deflated too quickly, it is possible that the pressure will not have returned to baseline, so that spuriously high systolic pressures may be recorded (8). Patients should therefore be

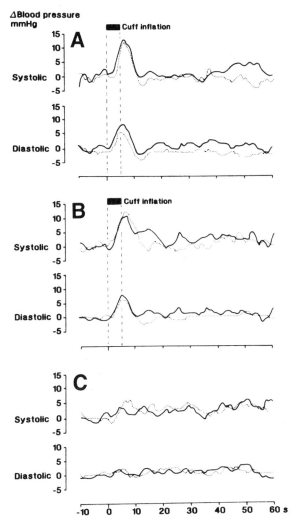

Fig. 1. Continuous noninvasive blood pressure recording from a Finapres monitor. Pressure changes are shown relative to baseline levels. (**A**) Effects of self-inflation of cuff worn on opposite arm; (**B**) Effects of self-inflation of cuff not worn by subject; (**C**) Effects of inflation of cuff by someone else. Reproduced with permission *(8)*.

instructed to inflate the cuff more than 30 mmHg above the expected systolic pressure and to deflate the cuff slowly.

DO PATIENTS PROVIDE
ACCURATE REPORTS OF THEIR READINGS?

Some years ago, a study of home glucose monitoring where patients were asked to keep a written record of their readings using a device that had a memory chip of which the patients were unaware found that there were substantial discrepancies between the readings reported by the patient and the actual readings stored in the devices memory, with a tendency to underreport extreme readings (9). The availability of oscillometric devices with memory chips such as the Omron IC has enabled the same type of study to be done with blood pressure readings, and so far, two publications have appeared describing its use. Both (10,11) found that although the average values reported by the patients were generally similar to the true readings, there were substantial numbers of patients in whom the average discrepancy was at least 10 mmHg systolic and 5 mmHg diastolic, with a greater tendency to underreport than to overreport the values (as had been observed with glucose monitoring).

DEMOGRAPHIC FACTORS INFLUENCING HOME BLOOD PRESSURE LEVELS

Gender

Home blood pressure is lower in women than men, as is true for clinic and ambulatory pressure. This has been well documented by the four large epidemiological studies (see Fig. 2) (12–15). However, the clinic–home differences are generally the same in men and women.

Age

Age also influences home blood pressure, with all studies that evaluated this showing an increase. In the largest population study to investigate this, conducted in Ohasama, Japan, the increase with age was surprisingly small: thus, the average home pressure was 118/71 mmHg for men aged 20–29 and 127/76 mmHg for men over 60 (Fig. 2) (13). The published results almost certainly underestimate the true changes, because subjects on antihypertensive medications were usually excluded and the prevalence of hypertension increases with age. Another age-related change is the increase of blood pressure variability, as shown by the Ohasama study. The day-to-day variability of systolic pressure increases markedly with age in both men and women, but diastolic pressure is little affected, and the variability of heart rate actually decreases.

ENVIRONMENTAL FACTORS INFLUENCING HOME BLOOD PRESSURE LEVELS

As with any other measure of blood pressure, the level of pressure that is recorded during home monitoring shows considerable variability and is likely to be influenced by a number of factors. These are summarized as follows (see Table 4).

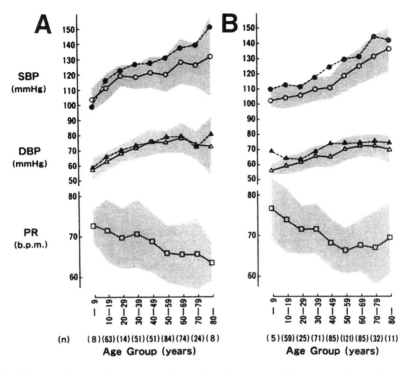

Fig. 2. Effects of age and gender on home blood pressure. Closed symbols show clinic readings; open symbols show home readings. Shaded areas show range (one standard deviation). (**A**) men; (**B**) women. SBP, DBP = systolic and diastolic pressure, respectively; PR = pulse rate. Reproduced with permission *(13)*.

Table 4
Factors Affecting Home Blood Pressure

Increase BP	Decrease BP
Winter	Summer
Caffeine	Exercise
Cigarets	
Stress	
Talking	

Season of the Year

Home blood pressure tends to be up to 5 mmHg higher in the winter than in the summer, at any rate in temperate climates *(16,17)*.

Time of Day

In studies in which morning and evening measurements were both taken, the evening readings tended to be higher for systolic pressure (by about 3 mmHg), but there were no consistent differences for diastolic pressure *(18–20)*. When pressures are recorded in the afternoon, they may be the highest of the day *(21)*. The pattern of blood pressure change over the day may vary considerably from one patient to another, depending on their daily routine.

Day of the Week

There is relatively little information as to whether pressures recorded on non-workdays are the same as on workdays. In a study using ambulatory monitoring of blood pressure, we found that the pressures at home in the evening were consistently higher if the patient had gone to work earlier in the day *(22)*.

Meals

In younger subjects, there is typically an increase of heart rate, a decrease of diastolic pressure, and little change of systolic pressure for up to 3 h after a meal *(23)*. In older subjects, there may be a pronounced fall of both systolic and diastolic pressure after food *(24)*.

Alcohol

Drinking alcohol may increase the heart rate, with small but variable effects on blood pressure in normal subjects, ranging from no significant change to an increase of 5/7 mmHg at 1 h after ingestion of alcohol in an amount equivalent to social drinking *(25–27)*. In hypertensives, blood pressure has been reported to increase within 1 h of drinking alcohol in moderate drinkers (by about 10/4 mmHg) but not in light drinkers. Studies of more prolonged drinking over several days have also shown variable effects in normotensives, with more consistent increases in hypertensives *(27,28)*.

Caffeine

Drinking coffee increases blood pressure but not heart rate. The increase of blood pressure begins within 15 min of drinking coffee and is maximal in about 1 h and may last for as much as 3 h. Typical increases are between 5/9 and 14/10 mmHg *(29,30)*. Drinking decaffeinated coffee produces little or no change *(29)*. These changes are dependent on the level of habitual caffeine intake: In people who do not use it regularly, the changes are much larger than in habitual users (12/10 versus 4/2 mmHg, respectively). Older subjects show greater increases of pressure than younger ones *(31)*.

Smoking

Smoking a cigaret raises both the heart rate and blood pressure. The effect on blood pressure is seen within a few minutes and lasts about 15 min. Coffee and cigarets are often taken together, and a study by Freestone and Ramsay showed that they may have an interactive effect *(32)*. As shown in Fig. 3, smoking a cigaret

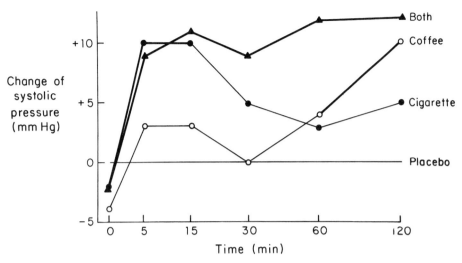

Fig. 3. Changes of systolic pressure occurring after drinking coffee and smoking cigarets, alone and in combination. Adapted with permission *(32)*.

elevated blood pressure for 15 min, whereas drinking coffee had no effect for 1 h, when there was a significant increase. When the cigaret and coffee were taken together, however, there was a significant increase of pressure of about 10 mmHg, which was seen within 5 min, and was still present 2 h later.

Talking

Talking is a potent pressor stimulus that has both physical and psychological components. Reading aloud produces an immediate increase of both systolic and diastolic pressure (by about 10/7 mmHg in normotensive individuals) and of heart rate, with an immediate return to baseline levels once silence is resumed *(33)*. However, reading silently does not affect the pressure. Speaking fast produces a larger increase than speaking slowly *(34)*. Although this is unlikely to be a factor in patients using a stethoscope to record their blood pressure, it could be relevant when a spouse is taking the readings.

Stress

Emotional stress can produce marked elevations of blood pressure that can outlast the stimulus. In a study in which people were asked to recall a situation that made them angry, we found that the blood pressure could increase by more than 20 mmHg and was still elevated by more than 10 mmHg 15 min later. In a survey of hypertensives who were monitoring their blood pressure at the time of the Hashin–Awaji earthquake in Japan in 1995, it was found those who lived within 50 km of the epicenter showed an increase of blood pressure of 11/6 mmHg on the day following the quake, which took a week to wear off, whereas those living farther away showed no change *(34)*.

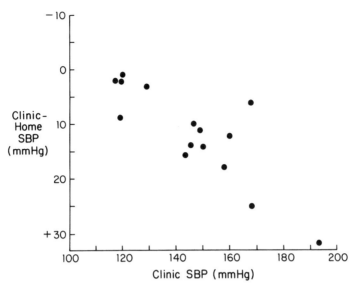

Fig. 4. Differences between systolic pressure between clinic and home in 10 studies; each point represents the average value for one group of subjects.

Exercise

Although blood pressure rises markedly during physical exercise, it rapidly returns to its baseline level when the exercise is completed, and there may be a period of several hours after a bout of heavy exercise when the pressure may remain below the pre-exercise level, a phenomenon described as postexercise hypotension.

COMPARISON OF HOME AND CLINIC PRESSURES

The original observation of Ayman and Goldshine that home pressures are usually much lower than clinic pressures has been confirmed in a number of studies, the results of some of which are plotted in Fig. 4. In patients with severe hypertension, clinic pressures may be 20/10 mmHg higher than home readings, and these clinic readings are also higher than readings taken in hospital by a nurse *(35)*. In mildly hypertensive subjects, the differences are usually smaller (e.g., approx 10/5 mmHg) *(36,37)*. In some cases, home pressures may show a progressive decline with repeated measurement *(19)*, but this is by no means, always seen *(38,39)*.

That the clinic–home difference is the result of the setting rather than the technique of blood pressure measurement can be demonstrated by having patients take readings both at home and in the clinic. In the clinic, it may be found that the patients' and the physicians' readings are very similar and higher than the

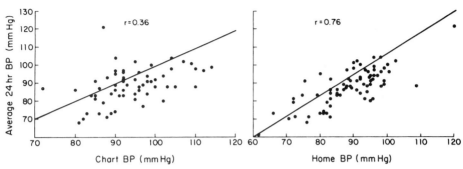

Fig. 5. Comparisons of clinic (chart), home, and 24-h average pressures in 93 patients. Lines of identity are shown. Reproduced with permission *(39)*.

home readings in both cases. In one study *(40)*, patient-measured home blood pressures and physician-measured clinic pressures were compared against intra-arterial pressure measured with the patients lying quietly, and it was found that the patients' measurements were closer to the intra-arterial pressure. Thus, it should not be assumed that when there is a discrepancy between the physician's and the patient's readings that the physician's readings are necessarily right, and the patient's wrong.

In normotensive subjects, the differences between clinic and home pressures are much smaller than in hypertensives *(see* Fig. 4) *(21)*. The discrepancy between home and clinic pressures raises the question of which is closer to the true pressure. As shown in Fig. 5, the home pressures are closer to the 24-h average than the clinic pressures *(39)*. Figure 5 also demonstrates the phenomenon seen in Fig. 10, namely that there is a progressively greater discrepancy between the clinic and the true pressure at higher levels of blood pressure. Other studies have also found that the correlation between home and ambulatory pressure is closer than for either of them with the clinic pressure *(41)*.

REPRODUCIBILITY OF HOME READINGS

Little information has been published on this issue, but it is important. In our study comparing the reproducibility of home, clinic, and ambulatory readings, all measured twice separated by an interval of 2 wk, we found that in hypertensive patients, there was a significant decline of systolic pressure in the clinic over this period, but the home and ambulatory pressures showed no significant change *(42)*. In normotensive subjects, there was no consistent change in any of the three measures of blood pressure. These findings support the notion that the fall of clinic pressure on successive visits is largely spurious and primarily the result of habituation to the clinic setting or regression to the mean. In another study, Jyothinagaram et al. measured clinic and home pressures 3 times over a 4-wk interval in 17 hypertensive patients *(43)*. The clinic pressure fell from 181/97 to

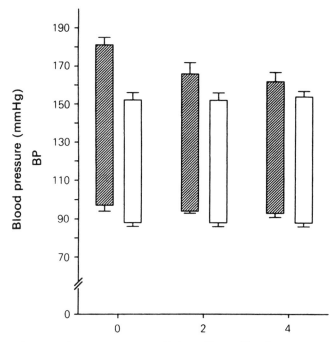

Fig. 6. Effect of repeated measurement on clinic and home blood pressure, each measured on three occasions over a 4-wk period. Despite a progressive decrease of clinic pressure, home pressure remains unchanged. Reproduced with permission *(43)*.

162/93 mmHg, and the home pressure showed no change (153/89 to 154/89 mmHg) (Fig. 6). The superior reproducibility of home and ambulatory measurements may be largely explained by the greater number of readings.

HOME BLOOD PRESSURE IN NORMAL SUBJECTS

As with ambulatory pressure, there is no universally agreed upon upper limit of normal home blood pressure, but there are several studies that have compared home and office levels of pressure, and others that have described average levels in normal populations. There have been four large epidemiological studies of home blood pressure that have attempted to define the normal ranges *(12–15)*.

WHAT IS A NORMAL HOME PRESSURE?

The distribution of blood pressure in the population is in the form of a Gaussian or bell-shaped curve, which tails off at the higher end. Any division into "normal" and "high" blood pressure is thus arbitrary, and this applies whichever measure of blood pressure is used. In practice, the need for such a dividing line is that it can be used as a treatment threshold. One common technique used to define the upper limit of a variable such as blood pressure, which is continuously distributed in the population, is to take the 95th percentile, which defines the upper 5% as being "abnormal." An obvious problem with this is that hypertension affects more than this number; another is that hypertensive individuals are often excluded from population surveys. Thus, if in the population studies described, the upper limit of normal home pressure was defined as the 95th percentile, which is approximately the same as the mean plus 2 standard deviations, the values would range from 137/86 to 152/99 mmHg, which are clearly too high.

An alternative method of defining the upper limit of normal home pressure is to estimate the home pressure equivalent to a clinic pressure of 140/90 mmHg, as has also been done for ambulatory pressure. This was done in the Dubendorf study, where the home reading corresponding to a clinic pressure of 140/90 mmHg was 133/86 mmHg *(12)*. The authors suggested that this should be the norm.

Another method was used by Mengden et al. *(41)*, who took 25 hypertensives with myocardial ischemia documented by thallium scans and found that although the home pressures were consistently lower than the clinic pressures, most were above 135/85 mmHg. They concluded that a cutoff level of 140/90 mmHg would have classified several of these patients as being normotensive.

The American Society of Hypertension recommended that an appropriate level for the upper limit of normal home blood pressure would be 135/85 mmHg *(44)*. This was based on the fact that home pressures tend to be somewhat lower than clinic pressures and is in accord with the findings of the Dubendorf study. It is also consistent with the prospective findings of the Ohasama study, in which home pressures above 138/83 mmHg were found to be associated with increased mortality *(45)*.

HOME MONITORING
FOR THE DIAGNOSIS OF HYPERTENSION

In principle, the prediction of individual risk could be improved by using additional measures of pressure taken outside the clinic setting, such as home or ambulatory readings. At the present time, the evidence supporting this view is supportive but not conclusive. There is substantial evidence that patients whose ambulatory pressures are low in relation to their clinic pressures ("white coat" hypertension) are at reduced risk in comparison with those who have high ambulatory pressure *(46)*. Home blood pressure readings contribute one-third to one-half of the ambulatory readings, depending on whether the nighttime recording is included. One pilot study (described later in this section) has suggested that home pressures may be more predictive than clinic pressures. By providing an inexpensive and convenient method for increasing the number of readings, home monitoring has the potential of reducing the error in assessing the patient's true blood pressure, which is likely to be high if only a few clinic readings are used.

It has been demonstrated that a better estimate of the true blood pressure can be obtained by taking a few readings on several different occasions than by taking a larger number on a single occasion *(1)*.

A potential problem with home pressures is that they usually represent the level of pressure at the lower end of the waking range, when the patient is relatively relaxed. Thus, they do not necessarily provide a good guide to what happens to the patient's pressure when undergoing the stresses of daily life, such as occur during work *(39)*. Although the majority of subjects do show a higher pressure at work than at home, we have encountered others whose pressure is the same or even higher at home. This is particularly true of women with children.

"White coat" hypertension is conventionally diagnosed by comparing the clinic and ambulatory (typically daytime) pressures. Whether or not self-monitored home pressures can be used as substitutes is unresolved. Larkin et al. found that 79% of patients would be classified the same way using either ambulatory or home readings, while the remaining 21% would not *(47)*.

As discussed earlier, clinic pressures tend to decrease with repeated visits. In a study by Padfield et al., clinic blood pressure was measured on three occasions over a period of 4 wk *(48)*. At the first visit, the patients were instructed in the use of home monitors and asked to measure their pressure over 3 d. The pressure at the first clinic visit was higher than the home pressures, but there was no consistent difference between the final clinic pressure and the home pressure. These authors concluded that home blood pressures can be used to predict the results of repeated clinic measurements and, hence, may be of use in making therapeutic decisions.

A potential concern with the use of self-monitoring of blood pressure is that it will increase the patient's anxiety about his or her condition. In practice, this usually has not been found to be the case: In one study, 70% of patients reported that they found the technique to be reassuring *(20)*. Nevertheless, there are some patients who become so obsessed with their blood pressure readings that self-monitoring becomes counterproductive.

HOW OFTEN SHOULD READINGS BE TAKEN?

The frequency of blood pressure readings can be varied according to the stage of the patient's evaluation. In the initial diagnostic period, frequent readings are desirable, but when the blood pressure is stable and well controlled, the frequency can decrease. It is desirable to get readings both in the morning and in the evening, both to detect diurnal variations in blood pressure in the untreated state and to assess the adequacy of treatment in patients who are taking medications. In the newly diagnosed patient, a typical recommendation would be to take three consecutive readings in the morning and three in the evening on 3 d a week for at least 2 wk. It is also helpful to get some readings on weekend days from

Table 5
Correlations Between Measures of Target Organ Damage (TOD)
and Blood Pressure Measured at Home or in the Clinic

			Clinic		Home	
Author (ref.)	*n*	*Measure of TOD*	*SBP*	*DBP*	*SBP*	*DBP*
Kleinert *(39)*	45	LV mass	0.22	0.07	0.45	0.40
Verdecchia *(50)*	34	LV mass	0.30	—	0.41	—
Abe *(51)*	100	Combined	0.42	0.34	0.42	0.33

patients who go out to work during the week, as they are often lower than readings taken on weekdays. It is often convenient to provide the patient with a form on which to enter the readings.

HOME BLOOD PRESSURES,
TARGET ORGAN DAMAGE, AND PROGNOSIS

One of the factors that has limited the acceptance of home blood pressures for clinical decision making has been the lack of prognostic data and, to date, only one large epidemiological study has shown that home blood pressures predict morbidity from cardiovascular disease any better or worse than clinic pressures. There is also limited evidence that home pressure correlates with measures of target organ damage, which can be regarded as surrogate measures for morbidity.

Home Blood Pressure and Target Organ Damage

In an early study of the effects of antihypertensive treatment on blood pressure and left ventricular hypertrophy (LVH), it was reported that regression of LVH evaluated by the electrocardiogram (ECG) correlated more closely with changes of home pressure than with clinic pressure *(49)*. Two studies have indicated that the correlation between echocardiographically determined LVH and blood pressure is better for home than for clinic readings, as shown in Table 5 *(39,50)*. A third study found that target organ damage (retinopathy, ECG–LVH, heart size on the chest X-ray, and serum creatinine) was less pronounced in patients whose home pressure was low in relation to the clinic pressure than in those in whom it was high *(51)*.

Home Blood Pressure and Prognosis

So far, the only study to have published data on the prognostic significance of home blood pressures is a prospective study of 1789 people living in the town of Ohasama, Japan, all of whom were evaluated in 1987 with clinic, home, and ambulatory recordings *(45,52,53)*. For each measure of blood pressure, the subjects were divided into quintiles. As shown in Fig. 7, the survival rate was significantly

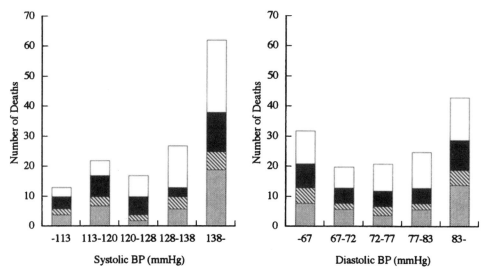

Fig. 7. Death rate according to home blood pressure level from the Ohasama study. Shaded bars = cerebrovascular disease; striped bars = heart disease; solid bars = cancer; open bars = other causes. Reproduced with permission *(52)*.

lower for people whose initial home pressure was above 138 mmHg systolic and 83 mmHg diastolic pressure *(52)*. As also shown in the figure, the consequences of a high clinic pressure were less clear. There was some suggestion from these data of a J-shaped curve, which is a paradoxical increase of mortality at low home blood pressures; the actual numbers were too small to be sure of this, however, and it was not observed for the screening blood pressures.

HOME MONITORING FOR THE EVALUATION OF ANTIHYPERTENSIVE TREATMENT

When patients have their antihypertensive medication initiated or changed, it is necessary to measure their blood pressure on repeated occasions. The validity of using home readings for monitoring the effects of treatment on blood pressure has been well established in a number of studies that have compared the response to treatment evaluated by clinic, home, and ambulatory pressures. It is important to stress that treatment does not eliminate the clinic–home difference ("white coat" effect). Home monitoring is also ideal for evaluating the time-course of the treatment response. As shown in Fig. 8, for a drug with a relatively rapid onset of action like enalapril, the maximal fall of blood pressure is seen within 1 d of starting the drug and the pressure returns to the pretreatment level quickly *(54)*.

Despite the general parallelism between clinic and home blood pressures during treatment, there may be a considerable discrepancy between the two in individual patients. In a study of 393 patients treated with trandalopril *(55)*, the

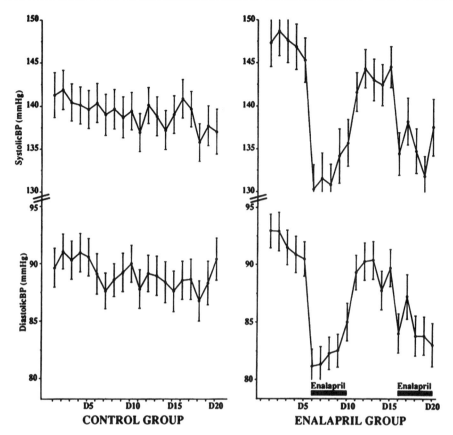

Fig. 8. Left-hand panel: Home blood pressure in a control group of patients with no intervention. Right-hand panel: Response to enalapril in one patient who took drug twice for 4 d each. Reproduced with permission *(54)*.

correlation coefficient between the clinic and home pressure response, although highly significant, was only 0.36. The slope of the line relating the two was also rather shallow and indicated that a decrease of 20 mmHg in clinic pressure was, on average, associated with a decrease of home pressure of only 10 mmHg. This discrepancy may, in part, be attributable to the inclusion of patients with "white coat" hypertension, in whom drug treatment tends to lower clinic pressure while having little or no effect on ambulatory or home pressures.

HOW MANY READINGS ARE NEEDED TO ESTABLISH THE EFFICACY OF TREATMENT?

It is helpful to know what the minimum number of home readings should be to establish a stable level when assessing the response to antihypertensive treatment, whether it be using medications or nonpharmacological treatment. To

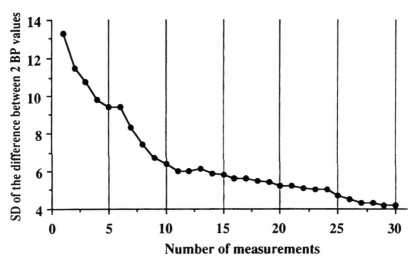

Fig. 9. Reduction of the SD of the difference between two mean levels of home blood pressure as a result of increasing the number of readings used to define each level. Reproduced with permission *(54)*.

determine the influence of the number of readings used to define the difference between two average blood pressure levels (which might be before and after treatment), Chatellier et al. instructed patients to take three readings in the morning and three in the evening over a period of 3 wk *(54)*. They then calculated the standard deviation of the difference between two means derived from increasing numbers of individual readings over two 10-d periods. As shown in Fig. 9, the standard deviation (SD) of the difference between the two means decreased progressively as larger numbers of individual readings were used to define each of the two means. About 80% of this reduction was obtained when 15 readings were used to define a mean, and including a larger number of readings brought little additional precision. The authors concluded that three readings taken over 5 d (preferably at the same time of day) should be sufficient to detect a drug-induced fall of blood pressure.

N-OF-1 TRIALS
FOR IDENTIFYING OPTIMAL TREATMENT

The increasing number of drugs available for the treatment of hypertension has done relatively little to improve the success of controlling hypertension in the population. In part, this may be because people vary widely in the degree to which they respond to any one drug, and there is no good way of predicting which drug is best for which patient. Thus, it is largely a matter of trial and error, which will require a large number of clinic visits. One potential way of improving this situation is using home monitoring for "*N*-of-1" trials, in which each patient is given a number of different medications given in sequence *(54)*. Because individual drugs vary in the time needed to achieve their full effect on blood pressure, it is likely that a minimum of 3 wk would be needed to test each drug, although the blood pressure readings need only be taken for the last few days of each period.

USE IN CLINICAL TRIALS

One of the advantages of using home monitoring rather than traditional clinic measurements in trials of antihypertensive drugs is that fewer patients should be needed to show an effect. The greater statistical power inherent in the use of home recordings rather than clinic recordings for the evaluation of antihypertensive medications was well illustrated in a study by Menard et al. *(56)*. It was estimated that in order to detect a treatment effect of 5 mmHg, 27 patients would be needed if clinic blood pressures were used for the evaluation, but only 20 patients if home pressures were used. Home monitoring can be a useful way of estimating the trough:peak (T:P) ratio. Morning readings are taken just before the dose (trough), and evening readings (or midday) approximate the peak effects for many long-acting drugs. Menard et al. used this procedure to evaluate the effects of enalapril and found a T:P ratio of 77%, which is similar to estimates made using ambulatory monitoring *(57)*.

EFFECTS ON COMPLIANCE

Several studies have examined the effects of home monitoring on compliance with medication *(58,59)*. This has been assessed both by pill counts and by blood pressure control. Although the results have been mixed, the general conclusion is that compliance is improved, particularly in patients who are least compliant in the beginning. Having a family member perform the monitoring may also help.

COST-EFFECTIVENESS OF HOME MONITORING

Appel and Stason, whose review formed the basis of the American College of Physicians Position Statement, stated that the societal cost of performing self-monitoring on all 50 million hypertensives in the United States (at a cost of $50 per test) would be $2.5 billion *(60)*. However, these figures assumed that there would be no savings resulting from these procedures, which is almost certainly not the case. There is some evidence that self-monitoring may be cost-effective. In a randomized study conducted by the Kaiser Permanente Medical Care Program in San Francisco *(61)*, 430 patients with mild hypertension, most of whom were taking antihypertensive medications, were randomized either to a usual care group or to use self-monitoring. At the end of 1 yr, the costs of care (which included physician visits, telephone calls, and laboratory test) were 29% lower in the self-monitoring group, and the blood pressure was slightly better controlled in the home monitoring group. The vast majority of both patients and their physicians considered that the self-monitoring procedure was worthwhile.

FUTURE TRENDS

It is likely that the use of self-monitoring using electronic devices for the routine evaluation of hypertensive patients will continue to grow in the foreseeable future. Because the readings are available in electronic form, there is, in principle, no reason why the patient should have to write them down at all. There are several ways by which readings can be stored and processed. Some devices have a printer attached, which at least avoids observer bias. Others have a memory, from which the data can be downloaded (e.g., into the physician's computer, as in the Omron IC) or transmitted by a telephone modem link to a central computer (62,63) or connected to the patient's own personal computer. The establishment of a two-way connection between the patient and the caregiver offers a whole new way of managing hypertensive patients, which is likely to revolutionize hypertension care over the next few years.

REFERENCES

1. Armitage P, Rose GA. The variability of measurements of casual blood pressure. I. A laboratory study. Clin Sci 1966;30:325–335.
2. Ayman P, Goldshine AD. Blood pressure determinations by patients with essential hypertension I. The difference between clinic and home readings before treatment. Am J Med Sci 1940; 200:465–474.
3. Bailey RH, Knaus VL, Bauer JH. Aneroid sphygmomanometers: an assessment of accuracy at a University Hospital and clinics. Arch Intern Med 1991;151:1409–1412.
4. Sesler JM, Munroe WP, McKenney JM. Clinical evaluation of a finger oscillometric blood pressure device. DICP 1991;25:1310–1314.
5. White WB, Berson AS, Robbins C, Jamieson MJ, Prisant LM, Roccella E, et al. National standard for measurement of resting and ambulatory blood pressures with automated sphygmomanometers. Hypertension 1993;21:504–509.
6. O'Brien E, Petrie J, Littler W, De Swiet M, Padfield PL, O'Malley K, et al. The British Hypertension Society protocol for the evaluation of automated and semiautomated blood pressure measuring devices with special reference to ambulatory systems [see comments]. J Hypertens 1990;8:607–619.
7. O'Brien E, Atkins N, Staessen J. State of the market. A review of ambulatory blood pressure monitoring devices. Hypertension 1995;26:835–842.
8. Veerman DP, Van Montfrans GA, Wieling W. Effects of cuff inflation on self-recorded blood pressure. Lancet 1990;335:451–453.
9. Mazze RS, Shamoon H, Pasmantier R, Lucido D, Murphy J, Hartmann K, et al. Reliability of blood glucose monitoring by patients with diabetes mellitus. Am J Med 1984;77:211–217.
10. Myers MG. Self-measurement of blood pressure at home: the potential for reporting bias. Blood Pressure Monit 1998;3(Suppl 1):S19–S22.
11. Mengden T, Hernandez Medina RM, Beltran B, Alvarez E, Kraft K, Vetter H. Reliability of reporting self-measured blood pressure values by hypertensive patients. Am J Hypertens 1998;11:1413–1417.

12. Weisser B, Grune S, Burger R, Blickenstorfer H, Iseli J, Michelsen SH, et al. The Dubendorf Study: a population-based investigation on normal values of blood pressure self-measurement. J Hum Hypertens 1994;8:227–231.

13. Imai Y, Satoh H, Nagai K, Sakuma M, Sakuma H, Minami N, et al. Characteristics of a community-based distribution of home blood pressure in Ohasama in northern Japan. J Hypertens 1993;11:1441–1449.

14. Staessen JA, Fagard R, Lijnen P, Thijs L, van Hulle S, Vyncke G, et al. Ambulatory blood pressure and blood pressure measured at home: progress report on a population study. J Cardiovasc Pharmacol 1994;23(Suppl 5):S5–S11.

15. Mejia AD, Julius S, Jones KA, Schork NJ, Kneisley J. The Tecumseh Blood Pressure Study. Normative data on blood pressure self-determination. Arch Intern Med 1990;150:1209–1213.

16. Minami J, Kawano Y, Ishimitsu T, Yoshimi H, Takishita S. Seasonal variations in office, home and 24 h ambulatory blood pressure in patients with essential hypertension. J Hypertens 1996;14:1421–1425.

17. Imai Y, Munakata M, Tsuji I, Ohkubo T, Satoh H, Yoshino H, et al. Seasonal variation in blood pressure in normotensive women studied by home measurements. Clin Sci (Colch) 1996;90: 55–60.

18. Welin L, Svardsudd K, Tibblin G. Home blood pressure measurements—feasibility and results compared to office measurements. The study of men born in 1913. Acta Med Scand 1982;211:275–279.

19. Laughlin KD, Fisher L, Sherrard DJ. Blood pressure reductions during self-recording of home blood pressure. Am Heart J 1979;98:629–634.

20. Burns-Cox CJ, Rees JR, Wilson RS. Pilot study of home measurement of blood pressure by hypertensive patients. Br Med J 1975;3:80.

21. Beckman M, Panfilov V, Sivertsson R, Sannerstedt R, Andersson O. Blood pressure and heart rate recordings at home and at the clinic. Evidence for increased cardiovascular reactivity in young men with mild blood pressure elevation. Acta Med Scand 1981;210:97–102.

22. Pieper C, Warren K, Pickering TG. A comparison of ambulatory blood pressure and heart rate at home and work on work and non-work days. J Hypertens 1993;11:177–183.

23. Kelbaek H, Munck O, Christensen NJ, Godtfredsen J. Central haemodynamic changes after a meal. Br Heart J 1989;61:506–509.

24. Peitzman SJ, Berger SR. Postprandial blood pressure decrease in well elderly persons. Arch Intern Med 1989;149:286–288.

25. Larbi EB, Cooper RS, Stamler J. Alcohol and hypertension. Arch Intern Med 1983;143:28–29.

26. Gould L, Zahir M, DeMartino A, Gomprecht RF. The cardiac effects of a cocktail. JAMA 1971;218:1799–1802.

27. Potter JF, Watson RDS, Skan W, Beevers DG. The pressor and metabolic effects of alcohol in normotensive subjects. Hypertension 1986;8:625–631.

28. Malhotra H, Mehta SR, Mathur D, Khandelwal PD. Pressure effects of alcohol in normotensive and hypertensive subjects. Lancet 1985;ii:584–586.

29. Smits P, Thien T, Van't Laar A. Circulatory effects of coffee in relation to the pharmacokinetics of caffeine. Am J Cardiol 1985;56:958–963.

30. Robertson D, Frolich JC, Carr RK. Effects of caffeine on plasma renin activity, catecholamines and blood pressure. N Engl J Med 1978;298:181–186.

31. Izzo JLJ, Ghosal A, Kwong T, Freeman RB, Jaenike JR. Age and prior caffeine use alter the cardiovascular and adrenomedullary responses to oral caffeine. Am J Cardiol 1983;52:769–773.

32. Freestone S, Ramsay LE. Effect of coffee and cigarette smoking on the blood pressure of untreated and diuretic-treated hypertensive patients. Am J Med 1982;73:348–353.

33. Lynch JJ, Long JM, Thomas SA, Malinow KL, Katcher AH. The effects of talking on the blood pressure of hypertensive and normotensive individuals. Psychosom Med 1981;43: 25–33.

34. Friedmann E, Thomas SA, Kulick-Ciuffo D, Lynch JJ, Suginohara M. The effects of normal and rapid speech on blood pressure. Psychosom Med 1982;44:545–553.
35. Corcoran AC, Dustan HP, Page IH. The evaluation of antihypertensive procedures, with particular reference to their effects on blood pressure. Ann Intern Med 1955;43:1161–1177.
36. Laughlin KD, Sherrard DJ, Fisher L. Comparison of clinic and home blood pressure levels in essential hypertension and variables associated with clinic–home differences. J Chronic Dis 1980;33:197–206.
37. Badskjaer J, Nielsen PE. Clinical experience using home readings in hypertensive subjects (indirect technique). Acta Med Scand 1982;670(Suppl):89–95.
38. Kenny RA, Brennan M, O'Malley K, O'Brien E. Blood pressure mesaurements in borderline hypertension. J Hypertens 1987;5(Suppl 5):483–485.
39. Kleinert HD, Harshfield GA, Pickering TG, Devereux RB, Sullivan PA, Marion RM, et al. What is the value of home blood pressure measurement in patients with mild hypertension? Hypertension 1984;6:574–578.
40. Kjeldsen SE, Moan A, Petrin J, Weder AB, Zweifler AJ, Julius S. Evaluation of self-measured home vs. clinic intra-arterial blood pressure. Blood Pressure 1993;2:28–34.
41. Mengden T, Schwartzkopff B, Strauer BE. What is the value of home (self) blood pressure monitoring in patients with hypertensive heart disease? Am J Hypertens 1998;11:813–819.
42. James GD, Pickering TG, Yee LS, Harshfield GA, Riva S, Laragh JH. The reproducibility of average ambulatory, home, and clinic pressures. Hypertension 1988;11:545–549.
43. Jyothinagaram SG, Rae L, Campbell A, Padfield PL. Stability of home blood pressure over time. J Hum Hypertens 1990;4:269–271.
44. Pickering T. Recommendations for the use of home (self) and ambulatory blood pressure monitoring. American Society of Hypertension Ad Hoc Panel. Am J Hypertens 1996;9:1–11.
45. Ohkubo T, Imai Y, Tsuji I, Nagai K, Ito S, Satoh H, et al. Reference values for 24-hour ambulatory blood pressure monitoring based on a prognostic criterion: the Ohasama Study. Hypertension 1998;32:255–259.
46. Verdecchia P, Porcellati C, Schillaci G, Borgioni C, Ciucci A, Battistelli M, et al. Ambulatory blood pressure. An independent predictor of prognosis in essential hypertension. Hypertension 1994;24:793–801. Erratum: 1995;25(3):462.
47. Larkin KT, Schauss SL, Elnicki DM. Isolated clinic hypertension and normotension: false positives and false negatives in the assessment of hypertension. Blood Pressure Monit 1998; 3:247–254.
48. Padfield PL, Lindsay BA, McLaren JA, Pirie A, Rademaker M. Changing relation between home and clinic blood-pressure measurements: do home measurements predict clinic hypertension? Lancet 1987;2:322–324.
49. Ibrahim MM, Tarazi RC, Dustan HP, Gifford RWJ. Electrocardiogram in evaluation of resistance to antihypertensive therapy. Arch Intern Med 1977;137:1125–1129.
50. Verdecchia P, Bentivoglia M, Providenza M, Savino K, Corea L. Reliability of home self-recorded arterial pressure in essential hypertension in relation to the stage of the disease. In: Germano G, ed. Blood Pressure Recording in the Clinical Management of Hypertension. Ediziono Pozzi, Rome, 1985, pp. 40–42.
51. Abe H, Yokouchi M, Saitoh F, Deguchi F, Kimura G, Kojima S, et al. Hypertensive complications and home blood pressure: comparison with blood pressure measured in the doctor's office. J Clin Hypertens 1987;3:661–669.
52. Tsuji I, Imai Y, Nagai K, Ohkubo T, Watanabe N, Minami N, et al. Proposal of reference values for home blood pressure measurement: prognostic criteria based on a prospective observation of the general population in Ohasama, Japan. Am J Hypertens 1997;10:409–418.
53. Imai Y, Ohkubo T, Tsuji I, Nagai K, Satoh H, Hisamichi S, et al. Prognostic value of ambulatory and home blood pressure measurements in comparison to screening blood pressure measurements: a pilot study in Ohasama. Blood Pressure Monit 1996;1(Suppl 2):S51–S58.

54. Chatellier G, Bobrc G, Menard J. Feasibility study of N-of–1 trials with blood pressure self monitoring in hypertension. Hypertension 1995;25:294–301.

55. Zannad F, Vaur L, Dutrey-Dupagne C, Genes N, Chatellier G, Elkik F, et al. Assessment of drug efficacy using home self-blood pressure measurement: the SMART study. Self Measurement for the Assessment of the Response to Trandolapril. J Hum Hypertens 1996;10:341–347.

56. Menard J, Serrurier D, Bautier P, Plouin PF, Corvol P. Crossover design to test antihypertensive drugs with self-recorded blood pressure. Hypertension 1988;11:153–159.

57. Menard J, Chatellier G, Day M, Vaur L. Self-measurement of blood pressure at home to evaluate drug effects by the trough: peak ratio. J Hypertens 1994;12(Suppl):S21–S25.

58. Johnson AL, Taylor DW, Sackett DL, Dunnett CW, Shimizu AG. Self-recording of blood pressure in the management of hypertension. Can Med Assoc J 1978;119:1034–1039.

59. Friedman RH, Kazis LE, Jette A, Smith MB, Stollerman J, Torgerson J, et al. A telecommunications system for monitoring and counseling patients with hypertension. Impact on medication adherence and blood pressure control. Am J Hypertens 1996;9:285–292.

60. Appel LJ, Stason WB. Ambulatory blood pressure monitoring and blood pressure self-measurement in the diagnosis and management of hypertension. Ann Intern Med 1993;118:867–882.

61. Soghikian K, Casper SM, Fireman BH, Hunkeler EM, Hurley LB, Tekawa IS, et al. Home blood pressure monitoring. Effect on use of medical services and medical care costs. Med Care 1992;30:855–865.

62. Mooney P, Dalton KJ, Swindells HE, Rushant S, Cartwright W, Juett D. Blood pressure measured telemetrically from home throughout pregnancy. Am J Obstet Gynecol 1990;163:30–36.

63. Menard J, Linhart A, Weber JL, Paria C, Herve C. Teletransmission and computer analysis of self-recorded measurements at home. Blood Pressure Monit 1996;1(Suppl 2):S63–S67.

2

Evaluation of Journals, Diaries, and Indexes of Worksite and Environmental Stress

Gary D. James, PhD

INTRODUCTION

Noninvasive ambulatory blood pressure monitors are being increasingly used in the clinical evaluation of hypertension. With this technology, blood pressures are measured at fixed time intervals over the course of a single day (up to 24 h) while the patient goes about typical daily activities, including sleep. There is a substantial intraindividual variation in ambulatory blood pressure measurements that is not cyclical or repetitive. It occurs as a consequence of homeostatic circulatory processes that act to maintain adequate blood flow to body tissues when changes in the internal physiological and external environmental conditions

From: *Contemporary Cardiology:*
Blood Pressure Monitoring in Cardiovascular Medicine and Therapeutics
Edited by: W. B. White © Humana Press Inc., Totowa, NJ

occur *(1,2)*. Thus, cardiovascular adjustments are continuously made every second of every day as people change their behavior to adapt to recurrent and sometimes patterned stressors that pervade and define their lifestyles. There are many behavioral and lifestyle factors that will increase the level of ambulatory blood pressure measurements *(1,3–6)*. If circumstances that raise blood pressure are experienced or sampled with a high frequency during an ambulatory monitoring in a patient with normal blood pressure, it is possible that they may be incorrectly diagnosed with hypertension *(2)*.

In clinically evaluating ambulatory blood pressures, it is critical to have appropriate and sufficient information about the conditions of measurement in order to differentiate adaptive physiological responses from true cardiovascular pathology. Much of this information is collected from diaries and questionnaires that are filled out at the time of the monitoring. The primary objective of this brief overview is to describe and evaluate the reported relationships between ambulatory blood pressure measurements and the psychological, behavioral, and environmental data collected in diaries and questionnaires during the course of ambulatory monitoring. How behavioral and environmental information can be usefully employed in evaluating ambulatory blood pressure measurements in the diagnosis and treatment of hypertension will also be briefly discussed.

DETERMINING THE CONDITIONS
OF AMBULATORY MEASUREMENTS

There are two ways to determine what the environmental conditions are during a noninvasive ambulatory blood pressure monitoring. The first is through direct observation. Specifically, a person other than the monitored patient continuously watches and records in a journal the ambient conditions of each individual blood pressure measurement. This approach is necessary when small children or demented elderly are being evaluated *(7)*, but it is really only practical when the patients are institutionalized. A drawback of this method of environmental assessment is that data concerning personal factors such as the patient's physiological or psychological state cannot be collected.

The second method involves having the patient self-report the conditions in a diary. In this scenario, the patient writes down the various parameters that are manifest when the blood pressure cuff inflates, including both personal and environmental factors. Several diary formats have been devised for patients to report the circumstances when their pressures are being taken (see, for example, refs. *1, 3, 4, 8,* and *9*).

For clinical (and analytic) purposes, the best diaries are those that are simple and straightforward and are easy for a patient to complete *(1)*. The reason is that every time the monitor takes a pressure, the patient is writing something down. If too much information is required or the form is overly complex, the informa-

NAME _____

Location Codes
H=Home
W=Work
M=Miscellaneous

Position Codes
S=Sitting
U=Upright/Standing
R=Reclining

Mood Codes
Place a number from 1 (low) to
10 (high) in the appropriate box
(Skip if mood is neutral)

| TIME | LOCATION | POSITION | MOOD | | | | ACTIVITIES |
			HAPPY	SAD	ANGRY	ANXIOUS	

Fig. 1. A useful ambulatory blood pressure diary for clinical practice.

tion gathered is likely to be spotty, incomplete, or may even affect the measurements themselves, in that filling out a complicated diary may itself be a stressor. An example of a diary that has been successfully used clinically over the past 15 yr in the Hypertension Center at Cornell Medical College is shown in Fig. 1.

Thorough patient instruction is also important in the use of diaries as a means for assessing the conditions of blood pressure measurements because insufficient or superfluous overreporting of the circumstances will affect the ability to properly analyze the blood pressure measurements. Pickering *(1)* has discussed several additional issues with ambulatory blood pressure diary design and use that are relevant to the evaluation of the data collected with them as well. These include the content and form of the diary, the validity and reliability of self-reported behavior, and the influence of self-reporting behavior on actual behavior. However, if adequate instruction is provided to the patient before the monitoring, the information collected in diaries should reasonably describe the approximate conditions of each ambulatory blood pressure measurement and should be useful in analyzing and interpreting the total data.

AMBULATORY BLOOD PRESSURE VARIATION AND PATHOLOGY DETERMINATION

Hypertension (high blood pressure) is defined from an arbitrary cut-point in the distribution of seated blood pressure measurements *(10,11)*. Although the definition has expanded to include severity *(11,12)*, its diagnosis is still confirmed from standardized seated blood pressure measurements that persistently exceed the threshold of 140/90 mmHg.

The variation in blood pressure measurements that occurs among patients as they go about their daily activity, even when sampled intermittently, can be viewed as an estimate of the cardiovascular adaptation to environmental challenges that are extant when the measurements are taken *(6)*. In evaluating the pathology in these ambulatory blood pressures, the question that should be asked is whether the magnitude of the measurements is appropriate for the circumstances, not whether or how often they transgress the arbitrary "hypertension Rubicon" (140/90 mmHg).

It is also not entirely appropriate to simply examine the average of all the measurements taken to see if it is excessive. As previously noted, in outpatients allowed to follow their daily routines, the average may be calculated from measurements taken under circumstances that tend to raise pressure; thus, the value on which a hypertension diagnosis would be based may actually be normal for the circumstances and not pathological. Interestingly, despite this fact, there are many efforts underway to find the normalcy–pathology dividing line with regard to ambulatory blood pressure averages *(13–16)*.

DETERMINING AMBULATORY BLOOD PRESSURE RESPONSES

Over the past 15 yr, many factors that form a part of daily life have been found to affect the diurnal variation of ambulatory blood pressure. Before presenting data on the effects of diary-reported circumstances on ambulatory blood pressure measurements, a brief discussion of methodological issues concerning how the blood pressure measurements are analyzed is needed. In a study sample (or, more generally, a population of subjects), every individual will have a different experience and mix of diary-reported factors (locations, postures, moods, and activities). Thus, in order to analyze this uneven data, certain statistical assumptions must be made *(3,4,17)*. Although nearly every study that has examined diary data for the purpose of estimating the effects of reported conditions has found similar results (remarkably), the exact estimates vary. This variation either occurs as a consequence of differences in the statistical assumptions about the data or, more likely, they occur because of differences in the populations studied *(3)*. The most problematic and contentious statistical issue in analyzing individual ambulatory blood pressure measurements is accounting for the between-person variance when estimating the effects of within-person parameters such as posture, location, and mood *(4,18,19)*. Person effects also need to be considered when evaluating the influence of risk factors such as gender and body mass index, which are characteristics of the person, not each individual blood pressure measurement *(4,20)*. A protracted detailed discussion of the merits of various statistical approaches is beyond the scope of this brief review, but it should be realized that every approach has its limitations. However, it is probably true that as long as reasonable assumptions concerning the partitioning of daily blood pressure variance are made and not violated, the estimates of the calculated factor effects will be valid.

A final consideration in evaluating the magnitude of the effects of various environmental, ecological, or psychological factors on any given blood pressure measurement is knowing the referent value from which the effect is calculated; that is, when one states that being at work elevates blood pressure by some amount, that amount will depend on the "standard value" with which it is being compared. Values that have been used include the average sleep blood pressure *(21)*, the average 24-h ambulatory pressure of the individual *(18)*, the average blood pressure of the entire population studied *(4)*, and the average seated blood pressure while at home *(20)*. Values presented in this discussion will be relative to the individual's average 24-h ambulatory pressure and will be calculated using the method of James et al. *(18)*, assuming a daily standard deviation of 10.

DIARY FACTORS ASSOCIATED WITH AMBULATORY BLOOD PRESSURE VARIATION

Virtually all the studies that have examined the effects of diary-reported factors on blood pressure have been conducted on sample groups from Western societies *(3)*. Most of the investigations that have examined the effects of work on ambulatory blood pressures (i.e., refs. *8*, *19*, and *22–27*) found that the average pressure at the place of employment is higher than the average pressure in all other daily venues. The work-related elevation in blood pressure is also independent of time of day, as the average pressure at the place of employment is elevated even in night-shift workers *(28–31)*.

Table 1
Average[a] Effects of Activity on Ambulatory
Blood Pressures (mmHg from 24-h Mean)

Activity	Systolic	Diastolic
Talking	5.1	5.9
Writing	3.3	6.7
Physical activity	8.6	7.4
Eating	6.3	7.0
Relaxing	−2.0	−3.6
Dressing	7.5	9.7
Traveling	6.5	5.5

[a]Assumes a 24-h standard deviation of 10.
Source: Modified from ref. *33.*

Reported posture has also been found to have a substantial effect on ambulatory blood pressures. Standing is associated with the highest pressures and reclining (while awake) with the lowest pressure during the day *(4,18,20,21,24).* Postural effects, however, covary with activity, as many activities occur in a single posture. Research examining the effects of reported activity on ambulatory pressure show that physical activities such as doing household chores tend to elevate pressures the most, whereas activities such as reading or writing, which require mental effort, or other activities such as eating, watching TV, or talking have less effect *(8,19,32,33,33a).* Table 1 presents estimates of the effects of several activities on blood pressure levels.

Personality may further interact with activity in affecting blood pressure such that individuals whose behavior is characterized as Type A *(34)* (manifested as impatience, chronic time urgency, enhanced competitiveness, aggressive drive, and an inclination toward hostility) may have larger diastolic pressure increases than other non-Type-A individuals during activities such as driving a car, talking, walking, desk work, and attending business meetings. Finally, in one study, physical activity was estimated from motion-sensing monitors instead of diary reports *(36).* The results showed that constant change in motion during the day accounted for about one-third of the variance among intermittently sampled ambulatory pressure measurements *(36).*

Blood pressure during the day is also influenced by the emotional state, with most emotions elevating both systolic and diastolic pressures to some extent *(4,18,21,37–39).* Happiness, however, may elevate pressure less than anger and anxiety *(4,18).* An important finding reported by Schwartz et al. *(4)* was the relative rarity of experienced anger. In their study, diary reports of anger during an ambulatory monitoring, when pressures were taken every 15 min while awake, occurred less than 1% of the time. As this emotional state has been thought to play an important role in the development of coronary disease and hypertension, the fact that it is rarely experienced suggests that it may contribute to these conditions more through its effect on the variability of blood pressure rather than on elevating the overall average daily pressure *(56)*. Finally, the location where emotions are experienced may further modify how high blood pressures rise *(21,33,39,40)*. For example, anxiety may have a greater effect when it occurs at work or some place other than home *(18)*.

The influence of location (i.e., work, home, sleep), posture, activity, and emotional state have been found to differ by gender *(18)*, by month of the year (winter or summer months) *(41)*, and, among men, by occupational classification *(33)*. In a study *(40)* comparing the effects of posture (standing, sitting, reclining), location (work, home, elsewhere), and emotional state (happy, angry, anxious) on the ambulatory blood pressures of 137 hypertensive men and 67 hypertensive women, the cumulative effects of location, posture, and reported emotions on the blood pressures of the women were found to be greater than the men. There were also gender differences in the way the emotions and situations affected blood pressure. Estimates of these effects are shown in Table 2.

The effects of posture, location, and emotional state (classified in the same way as in the previous gender study) were also found to differ among hypertensive patients measured in winter months (November–March) ($N = 101$) and summer months (May–September) ($N = 56$) in New York City *(41)*. Specifically, several effects were found to be more accentuated in the winter months. Estimates of these effects are shown in Table 3.

Emotional state may also affect the blood pressures of men in professional occupations (i.e., lawyers, physicians, scientists) differently than men employed in nonprofessional occupations (technicians and union laborers) *(33)*. Specifically, happiness and anxiety were found to have differing effects by occupational classification on blood pressures measured in locations such as bars and restaurants such that professional men had higher pressures when they were anxious, whereas nonprofessional men had higher pressures when they were happy. Estimates of these effects are shown in Table 4.

Finally, increased salt in the diet has also been found to increase the mean daily ambulatory blood pressure *(42–44)*, an effect that may be more accentuated in men than women *(44,45)*. However, the amount of dietary salt may also affect how blood pressure varies during the day with activity. In a study comparing ambulatory blood pressure variation in 19 hypertensive patients who consumed a low-salt (18 meq/day) and high-salt (327 meq/day) diet for a month each, the daily pressure variation associated with changing diary activities after a month on the low-salt diet tended to be higher than the variation after a month on the high-salt diet. Estimates of the posture, location, and activity effects on blood pressure measured on each diet are presented in Table 5 *(46)*.

In examining the estimated blood pressure changes associated with diary data in Tables 1–5, it is obvious that pressure is elevated (sometimes substantially)

Table 2
Comparison of the Average[a] Effects of Posture, Situation of Measurement, and Emotion on Systolic and Diastolic Pressure Between Men and Women (mmHg from 24-h Mean)

Posture	Situation		Women, emotion			Men, emotion		
			Happiness	Anger	Anxiety	Happiness	Anger	Anxiety
Sitting	Work	Systolic	4.1	3.3	5.8	2.9	10.9	6.6
		Diastolic	5.2	2.1	7.1	5.0	13.2	8.7
	Home	Systolic	0.3	6.4	5.2	0.8	5.0	1.4
		Diastolic	2.3	5.5	5.5	-0.1	8.4	3.0
	Elsewhere	Systolic	5.2	3.6	6.6	3.6	10.8	6.7
		Diastolic	2.5	0.8	7.4	3.8	10.6	6.4
Standing	Work	Systolic	11.7	18.2	16.6	3.4	10.6	7.1
		Diastolic	5.7	12.7	13.8	2.4	6.7	10.3
	Home	Systolic	6.2	5.3	7.0	4.2	4.3	3.9
		Diastolic	5.7	9.3	7.2	7.7	9.8	5.3
	Elsewhere	Systolic	11.9	9.2	7.9	5.3	6.9	12.9
		Diastolic	5.1	9.8	8.3	3.1	16.6	9.5

[a]Assumes a 24-h standard deviation of 10.
Source: Modified from ref. 40.

Table 3
Average[a] Effects of Emotions, Posture, and Situation of Measurement
on Systolic and Diastolic Pressure in Winter and Summer Months
(mmHg from 24-h Mean)

	Winter		Summer	
	Systolic pressure	Diastolic pressure	Systolic pressure	Diastolic pressure
Emotions				
Happiness	3.4	4.4	2.3	2.3
Anger	8.4	9.0	5.1	7.0
Anxiety	6.9	7.8	3.9	5.8
Posture				
Sitting	4.2	5.6	2.3	3.7
Standing	7.2	7.2	6.0	5.6
Situation				
Work	7.8	8.7	3.5	5.6
Home	3.3	4.8	1.2	3.1
Elsewhere	6.8	6.1	8.0	6.0

[a]Assumes a 24-h standard deviation of 10.
Source: Modified from ref. *41.*

under specific circumstances during an ambulatory monitoring. A closer examination of the effects of posture (activity), location, and emotional state on blood pressure show that the influence of these factors are more or less additive. Thus, being angry while standing at work will increase pressure substantially more than the experience of being angry or standing singularly. The effects of these factors are, to some extent, more accentuated (larger) in men than women, more accentuated when measurements are taken in winter (cold) months than in summer (warm) months, and also possibly elevated when the patient is on a low-salt diet. Indicators of social class such as occupation may also affect the magnitude of effects, particularly emotional states. Thus, factors such as gender, time of year, diet, and social class need to be considered when evaluating ambulatory blood pressure measurements for pathology.

JOB STRAIN
AND AMBULATORY BLOOD PRESSURE

Studies of employment-related stress and blood pressure have mostly focused on the concept of "job strain." These investigations have relied on the Job Content Survey, from which a measure of job strain has been developed *(47).* The presence of job strain is determined from elevated scores on two orthogonal subscales of the questionnaire: "psychological job demands," which measures the

Table 4
Average[a] Effects of Place of Measurement and Emotional State
on the Systolic and Diastolic Pressures in Two Occupational Groups
(mmHg from 24-h Mean)

Place	Emotion	Professional	Nonprofessional
Systolic pressure			
Work	Happy	2.0	2.9
	Angry	11.2	15.4
	Anxious	7.1	6.5
Home	Happy	−1.0	0.4
	Angry	5.7	2.4
	Anxious	1.6	−0.7
Elsewhere	Happy	0.6	10.5
	Angry	11.5	[b]
	Anxious	10.9	6.8
Diastolic pressure			
Work	Happy	3.1	5.4
	Angry	13.7	7.0
	Anxious	8.0	10.9
Home	Happy	−4.8	2.8
	Angry	7.4	9.8
	Anxious	1.8	−1.3
Elsewhere	Happy	−0.1	4.8
	Angry	10.1	−5.7
	Anxious	9.4	4.9

[a]Assumes a 24-h standard deviation of 10.
[b]Not estimable.
Source: Modified from ref. 33.

psychological workload of the job, and "decision latitude," which describes the degree of control that subjects perceive they have over their job (48,49). Schnall et al. (50) estimated that job strain tended to elevate work systolic pressure by 7 mmHg and diastolic pressure by 3 mmHg.

However, although some investigations show an effect of job strain on ambulatory blood pressure, others do not (51). It has been suggested that studies may get different results because researchers use different formulations in the index of job strain (51). However, the variation in results may also be affected by other independent factors that can influence whether or how job strain is perceived. A comparison of two studies in which job strain was indexed similarly illustrates this possibility. In the first, Van Egeren (35) studied 37 employees at Michigan State University (20 women and 17 men) and found that the women with high job strain had higher systolic blood pressure while at work than those with low job strain. The second study, conducted in North Carolina, included 34 white and 30 black women who worked for several different employers (25). There were no effects of job strain on the blood pressures of the women.

Table 5

Average[a] Effects of Activities, Postures, and Situations
on Systolic and Diastolic Pressure on High- and Low-Sodium Diets
(mmHg from 24-h Mean)

	High sodium		Low sodium	
	Systolic pressure	Diastolic pressure	Systolic pressure	Diastolic pressure
Activity				
Telephone/talking	6.7	3.3	2.6	5.0
Writing	5.6	4.6	4.5	8.5
Walking	6.2	3.3	7.1	4.8
Reading	0.8	0.4	1.8	1.3
Eating	3.7	5.9	1.1	4.1
Relaxing	2.1	0.7	−0.2	−2.2
TV	0.2	−2.1	−2.0	−4.2
Transportation	7.1	5.3	5.8	9.4
Distress	7.1	8.6	17.5	12.2
Dressing/washing	2.2	6.4	0.6	−0.5
Posture				
Standing	6.4	4.9	5.5	3.9
Sitting	3.5	1.7	2.4	4.9
Reclining	−1.5	−1.2	−1.2	−4.5
Situation				
Work	6.2	4.6	5.1	8.1
Home	1.4	0.0	−0.4	−0.3
Elsewhere	7.3	5.2	6.3	3.6

[a]Assumes a 24-h standard deviation of 10.
Source: Modified from ref. *46.*

Why were the results of these two studies at variance? One possibility is that the number of subjects in each study was small and nonrandomly selected; thus, the differences could be the result of sampling error. However, it is also possible that specific worksite factors were involved; that is, there is a fundamental difference in the nature of the worksites sampled in the two studies. The Michigan study consisted of women from the same workplace, whereas the North Carolina study includes women from a cross-section of occupations in several work settings. As Schlussel et al. *(52)* have shown, the actual workplace has a marked effect on work blood pressures. Specifically, they showed that people with the same occupational title (job) but who work in different companies had significantly different blood pressures. Because all the women in the Michigan study were from the same worksite, the place of employment has an equal effect on all the study subjects and, thus, was unlikely to affect the job strain effect. However, the North Carolina study sample was selected from several workplaces. Therefore, it is possible that differing environments in the different workplaces could dilute the job strain effects examined in the overall study. Finally, a third possibility is that the results vary because of local cultural, climatic, and demographic factors that differ between the states of Michigan and North Carolina *(49)*. These factors may affect how people view the stressfulness of their jobs. This possibility is supported by the fact that many intra-populational studies show that climate and subtle cultural variation among population subgroups are associated with differences in blood pressure (e.g., refs. *53–55*).

Finally, in examining the impact of job strain and other psychosocial or psychological constructs on blood pressures in differing venues, it is difficult to know whether they directly affect blood pressure or whether they are reflecting the increasing effects of emotional state, posture, activity, and their interactions; that is, it is possible that the perception of job experience is dictated by how often intense emotional arousal or long periods of standing or doing errands occur. This issue is an important one from a clinical standpoint in that the clinician needs to know whether diary data alone is sufficient to interpret the blood pressure variation properly during the day or whether a battery of psychometric questionnaires that measure complex behavioral constructs are needed as well. Anecdotally, one would expect that for most patients, the diary data will be sufficient.

HOME STRESS
AND AMBULATORY BLOOD PRESSURE

In further studies of women employed in wage jobs outside the home, stress in the home environment has been found to influence blood pressure as much or more during the day than stress experienced at work *(26,56–58)*. Specifically, if the home environment experience is as stressful or more stressful than the work environment, ambulatory blood pressures measured at home may be as high or higher than those measured at work *(26,58,59)*. The home stress effects found among women have been related to factors associated with the family, such as being married or the number of children *(26,57)*. In fact, it was estimated that women with children experience a 3 mmHg increase in both systolic and diastolic pressures at home for each child they have. Thus, for women, it may be important to know whether they have dependent children at home, as they could tend to raise pressure during a time when one might clinically expect it to fall. However, it is probably also true that this information will likely be reflected in diary reported data as well.

ETHNICITY AND BLOOD PRESSURE VARIATION

The literature examining ethnicity and blood pressure variation during the day is sparse, meaning that few studies have examined whether diary-reported conditions influence blood pressure differently in different ethnic groups. Gerber et al. *(20)* evaluated whether ethnic groups (white, African-American, Hispanic) were different with regard to the effects of posture and location on blood pressure and found no differences. However, in a recent study examining factors affecting the daily variation of blood pressure in Filipino-American and white women employed as nurses in Hawaii, Brown et al. *(60)* found that the Filipino-American women reported negative moods more frequently, had a greater proportion of readings taken while standing at work, and had different blood pressure responses than white women to specific activities, such as household chores. They suggested that blood pressure variation in daily life may be significantly influenced by the cultural background of the individual. From a clinical standpoint, the question is: Should the ethnic background of the patient be considered as a factor when evaluating how diary-reported data influence daily blood pressures? Because there are so few studies on which to base a judgment, this inquiry cannot be answered. Further research is needed to make this assessment.

WHAT DOES IT ALL MEAN?

Realistically, when evaluating ambulatory blood pressure measurements for the purpose of treatment, the individual values of patients with low averages over 24 h (i.e., less than 120/80 mmHg) do not need to be scrutinized because whatever they are doing is not excessively raising their pressure. Likewise, patients whose average ambulatory pressures are very high (i.e., more than 170/110 mmHg) do not require a close evaluation of every pressure either, in that even after adjusting their pressures for their activities and situations, their averages would still probably exceed 150/100 mmHg. The evaluation of what people are doing is most useful in the "borderline" patients. As previously reported *(2)*, a patient with an ambulatory average of 145/92 mmHg may be perfectly normal if the mix and duration of behaviors were such that they tended to raise pressure. The same values may also indicate the need for treatment if the reported behaviors were ones that had a minimal effect on pressure or tended to lower it.

In summary, because behavior can strongly influence the blood pressure of patients, it probably needs to be considered when assessing ambulatory blood pressures for the determination of treatment for hypertension. Thus, clinicians should examine the diary data that are collected during an ambulatory monitoring and compare it to the measurements collected, particularly among patients whose pressures are "borderline." Ignoring behavior in the evaluation of the ambulatory blood pressures might be considered as clinically incorrect as confirming a diagnosis of hypertension based on a single blood pressure measurement of 140/90 mmHg at a single office visit.

REFERENCES

1. Pickering TG. Ambulatory Monitoring and Blood Pressure Variability, Science, London, 1991.
2. James GD, Pickering TG. The influence of behavioral factors on the daily variation of blood pressure. Am J Hypertens 1993;6:170S–174S.

3. James GD. Blood pressure response to the daily stressors of urban environments: methodology, basic concepts and significance. Yrbk Phys Anthropol 1991;34:189–210.

4. Schwartz JE, Warren K, Pickering TG. Mood, location and physical position as predictors of ambulatory blood pressure and heart rate: application of a multilevel random effects model. Ann Behav Med 1994;16:210–220.

5. Pickering TG, Schwartz JE, James GD. Ambulatory blood pressure monitoring for evaluating the relationships between lifestyle, hypertension and cardiovascular risk. Clin Exp Pharmacol Phys 1995;22:226–231.

6. James GD, Brown DE. The biological stress response and lifestyle: catecholamines and blood pressure. Annu Rev Anthropol 1997;26:313–335.

7. Harper GJ. Stress and adaptation among elders in life care communities, PhD thesis, Department Anthropology, The Ohio State University, 1998.

8. Van Egeren LF, Madarasmi S. A computer assisted diary (CAD) for ambulatory blood pressure monitoring. Am J Hypertens 1988;1:179S–185S.

9. Chesney MA, Ironson GH. Diaries in ambulatory monitoring. In: Schneidermann N, Weiss SM, Kaufman PG, eds. Handbook of Research Methods in Cardiovascular Behavioral Medicine. Plenum, New York, 1989, pp. 317–332.

10. Kaplan NM. Clinical Hypertension, 5th ed. Williams & Wilkens, Baltimore, 1990.

11. Pickering TG. Modern definitions and clinical expressions of hypertension. In: Laragh JH, Brenner BM, eds. Hypertension: Pathophysiology Diagnosis and Management. Raven, New York, 1995, pp. 17–21.

12. Joint National Committee. The Sixth Report of the Joint National Committee on Prevention, Detection, Evaluation, and Treatment of High Blood Pressure. Arch Intern Med 1997;157: 2413–2446.

13. Baumgart P, Walger P, Jurgens U, Rahn KH. Reference data for ambulatory blood pressure monitoring: What results are equivalent to the established limits of office blood pressure? Klin Wochenschr 1990;68:723–727.

14. Mancia G, Sega R, Bravi C, DeVito G, Valagussa F, Cesana G, et al. Ambulatory blood pressure normality: results from the PAMELA Study. J Hypertens 1995;13:1377–1390.

15. Pickering TG, Kaplan NM, Krakoff L, Prisant LM, Sheps S, Weber MA, et al. for the American Society of Hypertension Expert Panel. Conclusions and recommendations on the clinical use of home (self) and ambulatory blood pressure monitoring. Am J Hypertens 1996;9: 1–11.

16. Imai Y, Ohkubo T. Ambulatory blood pressure normality: experience in the Ohasama Study. Blood Pressure Monit 1998;3:185–188.

17. Schwartz JE, Stone AA. Strategies for analyzing ecological momentary assessment data. Health Psychol 1998;17:6–16.

18. James GD, Yee LS, Harshfield GA, Blank S, Pickering, TG. The influence of happiness, anger and anxiety on the blood pressure of borderline hypertensives. Psychosom Med 1986;48: 502–508.

19. Clark LA, Denby L, Presibon D, Harshfield GA, Pickering TG, Blank S, et al. A quantitative analysis of the effects of activity and time of day on the diurnal variations of blood pressure. J Chronic Dis 1987;40:671–681.

20. Gerber LM, Schwartz JE, Pickering TG. Does the relationship of ambulatory blood pressure to position and location vary by age, sex, race/ethnicity or body mass index? Am J Hum Biol 1998;10:459–470.

21. Gellman M, Spitzer S, Fronson G, Llabre M, Saab P, et al. Posture, place and mood effects on ambulatory blood pressure. Psychophysiology 1990;27:544–551.

22. Pickering TG, Harshfield GA, Kleinert HD, Blank S, Laragh JH. Blood pressure during normal daily activities, sleep and exercise. Comparison of values in normal and hypertensive subjects. J Am Med Assoc 1982;247:992–996.

23. Harshfield GA, Pickering TG, Kleinert HD, Blank S, Laragh JH. Situational variation of blood pressure in ambulatory hypertensive patients. Psychosom Med 1982;44:237–245.

24. Llabre MM, Ironson GH, Spitzer SB, Gellman MD, Weidler, DJ, Schneiderman N. How many blood pressure measurements are enough?: an application of generalizability theory to the study of blood pressure reliability. Psychophysiology 1988;25:97–106.

25. Light KC, Turner JR, Hinderliter AL. Job strain and ambulatory work blood pressure in healthy young men and women. Hypertension 1992;20:214–218.

26. James GD, Schlussel YR, Pickering TG. The association between daily blood pressure and catecholamine variability in normotensive working women. Psychosom Med 1993;55:55–60.

27. Light KC, Brownley KA, Turner JR, Hinderliter AL, Girdler SS, Sherwood A, et al. Job status and high-effort coping influence work blood pressure in women and blacks. Hypertension 1995;25:554–559.

28. Sundburg S, Kohvakka A, Gordin A. Rapid reversal of circadian blood pressure rhythm in shift workers. J Hypertens 1988;6:393–396.

29. Baumgart P, Walger P, Fuchs G, Dorst KG, Vetter H, et al. Twenty-four-hour blood pressure is not dependent on endogenous circadian rhythm. J Hypertens 1989;7:331–334.

30. Broege PA, James GD, Peters M. Anxiety coping style and daily blood pressure variation in female nurses. Blood Pressure Monit 1997;2:155–159.

31. Yamasaki F, Schwartz JE, Gerber LM, Warren K, Pickering TG. Impact of shift work and race/ ethnicity on the diurnal rhythm of blood pressure and catecholamines. Hypertension 1998;32: 417–423.

32. Harshfield GA, Pickering TG, James GD, Blank SG. Blood pressure variability and reactivity in the natural environment. In: Meyer-Sabellek W, Anlauf M, Gotzen R, Steinfield L, eds. Blood Pressure Measurements. New Techniques in Automatic and 24-Hour Indirect Monitoring. Springer-Verlag, New York, 1990, pp. 241–225.

33. James GD, Pickering TG. Ambulatory blood pressure monitoring: assessing the diurnal variation of blood pressure. Am J Phys Anthropol 1991;84:343–349.

33a. Van Egeren LF, Sparrow AW. Ambulatory monitoring to assess real-life cardiovascular reactivity in type A and B subjects. Psychosom Med 1990;52:297–306.

34. Rosenman RH. The interview method of assessment of the coronary-prone behavior pattern. In: Dembrowski TM, Weiss SM, Sheilds JL, Haynes SG, Feinlab M. eds. Coronary-Prone Behavior. Springer-Verlag, Berlin, 1978, pp. 55–69.

35. Van Egeren LF. The relationship between job strain and blood pressure at work, at home and during sleep. Psychosom Med 1992;54:337–343.

36. Gretler DD, Carlson GF, Montano AV, Murphy MB. Diurnal blood pressure variability and physical activity measured electronically and by diary. Am J Hypertens 1993;6:127–133.

37. Sokolow M, Werdegar D, Perloff DB, Cowan RM, Brenenstuhl H. Preliminary studies relating portably recorded blood pressures to daily life events in patients with essential hypertension. Bibl Psychiatrica 1970;144:164–189.

38. Southard DR, Coates TJ, Kolodner K, Parker C, Padgett NE, et al. Relationship between mood and blood pressure in the natural environment: an adolescent population. Health Psychol 1986;5:469–480.

39. Brondolo E, Karlin W, Alexander K, Bobrow A, Schwartz J. Workday communication and ambulatory blood pressure: Implications for the reactivity hypothesis. Psychophysiology 1999;36:86–94.

40. James GD, Yee LS, Harshfield GA, Pickering TG. Sex differences in factors affecting the daily variation of blood pressure. Soc Sci Med 1988;26:1019–1023.

41. James GD, Yee LS, Pickering TG. Winter-summer differences in the effects of emotion, posture and place of measurement on blood pressure. Soc Sci Med 1990;31:1213–1217.

42. Gerdts E, Myking OL, Omivik P. Salt sensitive essential hypertension evaluated by 24-hour ambulatory blood pressure. Blood Pressure 1994;3:375–380.

43. Overlack A, Ruppert M, Kolloch R, Kraft K, Stumpe KO. Age is a major determinant of the divergent blood pressure responses to varying salt intake in essential hypertension. Am J Hypertens 1995;8:829–836.

44. James GD, Pecker MS, Pickering TG. Sex differences in casual and ambulatory blood pressure responses to extreme changes in dietary sodium. Blood Pressure Monit 1996;1:397–401.

45. Moore TJ, Halarick C, Olmedo A, Klein RC. Salt restriction lowers resting but not 24-h ambulatory pressure. Am J Hypertens 1991;4:410–415.

46. James GD, Pecker MS, Pickering TG, Jackson S, DiFabio B, et al. Extreme changes in dietary sodium effect the daily variability and level of blood pressure in borderline hypertensive patients. Am J Hum Biol 1994;6:283–291.

47. Karasek R, Baker D, Marxer F, Ahlom A, Theorell T. Job decision latitude, job demands and cardiovascular disease: a prospective study of Swedish men. Am J Public Health 1981;71: 694–705.

48. Pickering TG, James GD, Schnall PL, Schlussel YR, Pieper CT, Gerin W, et al. Occupational stress and blood pressure: studies in working men and women. In: Frankenhaeuser M, Lundberg U, Chesney M, eds. Women, Work and Health: Stress and Opportunities. Plenum, New York, 1991, pp. 171–186.

49. James GD, Broege PA, Schlussel YR. Assessing cardiovascular risk and stress-related blood pressure variability in young women employed in wage jobs. Am J Hum Biol 1996;8:743–749.

50. Schnall PL, Schwartz JE, Landsbergis PA, Warren K, Pickering TG. Relation between job strain, alcohol and ambulatory blood pressure. Hypertension 1992;19:488–494.

51. Landesbergis PA, Schnall PL, Warren K, Pickering TG, Schwartz JE. Association between ambulatory blood pressure and alternative formulations of job strain. Scand J Work Environ Health 1994;20:349–363.

52. Schlussel YR, Schnall PL, Zimbler M, Warren K, Pickering TG. The effect of work environments on blood pressure: evidence from seven New York organizations. J Hypertens 1990;8: 679–685.

53. James GD, Baker PT. Human population biology and blood pressure: evolutionary and ecological considerations and interpretations of population studies. In: Laragh JH, Brenner BM, eds. Hypertension: Pathophysiology, Diagnosis and Management, 2nd ed. Raven, New York, 1995, pp. 115–126.

54. Schall JI. Sex differences in the response of blood pressure to modernization. Am J Hum Biol 1995;7:159–172.

55. McGarvey ST, Schendel DE. Blood pressure of Samoans. In: Baker PT, Hanna JM, Baker TS, eds. The Changing Samoans: Behavior and Health in Transition. Oxford University Press, New York, 1986, pp. 350–393.

56. Pickering TG, Devereux RB, Gerin W, James GD, Pieper C, Schlussel YR, et al. The role of behavioral factors in white coat and sustained hypertension. J Hypertens 1990;8(Suppl 7): S141–S147.

57. James GD, Cates EM, Pickering TG, Laragh JH. Parity and perceived job stress elevate blood pressure in young normotensive women. Am J Hypertens 1989;2:637–639.

58. James GD, Moucha OP, Pickering TG. The normal hourly variation of blood pressure in women: average patterns and the effect of work stress. J Hum Hypertens 1991;5:505–509.

59. James, GD. Race and perceived stress independently affect the diurnal variation of blood pressure in women. Am J Hypertens 1991;4:382–384.

60. Brown DE, James GD, Nordloh L. Comparison of factors affecting daily variation of blood pressure in Filipino-American and Caucasian nurses in Hawaii. Am J Phys Anthropol 1998; 106:373–383.

3

Electronic Activity Recording in Cardiovascular Disease

George A. Mansoor, MD, MRCP

CONTENTS

INTRODUCTION

Electronic activity recording is a noninvasive technique to monitor human physical movements without any direct input from the subject. The motion-sensing technology has many types but actigraphy has been sufficiently developed that commercially available devices are small, compact, and technologically sophisticated although standardization of data collection is lacking. Actigraphy continues to be used widely in psychology and sleep research *(1)* and it shows promise in becoming a useful tool in cardiovascular disease research. Unlike the guidelines for its use in sleep research *(2,3)*, there are no standards or guidelines in its use in cardiovascular-related diseases.

From: *Contemporary Cardiology:*
Blood Pressure Monitoring in Cardiovascular Medicine and Therapeutics
Edited by: W. B. White © Humana Press Inc., Totowa, NJ

EQUIPMENT,
MODES OF OPERATION, AND LIMITATIONS

Several types of actigraphs are available from different manufacturers; two commonly used in research are the Mini-MotionLogger Actigraph from Ambulatory Monitoring (Ardsley, NY) and the Activity Monitor from Gaehwiler Electronic (Hombrechtikon, Switzerland). These activity monitors contain a sensor that generates a voltage on experiencing a movement exceeding a certain threshold. This voltage is then sent through an analog circuit, the signal is filtered and amplified and then compared to a reference. This comparison is performed and kept in temporary memory for the duration of time called an epoch (e.g., 1 min) set by the user. A few devices have an event marker that the patient can activate to define a particular event, such as arising out of bed or removal of the actigraph for showering.

The units of activity are somewhat arbitrary and are instrument-specific. They reflect our limited understanding of optimal methods to define and measure complex human motion *(1)*. Because of these differences, it is necessary for researchers to be familiar with the way each unit works and the differing modes of data collection. For example, the Motionlogger offers at least two modes of data collection; the zero crossing mode (ZCM) and the time above threshold mode (TAT). The ZCM estimates frequency of movement by accumulating the number of times the signal voltage crosses the reference voltage during an epoch, whereas the TAT estimates the duration of movement by accumulating the time (as units of tenths of a second) spent above the reference voltage. Other modes of collection that have been developed include area under the curve of activity or some variant. In general, it is recommended that the ZCM mode be used for sleep studies because most validation studies of sleep scoring algorithms have used this mode. Commercial devices can collect data for periods of up to 30 d and manufacturers allow the user to modify the instruments' sensitivity and sampling frequency as well as the option of using filters. A typical 48-h actigraphic study using a Mini-MotionLogger unit is shown in Fig. 1.

It is important to be aware of the limitations of current actigraphic devices. A very significant limitation is that the data generated by actigraphic devices from different manufacturers are not interchangeable nor readily comparable. This is illustrated in a recent study *(4)* of two popular activity recorders in which possibly important differences in performance and sensitivity were found. The authors compared the Mini-MotionLogger Actigraphs (Model 20000, Ambulatory Monitoring, Inc.) and the Activity Monitor (Model Z80-32K V1, Gaehwiler Electronics) in five subjects who underwent a total of eight separate recordings of durations of 7–92 h. They also compared two devices of the same type in similar fashion. The devices were worn one above the other and the positions reversed in the middle of the recording. Within-actigraph-type comparisons indicated

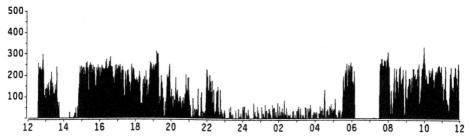

Fig. 1. An actual actigraphic tracing (Mini-MotionLogger Actigraph [Ambulatory Monitoring, Ardsley, NY]) starting at midday and showing a marked reduction in activity during sleep (2300 hours to 0530 hours). The activity units are in units per minute.

excellent correlations ($r > 0.98$). When the two types of recorders were compared, interesting similarities and differences were discovered. Both activity recorders detected circadian activity patterns of day and night adequately as inferred from the activity recordings. The Gaehwiler actigraph, however, frequently recorded zeros when the Mini-MotionLogger recorded movement, indicating a lower sensitivity of the former instrument (4). However, even the Mini-Motionlogger had limited sensitivity during certain activities, as judged by the relatively frequent zero readings. Therefore, the two instruments were comparable to globally assess circadian activity but were not comparable when the objective was low-level activity or sleep data analysis.

There are also differences in the data generated when the different modes of operation are used. A direct comparison of the ZCM and the TAT modes of the Mini-MotionLogger was performed by Leidy in 20 healthy volunteers of mean age 36 yr (5). These volunteers wore a dual-mode actigraph twice on the nondominant wrist and performed specified common tasks representing three graded levels of activity: light (1–2 metabolic equivalents or METs), moderate (3–4 METs), and heavy (4–6 METs). These three levels of activity were designed to include tasks commonly performed by subjects in their home environment. Both modes successfully distinguished between light and moderate, and light and heavy activities. However, neither mode was able to distinguish between moderate- and heavy-level activities, indicating the possibility of a saturation effect of moderate exercise on the instruments' scoring of activity. Reproducibility correlations across activity levels were 0.80 and 0.66 for the ZCM and TAT modes, respectively. Interestingly, the authors also found that average movement duration, which is calculated as the TAT divided by the ZCM, was less useful in distinguishing the activity level and was only able to distinguish light and heavy activity levels. It is likely that each mode of data collection may be particularly suited to certain types of activity monitoring and the two modes should be further studied in various types of activity.

An additional limitation is the lack of a consensus regarding the optimal body site for attachment of actigraphs during research studies *(2)*. It is not difficult to conceive of certain movements during which the upper limbs or the trunk are moved more than the lower limbs and vice versa. Nevertheless, most research studies have attached the actigraph to the nondominant or dominant wrist, unless the activity being monitored is walking *(6)* or the study subject is an infant, in which case the waist or ankle may be preferable. In cardiovascular disease research, where ambulatory blood pressure or heart-rate-monitoring equipment is already attached to the patients nondominant side, logistical issues arise about the preferable attachment site. In our experience, most patients can comfortably wear the actigraphs on either wrist without problems and both sites provide similar data. However, consistent site placement is needed in methodological studies to assess the performance of these devices in clinical settings. As discussed in the position paper on actigraphy in sleep disorders *(2)*, artifacts as well as sleeping conditions may affect the actigraphic tracing.

RELATIONSHIP AMONG PHYSICAL ACTIVITY, BLOOD PRESSURE, AND HEART RATE

One of the first areas in cardiovascular medicine in which electronic activity monitoring has been used is the study of the relationship among overall physical activity, blood pressure, and heart rate. There is undoubtedly an appreciable but complex influence of physical activity on blood pressure variability, as illustrated in Fig. 2. Van Egeren *(7)* pioneered the study of actigraphic wrist motion and ambulatory blood pressure by studying 82 healthy normotensive employed subjects. Most of his study subjects were found to have a moderate correlation (averaged $r = 0.50$) of blood pressure with activity (counts for the 10 min before each blood pressure reading was taken). This positive linear relationship of physical activity to blood pressure was not significantly influenced by any other clinical factor. Similarly, Gretler and colleagues *(8)* performed a study in 10 healthy young (mean age, 32 yr) normotensive volunteers. Interestingly, in this study, each subject wore four activity monitors: on both wrists, the waist, and the left ankle. The authors then calculated the activity level 30 s and 2, 5, 10, 15, and 30 min prior to each valid blood pressure reading and correlated it with blood pressure. Activity data correlated significantly with both blood pressure and heart rate in every subject, although there was a wide range of correlation coefficients. The authors also determined that the dominant wrist site provided the best correlation with activity measured 2–10 min just prior to a reading. Actigraphic physical activity accounted for 18–69% of the systolic blood pressure variability and they suggested that ambulatory blood pressure data should be interpreted in association with concomitant physical activity measures. Stewart and co-authors *(9)* reported similar findings in a group of 30 middle-aged patients (mean age 52 yr)

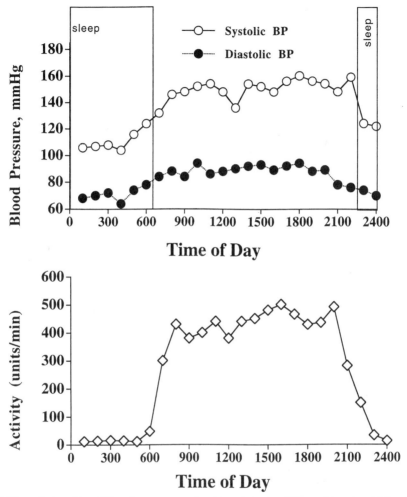

Fig. 2. The relationship of blood pressure and wrist activity in a 36-yr-old male with border-line hypertension. Data for blood pressure and activity is shown as hourly averages. Blood pressure is in mmHg and activity is in average units per hour. A decrease in blood pressure and activity is seen during the sleep period (boxed portion of blood pressure curve).

and were able to ascribe 20% of systolic blood pressure variation to actigraph-ically measured activity. These findings are consistent with the finding that a relatively flat blood pressure profile is seen if patients are kept in bed or hospi-talized, indicating that a major determinant of blood pressure and the circadian profile is caused by variations in daily physical activity *(10)*.

However, the above-described findings between physical activity and ambu-latory blood pressure must be considered preliminary because they were done primarily in healthy volunteers and few studies have been done in older patients or in subjects with cardiovascular or hypertensive disease. For example, Shapiro

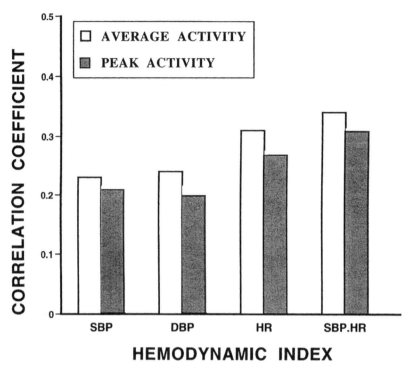

Fig. 3. The relationship of average and peak activity (5 min before each reading) to ambulatory blood pressure, heart rate, and the rate–pressure product. The strongest correlation was with the rate–pressure product.

and colleagues found little or no relationship between activity and ambulatory blood pressure and heart rate in 119 older healthy subjects (mean age 67 yr, 68% were retired) *(11)*. They concluded that activity monitoring was not likely to improve the ambulatory blood pressure data reproducibility. Our own work *(12)* in untreated essential hypertensive subjects reveals that there is considerable interperson variability in the effects of activity on ambulatory blood pressure and heart rate. We studied a group of 39 untreated hypertensive subjects of average age 57 yr using actigraphy and ambulatory blood pressure monitoring. Our analyses included both average activity for 5 min and peak activity during that time prior to each valid blood pressure and heart reading. We found that there was substantial variability in the correlation of 5-min activity with blood pressure and heart rate. Indeed, in some patients, there was no correlation. We also found that there was a trend that the strength of the correlation was higher in younger subjects. Furthermore, the best correlate of average and peak 5-min activity was the heart rate–blood pressure product (Fig. 3). It seems that considerable disagreement remains about whether ambulatory blood pressure data need to be adjusted for activity levels. Additional work in hypertensive subjects is needed to study the effects of average physical activity on blood pressure and heart rate.

PHYSICAL ACTIVITY, SLEEP,
AND CIRCADIAN BLOOD PRESSURE

Apart from the study of the relationship of day-to-day activity on blood pressure and heart rate, actigraphy can play a role in defining sleep and wake times as well as possibly explain the effects of sleep quality on dipper and nondipper status. The normal blood pressure and heart rate pattern is one of relatively higher blood pressure during the day with lower readings during sleep and then a sharp rise in the early morning on awakening *(13)*. The decline in blood pressure and heart rate during sleep has been ascribed to both an endogenous rhythm and the relative effects of physical inactivity during sleep. Irrespective of the cause, there are several pathophysiological implications of blood pressure variability. First, a small but significant group of subjects do not have the expected decline of blood pressure during sleep. These "nondipper' hypertensive patients have been observed to be generally older patients and to have a higher prevalence of secondary hypertension. This "nondipping" pattern may not be an academic curiosity because it has been shown to be a contributing factor in increasing left ventricular mass *(14)*, ischemic cerebrovascular damage *(15)*, and cardiovascular events *(16)*.

Furthermore, systematic study *(17,18)* has revealed that there is a definite excess of cardiovascular events in the early to mid-morning period, the time of the largest increase in blood pressure and heart rate. Several large studies have shown that acute myocardial infarction, sudden death, arrhythmias, and stroke (both ischemic and hemorrhagic) all have excessive rates in the morning period *(17–19)*. These findings have led to the hypothesis that both hemodynamic (sharp rise in blood pressure and heart rate) and other changes in blood hemostatic and neurohumoral mechanisms may be responsible for these excess events. Researchers are, therefore, very interested in understanding the factors responsible for the sleep blood pressure decline and the factors contributing to the excess cardiovascular events in the early morning.

Electronic activity monitoring by its ability to monitor activity and the sleep–wake cycle continuously complements chronotherapeutics research. Actigraphy has been used in this area to identify sleep and awake periods accurately, the time of awakening, and sleep quality. Automated scoring of sleep quantity and quality as well as the presence of a circadian character to sleep is possible from the actigraphic data. Such algorithms have been validated prospectively against polysomnography *(20)*. The method correctly distinguished sleep from wakefulness with over 88% accuracy. However, the two methods are not completely identical, with actigraphy slightly overestimating sleep times. Furthermore, actigraphy cannot provide any information on sleep stages that can be obtained from polysomnography.

A promising application of actigraphy appears to be in the noninvasive determination of sleep times during ambulatory blood pressure monitoring. It is generally accepted that daytime or awake averages should be separated from nighttime or sleep periods for the calculation of average blood pressure and blood pressure loads. Traditionally, several different methods of defining these two periods have been used; the more commonly used is to divide the 24-h period using a fixed arbitrary time for sleep (e.g., 10 PM to 6 AM) or by use of a patient-kept diary. Although the difference in blood pressure when calculated by these two methods is small, moderate differences have been observed in some subjects especially during sleep *(21)*. Furthermore, the definition of the sleep-associated decline in blood pressure implies accurate sleep time recognition. Several groups of researchers have reported that the diary method of defining sleep is superior to the arbitrary fixed-time methods in which an arbitrary sleep time is imposed on all subjects *(21–25)*. It appears that based on current data, the best methods for dividing ambulatory blood pressure data for research purposes is by the use of diary times and/or actigraphically determined sleep times. Cusum analysis, which is a statistical method for analyzing trends in timed data, can give similar information but may be impractical for routine use *(25)*.

Several problems remain in the use of actigraphy as a tool to identify sleep times during ambulatory blood pressure monitoring. No consensus has been reached on the best actigraphic criteria to identify sleep onset or awakening. Several different methods could theoretically be used, including event markers, built-in sleep algorithms, or arbitrary manual-scoring criteria. Furthermore, it is not clear what should be done about blood pressure readings taken during periods of sleep when significant activity is detected by the actigraph.

It is tempting to speculate that one reason for the so-called nondipping blood pressure profile is sleep interference by the blood pressure monitor itself. A recent article *(26)* used actigraphy to compare sleep activity levels among age- and weight-matched normotensives and essential hypertensives. The authors found that hypertensives fell asleep later, slept less, and had more sleep disturbance and nocturnal activity than their normotensive counterparts. The hypertensive group had significantly smaller reductions of blood pressure during sleep than their normotensive controls. The authors suggested that this may be the result of the higher cuff inflation experienced by hypertensive patients undergoing blood pressure monitoring. Our group *(27)* recently reported in abstract form that nondippers, in general, have more sleep activity than dippers among a group of hypertensives. In this study, diary times were used to define sleep times. Additional study is clearly needed to evaluate the causes of this increased activity and whether it relates to poor sleep.

Actigraphy may also be useful for researchers to define better the early morning period after awakening *(23)*. Recent studies *(19)* have examined the hemodynamic and neurohormonal changes of the early morning period and a novel form of antihypertensive drug therapy has been developed targeting this time period *(28)*. Therefore, accurate determination of wake-up time is essential. In one study *(23)*, actigraphy and diary times of awakening provided similar early morning blood pressure averages to diary and arbitrary times, indicating that the least favorable method would be the imposition of a fixed wake-up time on all study participants. Khoury et al. *(29)*, by monitoring blood pressure and actual wake up times, found that the act of physically getting out of bed was the main reason for the steep rise in blood pressure and heart rate.

ACTIGRAPHY IN ASSESSING SLEEP QUALITY AFTER CORONARY ARTERY BYPASS SURGERY

Sleep quality has been assessed in a number of studies related to cardiac disease. For example, the effects of coronary artery bypass surgery on actigraphically determined sleep both in the short term (1 wk) and the long term (6 mo) have been reported *(30,31)*. The authors described significant sleep fragmentation in the first week after coronary artery bypass grafting, which improved over long-term follow-up. Furthermore, an increase in overall physical activity and restoration of a circadian sleep rhythm was seen over the study period. This type of information regarding sleep can allow intelligent therapeutic intervention to improve sleep hygiene in the postoperative and rehabilitative phases of recovery after cardiac surgery.

All of these uses of actigraphy use data collected on physical activity to make inferences about sleep onset, termination, duration, quality, and rhythmicity.

VALIDATION OF AMBULATORY BLOOD PRESSURE MONITORS

Traditionally, validation of ambulatory blood pressure monitors is done according to the American Association of Medical Instrumentation guidelines or the British Hypertension Society Protocols *(32,33)*. It has been reported that physical activity increases errors during ambulatory blood pressure monitoring *(34)*. Therefore, if very sedentary individuals are included in the validation protocol, then the real-life performance of the monitor is not being tested. In one validation study of an ambulatory blood pressure monitor *(35)*, a significantly higher reading rejection rate was noted in the highest tertile of physical activity compared to the lowest tertile of activity. Clinically, the groups were similar and no other clinical factor could explain the differences seen. The authors suggested that electronic activity monitoring be incorporated into validation protocols of ambulatory blood pressure monitoring equipment to ensure that the subjects participating in validation of monitors maintain an average level of physical activity.

ACTIGRAPHY AND SLEEP APNEA SYNDROME

Sleep apnea is commonly found in association with hypertension and coronary artery disease *(36)*. It has also been observed that treatment of sleep apnea can improve blood pressure levels *(37)*. It is possible that the frequent waking episodes leading to sleep fragmentation may be detectable by actigraphy and the technique may become a simple screening tool for the disorder. Nevertheless, the clinical standard for the diagnosis remains polysomnography in the sleep laboratory. Aubert-Tulkens et al. *(38)* tried to determine if any actigraphically determined sleep index could distinguish sleep apnea patients. They compared a movement index (a percentage of time with movement divided by total sleep time) and fragmentation index (ratio of the number of phases of 1-min immobility to the total number of immobility phases of all duration expressed as a percentage) between 18 subjects with sleep apnea and 22 control subjects. Sleep apnea was diagnosed in the study subjects with polysomnography. Half of these subjects were hypertensive. The sleep apnea patients had a significantly higher movement index and fragmentation index than controls. Similarly, Sadeh et al. *(39)*, using activity measures, reported that sleep apnea patients were distinguishable from controls. However, Middelkoop et al. *(40)* did not confirm these data in a study of 116 community-based subjects suspected of sleep apnea (snoring and daytime sleepiness). Using an ambulatory monitor of respiration (oronasal flow thermistry) and an activity wrist recorder, they evaluated the use of actigraphic activity indices during sleep to determine the presence of sleep apnea syndrome. This study must be interpreted with caution, however, because of the large number of failed recordings and the low overall number of patients with confirmed sleep apnea syndrome. Further work is needed in this area, as actigraphy remains a promising tool to screen for sleep apnea.

CONCLUSIONS

Actigraphy is a potentially useful tool for the study of overall physical activity and its relationship to blood pressure and heart rate. This method of activity monitoring promises to provide noninvasive measures of sleep quality and duration for a variety of uses, including their relationship to a variety of diseases states. However, much work is needed in the standardization of equipment, sites of attachment, criteria, and consistency of sleep determination. Undoubtedly, there will be more use of actigraphy in the diagnosis and treatment of a variety of cardiovascular disorders.

REFERENCES

1. Tryon WW. Activity Measurement in Psychology and Medicine. Plenum, New York, 1991.
2. An American Sleep Disorders Association Report. Practice parameters for the use of actigraphy in the clinical assessment of sleep disorders. Sleep 1995;18:285–287.
3. Sadeh A, Hauri PJ, Kripke DF, Lavie P. The role of actigraphy in the evaluation of sleep disorders. Sleep 1995;18:288–302.
4. Pollak CP, Stokes PE, Wagner DR. Direct comparison of two widely used activity recorders. Sleep 1998;21:207–212.

5. Leidy NK, Abbott RD, Fedenko KM. Sensitivity and reproducibility of the dual-mode actigraph under controlled levels of activity intensity. Nurs Res 1997;46:5–11.
6. Sleminski DJ, Gradner AW. The relationship between free-living daily physical activity and the severity of peripheral arterial occlusive disease. Vasc Med 1997;2:286–291.
7. Van Egeren LF. Monitoring activity and blood pressure. J Hypertens 1991;9:S25–S27.
8. Gretler DD, Carlson GF, Montano AV, Murphy MB. Diurnal blood pressure variability and physical activity measured electronically and by diary. Am J Hypertens 1993;6:127–133.
9. Stewart MJ, Brown H, Padfield PL. Can simultaneous ambulatory blood pressure and activity monitoring improve the definition of blood pressure. Am J Hypertens 1993;6:174S–178S.
10. Young MA, Rowlands DB, Stallard TH, Watson RDS, Littler WA. Effect of environment on blood pressure: home versus hospital. Br Med J 1983;286:1235–1236.
11. Shapiro D, Goldstein IB. Wrist actigraph measures of physical activity level and ambulatory blood pressure in healthy elderly persons. Psychophysiology 1998;35:305–312.
12. Mansoor GA, White WB. The influence of electronically-measured physical activity on ambulatory blood pressure, heart rate, and the rate pressure product. Am J Hypertens 2000;13:262–267.
13. Littler WA, Honour AJ, Carter RD, Sleight P. Sleep and blood pressure. Br Med J 1975;3:346–348.
14. Verdecchia P, Schillachi G, Guerrieri M, Gatteschi C, Benemio G, Boldrini F. Circadian blood pressure changes and left ventricular hypertrophy in essential hypertension. Circulation 1990;81:528–536.
15. Shimada K, Kawamoto A, Matsubayashi K, Nishinaga M, Kimura S, Ozawa T. Diurnal blood pressure variations and silent cerebrovascular damage in elderly patients with hypertension. J Hypertens 1992;10:875–878.
16. Verdecchia P, Schillaci G, Borgioni C, Ciucci A, Gattobiogi R, Porcellati C. Nocturnal pressure is the true pressure. Blood Pressure Monit 1996;1:S81–S85.
17. Muller JE, Stone PH, Turi ZG, et al. Circadian variation in the frequency of onset of acute myocardial infarction. N Engl J Med 1985;313:1315–1322.
18. Goldberg RJ. Epidemiological aspects of circadian patterns of cardiovascular disease and triggers of acute cardiac events. Cardiol Clin 1996;14:175–184.
19. Anis Y, White WB. Chronotherapeutics for cardiovascular disease. Drugs 1998;55:631–643.
20. Cole RJ, Kripke DF, Gruen W, Mullaney DJ, Gillin JC. Automatic sleep/wake identification from wrist activity. Sleep 1992;15:461–469.
21. Peixoto AJ, Mansoor GA, White WB. Effects of actual versus arbitrary awake and sleep times on analyses of 24-h blood pressure. Am J Hypertens 1995;8:676–680.
22. Va Ittersum FJ, Ijzerman G, Stehouwer CDA, Donker AJM. Analysis of twenty four hour ambulatory blood pressure monitoring: what time period to assess blood pressures during waking and sleeping? J Hypertens 1995;13:1053–1058.
23. Mansoor GA, Peixoto AJ, White WB. Effects of three methods of analysis on ambulatory blood pressure indices and the early morning rise in blood pressure. Blood Pressure Monit 1996;1:355–360.
24. Robinson T, James M, Ward S, Potter J. What method should be used to define "night" when assessing diurnal systolic blood pressure variation in the elderly. J Hum Hypertens 1995;9:993–999.
25. Youde JH, Robinson TG, James MA, Ward S, Potter JF. Comparison of diurnal systolic blood pressure change as defined by wrist actigraphy, fixed time periods and cusums. Blood Pressure 1996;5:216–221.
26. Leary AC, Murphy MB. Sleep disturbance during ambulatory blood pressure monitoring of hypertensive patients. Blood Pressure Monit 1998;3:11–15.
27. Mansoor GA, White WB. Nondippers with essential hypertension have greater sleep activity than dippers. Am J Hypertens 1999;11:38A.

28. White WB, Anders RJ, MacIntyre JM, Black HR, Sica DA, and the Verapamil Study Group. Nocturnal dosing of a novel delivery system of verapamil for systemic hypertension. Am J Cardiol 1995;76:375–380.
29. Khoury AF, Sunderajan P, Kaplan NM. The early morning rise in blood pressure is related mainly to ambulation. Am J Hypertens 1992;5:339–344.
30. Redeker NS, Mason DJ, Wykpisz E, Glica B. Women's patterns of activity over 6 months after coronary artery bypass surgery. Heart Lung 1995;24:502–511.
31. Redeker NS, Mason DJ, Wykpisz E, Glica B. Sleep patterns in women after coronary artery bypass surgery. Appl Nurs Res 1996;9:115–122.
32. White WB, Berson AS, Robbins C, Jamieson MJ, Prisnat LM, Rocella E, et al. National standards for measurment of resting and mabulatory blood pressures with automated sphygmomanometers. Hypertension 1993;21:504–509.
33. O'Brien E, Petrie J, Littler W, De Swiet M, Padfield PL, O'Malley K. et al. An outline of the revised British Hypertension Society protocol for the evaluation of blood pressure measuring devices. J Hypertens 1993;11:677–679.
34. White WB, Lund-Johansen P, Omvik P. Assessment of four ambulatory blood pressure monitors and measurements by clinicians versus intraarterial blood pressure at rest and during exercise. Am J Cardiol 1990;65:60–66.
35. O'Shea JC, Murphy MB. Factors confounding assessment of ambulatory blood pressure monitors, studied during formal evaluation of the Tycos Quiet-Trak. Am J Hypertens 1997;10: 175–180.
36. Shepard JW. Hypertension, cardiac arrhythmias, myocardial infarction, and stroke in relation to obstructive sleep apnea. Clin Chest Med 1992;13:437–458.
37. Lund-Johansen P, White WB. Central hemodynamics and 24-hour blood pressure in obstructive sleep apnea syndrome: effects of corrective surgery. Am J Med 1990;88:678–682.
38. Aubert-Tulkens G, Culee C, Rijckevorsel HV, Rodenstein DO. Ambulatory evaluation of sleep disturbance and therapeutic effects in sleep apnea syndrome by wrist activity monitoring. Am Rev Respir Dis 1987;136:851–856.
39. Sadeh A, Alster J, Urbach D, Lavie P. Actigraphically based bedtime sleep wake scoring; validity and clinical applications. J Ambul Monit1989;2:209–216.
40. Middelkoop HAM, Neven AK, Hilten JJ, Ruwhof CW, Kamphuisen HAC. Wrist actigraphic assessment of sleep in 116 community based subjects suspected of obstructive sleep apnea syndrome. Thorax 1995;50:284–289.

4 Ambulatory Monitoring of Blood Pressure

Devices, Analysis, and Clinical Utility

Yusra Anis Anwar, MD
and William B. White, MD

INTRODUCTION

Ambulatory blood pressure (ABP) monitoring has been available for over 30 yr but has been utilized primarily in research trials. Recently though, ambulatory blood pressure monitors have become increasingly popular in clinical medicine. Among the numerous benefits include the avoidance of potential BP measurement errors such as observer bias and terminal digit preference *(1)* and provision of more comprehensive information on BP behavior than is possible with office or home BP.

From: *Contemporary Cardiology:*
Blood Pressure Monitoring in Cardiovascular Medicine and Therapeutics
Edited by: W. B. White © Humana Press Inc., Totowa, NJ

Blood pressure varies reproducibly over a 24-h cycle with a number of well-recognized patterns. Most patients are "dippers": These individuals are characterized by at least a 10% decline in nocturnal BP compared to their awake BP *(2)*. Some patients may have an exaggerated drop in nocturnal pressures of >20% and have been referred to as "extreme" dippers *(3)*. Kario and co-workers *(3)* conducted a study that demonstrated that extreme dippers were more likely to have ischemic lesions on magnetic resonance imaging compared to dippers. Approximately 10–30% of patients are "nondippers," where the blood pressures decline is blunted or absent during sleep *(4,5)*. This may be the result of a variety of types of autonomic dysfunction or certain causes of secondary hypertension *(6)*. A small proportion of patients exhibit an "inverse" dipping pattern *(7)*. Here, the nocturnal blood pressures do not fall during sleep and, in some cases, may actually be higher than the daytime readings. Other 24-h BP patterns that have been observed resulting from the advent of ABP include "white coat" hypertension or the "white coat" effect *(8)*. In these patients office blood pressures are substantially higher than ambulatory awake BP averages. There are also some individuals who may present with a "white coat" normotensive pattern, where ambulatory blood pressure is elevated but office BP is normal *(9)*. This phenomenon may, in part, be the result of factors not present in the physician's office (e.g., smoking cigarets, mental stress, or excessive physical activity). Lui and colleagues *(10)* recently reported that "white coat" normotensives are as likely to have left ventricular hypertrophy and carotid artery intimal–medial thickening as those patients with definite hypertension.

Most research has shown that the clinic blood pressure reading is not as comprehensive an indicator of the overall hypertension burden, as it is only one point in time on a patient's 24-h blood pressure profile. Ambulatory blood pressure monitors overcome this problem by obtaining multiple readings over the 24-h period and capturing the blood pressure variability. Numerous studies have also shown that clinic blood pressures have a less predictive value for hypertensive target end-organ damage compared with 24-h blood pressure averages or loads.

This chapter will focus on the ABP monitoring devices and their validation as well as the clinical utility of the method in patients with hypertension.

AMBULATORY BLOOD PRESSURE MONITORING DEVICES: AUSCULTATORY AND OSCILLOMETRIC

Ambulatory blood pressure monitors are automated and programmable devices that detect blood pressure either by the auscultatory method or the oscillometric route. Some devices have the option of both techniques. Each method has its own advantages and limitations. The auscultatory devices employ the use of a microphone to detect the Korotkoff sounds. Unfortunately, auscultatory devices are also sensitive to external artifactual noise and may be also less precise in the obese

Table 1
Advantages and Disadvantages of ABPM Compared to Clinic Blood Pressures

Advantages	Disadvantages
Elimination of observer bias/error	Cost
Elimination of the "white coat" effect	Time commitment on behalf of patient
More comprehensive assessment of antihypertensive therapy	Disturbed sleep
Superior prognostic indicator	Cuff discomfort
Calculation of blood pressure loads	Inaccurate in atrial fibrillation
Evaluation of dipping/nondipping status	
Ability to better assess BP variability	
More reproducible over time	

upper extremity. In some devices, these limitations are overcome by synchronizing the Korotkoff sounds with the R-wave of the electrocardiogram (ECG gating) *(11)*. The oscillometric technique is less affected by an external artifact, as it detects initial and maximal arterial vibrations or the *mean* arterial blood pressure. The systolic and diastolic BP values are actually computed via set algorithms. Hence, the more sensitive the algorithm, the more accurate the device. Extremes in blood pressures increase the likelihood of error of the oscillometric device *(12)*.

Modern ABP recorders are compact, lightweight monitors that can be programmed to take blood pressure readings at various intervals (e.g., every 15 min during the day and every 30 min at night). In most devices, the bleed rates of deflation of the cuff and maximal inflation pressures can be programmed; some devices also have a patient-initiated event button (to monitor symptoms). Most devices have algorithms to screen out erroneous readings (to a certain extent) and will perform a repeat of the blood pressure measurement within 1–2 min.

Prior to initiation and again at the termination of the study, the ABP device should be calibrated against a mercury-column sphygmomanometer to verify that the SBP and DBP agree within about 5 mmHg. Patients should be educated regarding the use of the ABPM at device hookup. For example, the patient needs to be aware that when the actual readings are being measured, the arm should be held motionless to avoid artifact and repetitive readings *(13)*. Excessive heavy physical activity should be discouraged, as it usually interferes with the accuracy of the measurements. A diary that records wake-up and sleep times, time of medication administration, meals, and any occurrence of symptoms (the ability to manually initiate an additional reading out of sequence must be stressed at ABP hookup) should be maintained. The ABPM study should be performed on a regular working day rather than a non-working day or on the weekend to obtain the most representative BP values. A study conducted by Devereux and co-workers *(14)* demonstrated that daytime (work) BPs were a more sensitive determinant of left ventricular mass index than to daytime values taken at home.

The clinical advantages of ABPM studies are many and the disadvantages are few (Table 1). Ambulatory blood pressure monitoring eliminates observer error as well as the "white coat" effect and it allows for a more comprehensive assessment of antihypertensive therapy. In addition, ABP is a superior prognostic indicator for hypertensive target end-organ damage as compared to clinical blood pressures. The potential limitations of ABP devices include poor technical results in patients with atrial fibrillation or frequent ectopic beats or in those patients with an obese or muscular upper extremity that exceeds a mid-bicep circumference of 40 cm. Imprecise data may be recorded in patients with weak pulses or an auscultatory gap. The devices are usually well tolerated by patients, but, occasionally, there may be bruising or petechiae at the upper or distal arm. Some subjects may experience a lack of sleep at night or poor sleep quality because of the repeated cuff inflations.

VALIDATION OF AMBULATORY BLOOD PRESSURE MONITORS

The importance of the accuracy of ABP monitors has long been recognized by the Association for the Advancement of Medical Instrumentation (AAMI). A protocol was developed for the assessment of device accuracy and reliability in 1987 *(15)*. The AAMI protocol was followed by a more complex method of independent validation from the British Hypertension Society (BHS) in 1990 *(16)*. Although the protocols differed, their aim was to establish minimum accuracy standards of these devices in order for them to be considered reliable clinical tools. Since then, revisions have been made to both protocols *(17,18)*. In addition to clinical testing, the protocols include recommendations such as labeling information, details for environmental performance and stability, and safety requirements.

In an updated version in 1992, the Association for the Advancement of Medical Instrumentation *(17)* advised that BP should be measured at the onset and conclusion of the validation study in three positions (supine, seated, and standing) and the difference between the ABPM versus the reference standard should not be more than 5 mmHg with a standard deviation of ±8 mmHg. Additionally, the disparity between the ABPM and the reference sphygmomanometer should be assessed in 20 subjects at the beginning and the end of a 24-h BP study. This difference should not exceed 5 mmHg in at least 75% of the readings. For reliability testing, 3 different instruments should be assessed in a minimum of 10 subjects for a total of 30, 24-h ABP studies. It is recommended that a minimum of 75 readings in each of the 24-h studies be obtained with 15-min intervals during the awake period and 30-min intervals during sleep. The number of satisfactory readings (i.e., no error codes) should exceed 80% of the total number of readings programmed for the day.

The BHS protocol is a more complex validation protocol that has the grading system outlined in Table 2. The BHS protocol calls for five phases of validation: (I)

Table 2
British Hypertension Society Grading Criteria

| | Absolute difference between standard and test device (mmHg) | | |
Grade	≤5	≤10	≤15
A	60%	85%	95%
B	50%	75%	90%
C	40%	65%	85%
D		Worse than C	

Note: Grades are derived from percentages of readings within 5, 10, and 15 mmHg. To achieve a grade, all three percentages must be equal to or greater than the tabulated values.
Source: ref. *16*, with permission. © 1990 Lippincott-Williams & Wilkins.

Table 3
Validated Ambulatory Blood Pressure Monitors

Device	AAMI	BHS Grade
CH-DRUCK	Pass	A/A
Profilomat	Pass	B/A
Nissei DS- 240	Pass	B/A
Quiet Trak	Pass	B/B
Space Lab—SL 90202	Pass	B/B
Space Lab—SL 90207	Pass	B/B
A&D TM-2420 model 6	Pass	B/B
A&D TM-2420 model 7	Pass	B/B
A&D TM-2421	Pass	B/A

Note: For fulfillment of BHS protocol, the device must achieve at least grade B/B (where A indicates best agreement with mercury standard sphygmomanometer and D indicates worst agreement). For fulfillment of the AAMI standard, the mean difference ≤5 ± 8 mmHg.
Source: ref. *19*, with permission.

before use device validation, (II) in-use (field) assessment, (III) after-use device calibration, (IV) static device calibration where the device is rechecked after 1 mo of usage, and (V) report of evaluation. Each phase has its own passing criteria *(18)*.

A recent state of the market review on ABP monitoring devices by O'Brien and colleagues identified 43 devices available for clinical use at the time of publication in 1995 *(19)*. The review found that just 18 of the 43 devices had been subjected to an independent validation study (i.e., 9/31 of the suppliers). Of the recorders that underwent validation, only nine devices fulfilled both the AAMI and BHS criteria for accuracy (i.e., a maximum difference of 5 ± 8 mmHg between ABPM and reference sphygmomanometer or a grade of B/B for both systolic and diastolic BP, respectively). These independently validated ABP monitors (up until 1995) are shown in Table 3.

Table 4
Suggested Upper Limits of Normal
of Average Ambulatory Blood Pressure and Load

BP Measure	Probably normal	Borderline	Probably abnormal
Systolic average			
Awake	<135	135–140	>140
Asleep	<120	120–125	>125
24 h	<130	130–135	>135
Diastolic average			
Awake	<85	85–90	>90
Asleep	<75	75–80	>80
24 h	<80	80–85	>85
Systolic load (%)			
Awake	<15	15–30	>30
Asleep	<15	15–30	>30
Diastolic load (%)			
Awake	<15	15–30	>30
Asleep	<15	15–30	>30

Source: ref. *20*, with permission. © 1996 American Journal of Hypertension, Ltd.

ANALYSIS OF AMBULATORY BLOOD PRESSURE MONITORING DATA

Upon completion of the 24-h ABP recording, the data are downloaded and analyzed statistically to calculate blood pressure averages (i.e., 24 h, awake or daytime, and sleep or nighttime) as well as blood pressure loads (see below). Approximately 75–80 valid readings should be obtained. The American Society of Hypertension has proposed limits of normal blood pressure and blood pressure loads as depicted in Table 4 *(20)*.

Descriptive Blood Pressure Data from ABPM

Data are reported separately for the 24-h, daytime, and nighttime periods. These averages should be accompanied by the standard deviations as a simple indicator of blood pressure variability. Some studies have indicated that there is a significant relationship between blood pressure variability and target end-organ damage *(21)*, especially with beat-to-beat intra-arterial data. Frattola and co-workers conducted a study on 73 essential hypertensives who underwent intra-arterial blood pressure monitoring at the initiation of the study *(22)*. Subsequently, echocardiography was performed to assess left ventricular mass on subjects at the onset and at the conclusion of the study 7 yr later. The standard deviations were obtained and the average blood pressure variability for the group was calculated as 10.8 mmHg. The authors observed that end-organ damage was significantly higher in patients who had a greater than average BP variability (for

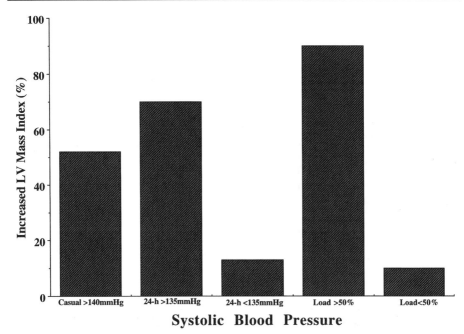

Systolic Blood Pressure

Fig. 1. The bars show the percentage of increased LV mass in subjects with elevated systolic blood pressures (both clinical and ambulatory) and systolic blood pressure loads. Reproduced with permission from Am J Hypertens **11,** Mochizuki Y, et al. Limited reproducibility of circadian variation in blood pressure dippers and nondippers, 403–409, © 1998, with permission from Elsevier Science.

the group as a whole) given that the 24-h mean arterial pressure was similar in both groups. Unfortunately, 24-h BP monitoring was not conducted at the end of the study to confirm if the same level of BP variability persisted.

Blood Pressure Loads

The BP load is calculated as the proportion of BPs >140/90 mmHg during the awake period and >120/80 mmHg during the sleep hours. White and colleagues were one of the first groups to introduce the concept of blood pressure loads *(23)*. They conducted a study in 30 previously untreated hypertensives and observed that the blood pressure load was a sensitive predictor of indices of hypertensive cardiac involvement. The results demonstrated that when the systolic or diastolic blood pressure loads were less than 30%, the likelihood of left ventricular hypertension (LVH) was negligible. However, with a systolic BP load exceeding 50%, the incidence of LVH approximated 90%, and with the diastolic BP load over 40%, LVH occurred in 70% of the subjects (Fig. 1) *(24)*.

"White Coat" Hypertension and "White Coat" Effect

"White coat" hypertension occurs when the patient's 24-h blood pressure is within normal limits, but BP in the clinic is persistently elevated (Fig. 2). In

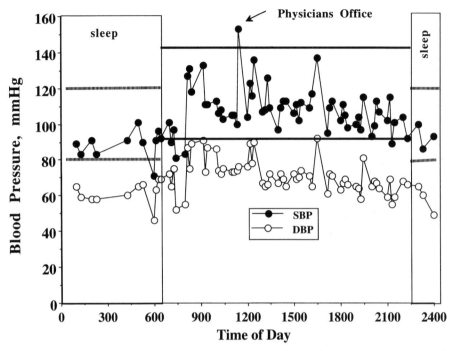

Fig. 2. The plot shows a 24-h blood pressure curve depicting WCH and dipping status. The patient's BP in the physician's office is 153/76 mmHg. The daytime ambulatory average is normal at 108/71 ± 13/9 mmHg. The subject has WCH with a 45/5 mmHg rise in BP in the physician's office. The patient also has a normal drop in nocturnal pressures, with a nighttime average of 90/60 ± 7/6 mmHg.

contrast, the "white coat" effect is defined as that additional pressor response in the established hypertensive subject causing an overestimation of the real BP (Fig. 3).

Dipping/Nondipping

Blood pressure normally has a circadian pattern in which BP drops during sleep and is higher during the awake hours of the day. This pattern is referred to as "dipping" (Fig. 2). The dipping status can be determined by evaluating awake and asleep blood pressure and calculating differences between the two averages. The percentage "dip" is then determined by dividing this difference by the awake average. The degree of decline in blood pressure varies from person to person, but a general, arbitrary consensus is that ≥10% drop in blood pressure during sleep is "normal." The patient who has *less* than a 10% drop in BP at night is referred to as a "nondipper" (Fig. 3).

Reporting of Ambulatory Blood Pressure Data

Using all of the above-referenced values in an informative report can be generated indicating the status of the patient's blood pressure. The reports should

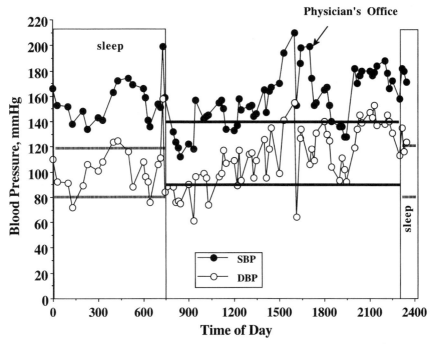

Fig. 3. The plot shows a 24-h blood pressure curve depicting WCE and nondipper status. The patient is hypertensive with a daytime average of 158/110 ± 21/23 mmHg. The nighttime BP does not drop significantly (157/105 ± 15/16 mmHg). The patient, in addition to his hypertension, has a significant WCE in which the BP is 216/98 mmHg in the physician's office.

include demographics, all medications taken during the study, the number of accurate readings obtained, the sleep times, and any symptoms that were experienced. The clinical report could also graphically depict blood pressures and heart rates over the 24 h, as shown in Figs. 1–3.

REPRODUCIBILITY OF ABPM

The majority of clinical trials conducted to evaluate ABP reproducibility confirm both superior short-term (<1 yr) (25,26) and long-term (>1 yr) (27–29) reproducibility of ABPM as compared to the clinical BP measurement. A recent substudy from the Systolic Hypertension in Europe (SYST-EUR) trial evaluated 112 patients who were randomized to receive placebo (27). Clinic and ABPM readings done at baseline were repeated after 1 mo in 51 subjects and a full year in 112 subjects. The results indicated that differences in 24-h ambulatory systolic BP (2.4 ± 10.7 mmHg [$p < 0.05$]) were far less than for clinical systolic BP (6.6 ± 15.9 mmHg [$p < 0.001$]) taken at 1 yr (Fig. 4). Another large-scale trial that also observed better reproducibility for ABP monitoring than clinical BP was the Hypertension and Ambulatory Recording Study (HARVEST), in which

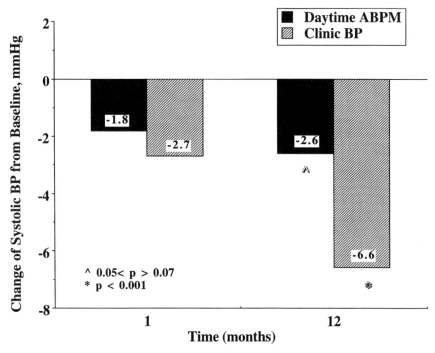

Fig. 4. The bars show the superior reproducibility of ambulatory BP versus clinic/office BP from the SYST-EUR trial (*n* = 112). Blood pressures were measured 1 mo and 12 mo after baseline measurements. Reprinted from J Hypertens **12,** Staessen JA, et al., Ambulatory blood pressure decreases on long-term placebo in older patients with isolated systolic hypertension, 1035–1039, © 1994, with permission from Elsevier Science.

508 subjects were evaluated *(28).* Ambulatory blood pressure monitors were conducted at baseline and 3 mo later in the untreated state. A very modest difference in the two sequential ABPMs for the group as a whole was observed (−0.4/−0.7 mmHg).

Studies evaluating the reproducibility of the circadian rhythm have not had such promising results. For example, a recent study by Mochizuki and colleagues found that there was limited reproducibility of the circadian rhythm *(30).* In that study, 253 untreated essential hypertensives were monitored for 48 h. In these 2 d, 16% of dippers "converted" into nondippers and 13% of nondippers "converted" into dippers (Fig. 5). The authors suggested that 48-h ABP monitors be performed to assess the circadian BP profile of an individual *(31).* Although this will not solve the problem entirely, it should decrease the likelihood of error.

INDICATIONS OF ABPM

Ambulatory blood pressure monitoring has been recognized as an important clinical tool by a number of expert medical groups and societies. Foremost, the

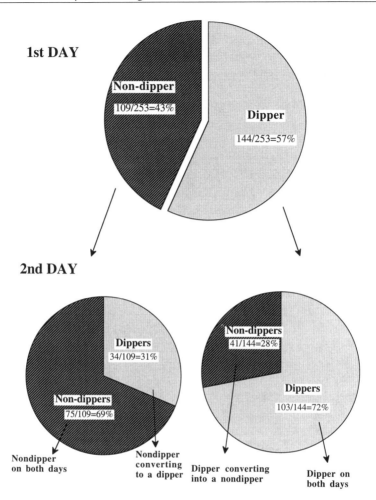

Fig. 5. The figure shows the limited reproducibility of the circadian rhythm (i.e., the dipping/nondipping status) with ABPM studies conducted over 48 h in 253 subjects. Reproduced with permission *(30)*. © 1998 American Journal of Hypertension, Ltd.

Joint National Committee (JNC VI) recommended ABP monitoring for a number of clinical situations (Table 5) *(32)*. Similar recommendations for ABPM have been made by the American Society of Hypertension and the American Society of Cardiology *(33)*. There is definite clinical benefit to be gained from ABP if the study is used judiciously. The section below briefly discusses the various clinical indications for this test.

"White Coat" Hypertension

"White coat" hypertension (WCH) is a result of the pressor response that patients experience when entering a medical environment. The patients have

Table 5
Primary Indications
for Ambulatory Blood Pressure Monitoring

Borderline hypertension
"White coat" hypertension
Drug-resistant hypertension
Hypotensive symptoms with antihypertensive therapy
Episodic hypertension
Autonomic dysfunction

Source: ref. 32.

a normal blood pressure outside of the doctor's office during activities of regular daily life. The prevalence has been estimated to be approximately 20% in untreated borderline hypertensives *(34)*. The prognostic significance of this diagnosis has been the subject of considerable debate. Verdecchia et al. prospectively followed 1187 subjects from the PIUMA registry, for up to 7.5 yr *(35)*. In their study, WCH was defined as an ambulatory daytime BP of <131/86 mmHg for women and <136/87 mmHg for men, and the clinic BP was >140/90 mmHg. No difference in cardiovascular morbidity was observed in the WCH population when compared to the normotensive control group. Follow-up of this database was later conducted with the use of a larger number ($n = 1500$) of patients *(36)*. The WCH patients were stratified into two subgroups. The first subgroup had a more restrictive and conservative definition of WCH (daytime ABP <130/80 mmHg), whereas the second group had more liberal limits for ABP (daytime ABP <131/86 mmHg for women and <136/87 mmHg for men). Cardiovascular morbid events in the first and more restrictive group was similar to the normotensive controls, but event rates in the more liberally defined group were significantly higher than the normotensive population. In the HARVEST trial, 722 hypertensive patients were evaluated using the more restrictive threshold levels to define WCH *(37)*. There was a significantly higher left ventricular (LV) mass index in the population with WCH (threshold <130/80 mmHg) when compared with the normotensive population (Fig. 6). Given the results of these rather large trials, WCH might be considered a prehypertensive state in some patients. Thus, monitoring and follow-up is required, and at some point, the institution of therapy may be needed. We believe that follow-up is necessary even in the 6–8% of true WCH patients with daytime ABP <130/80 mmHg.

Therapeutic Interventions

Accurate blood pressure measurement is the key to assessing the indication for antihypertensive therapy and to take it one step further, the efficacy and reliability of an antihypertensive drug. Ambulatory blood pressure monitoring can be used to assess both the need for or effectiveness of initial or additional antihypertensive therapy. To illustrate this benefit, a randomized prospective trial was con-

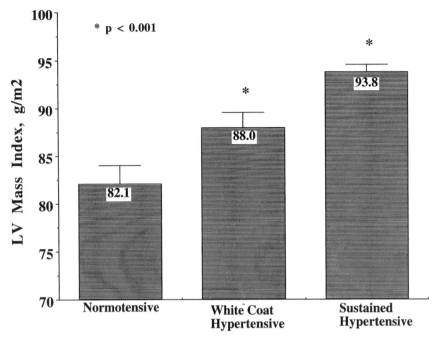

Fig. 6. The bars show the LV mass in three categories of patients (*n* = 722): the normotensive, those with WCH (threshold of <130/80 mmHg), and the sustained hypertensive (HARVEST trial). Reprinted from Hypertension **23,** Palatini P, et al., Factors affecting ambulatory blood pressure reproducibility, 211–216, © 1994, with permission from Lippincott-Williams & Wilkins.

ducted by Staessen and co-workers, who evaluated 419 untreated hypertensive patients over a course of approximately 6 mo using clinic versus ABP in therapeutic interventions *(38).* The Ambulatory Blood Pressure Monitoring and Treatment of Hypertension (APTH) trial randomized patients to an ambulatory blood pressure (ABP) arm versus a clinical blood pressure (CBP) arm. Drug treatment was adjusted in a stepwise fashion based on daytime ABP readings versus the average of three clinical measurements. At the end of the study, it was shown that more subjects in the ABP group discontinued antihypertensive drug therapy. Furthermore, fewer subjects in the ABP group had progressed to receive multiple antihypertensive drugs (Fig. 7). There were no significant differences in the final BP, LV mass, or reported symptoms between groups. Therefore, ambulatory blood pressure monitors can complement conventional approaches in determining optimal medication dosage and frequency of dosing.

Resistant Hypertension

Resistant hypertension has been defined as uncontrolled blood pressure despite triple drug therapy in near-maximal doses *(39).* Ambulatory blood pressure

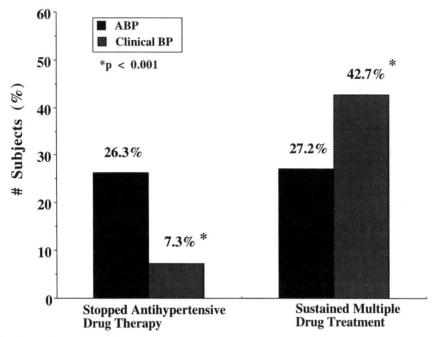

Fig. 7. The bars depict the percentage of subjects (*n* = 419) who stopped antihypertensive therapy and those who sustained multiple-drug therapy with the medication regimen being controlled either by ABPM results or by clinical measurements (APTH trial). Reproduced with permission *(38)*. © 1997 American Medical Association.

monitors are useful in the evaluation of those patients who do not appear to be responding to therapy or for those on complicated medication regimens. With an ABPM, the physicians can ascertain if and at what time additional therapy is needed or if it is needed at all. Mezzetti and co-workers evaluated 27 subjects with resistant hypertension by ABPM *(40)*. They observed that over 50% of the subjects showed a large "white coat" effect and were actually normotensive (<135/85 mmHg) on their current medication regimens. Conversely, Redon et al. conducted a larger study in 86 refractory hypertensives over 49 mo *(41)*. These patients were divided into tertiles of average diastolic BP from the ABPM. The *office* blood pressures were not different among the three groups. It was found that subjects in the highest tertile group (diastolic BP > 97 mmHg) had greater progression in hypertensive end organ compared to the lower two tertile groups. Thus, ABPM identified high-risk patients with refractory hypertension that was not apparent by office BP measurements alone.

Type of Therapy/Chronotherapuetics

It has been well documented that a majority of cardiovascular events occur in the morning hours because of a number of inciting hemodynamic, hormonal,

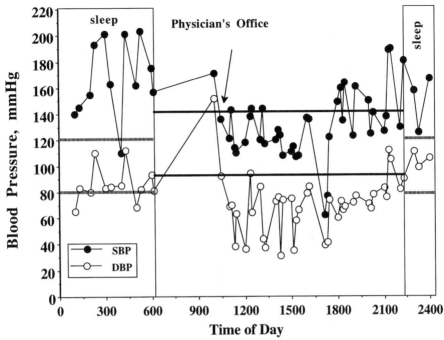

Fig. 8. The plot shows a 24-h blood pressure curve depicting autonomic dysfunction and inverse dipping. There is significant variability of blood pressure as seen by the standard deviation. The awake BP average is 132/71 ± 26/23 mmHg and the sleep average is 164/89 ± 28/15 mmHg. The sleep averages are higher than awake averages, indicating an inverse dipping pattern.

and hematological factors. Recently, Gosse and co-workers established in 181 patients that the *arising* blood pressure correlated with LV mass better than did the office blood pressures *(42)*. Hence, the higher the early morning blood pressure, the greater the LV mass. This rise in morning BP can best obtained by a 24-h ABPM. Another study conducted by Kuwajima and colleagues *(43)* in 23 elderly hypertensive subjects also demonstrated, with the help of combined ABP monitoring and activity monitors, that the change in systolic blood pressure after arising from bed significantly correlated with the LV mass index. Of note, there was no correlation with the change in systolic pressure *before* rising from bed and LV mass.

Orthostatic Hypotension/Autonomic Dysfunction

Individuals with autonomic dysfunction (e.g., diabetics) or orthostatic hypotension tend to lose the normal circadian variation in BP and may even demonstrate an inverse dipping phenomenon (Fig. 8). The Ohasama, Japan study clearly demonstrated in 1542 subjects that patients with inverse dipping had a significantly worse cardiovascular outcome as compared to the other patient groups (Fig. 9) *(7)*. Generally, there is also considerable variability of BP noted in the

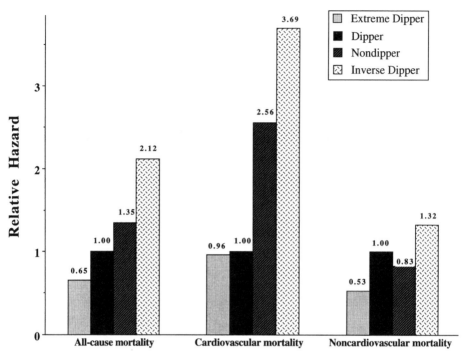

Fig. 9. The bars show the relative hazard of all cause mortality, cardiovascular mortality, and noncardiovascular mortality in four subsets of patients (*n* = 1542): the extreme dipper, the dipper, the nondipper, and the inverse dipper (Ohasama trial). Reproduced with permission *(7)*.

inverse-dipping patient population. Patients with inverse dipping may benefit from short-acting medications that can be taken at bedtime to reduce the nighttime BP average. In addition, some complicated patients with idiopathic orthostatic hypotension may be severely hypertensive in the supine position and markedly hypotensive in the upright position. Medication regimens can be tailored individually for these patients via the detailed BP information obtained through a 24-h ABPM.

Other indications for an ABPM study, as outlined by the JNC VI committee, include evaluation of symptoms and episodic hypertension. With the help of a patient-initiated event button, the physician can determine if the symptoms correlate with either a hypertensive (in the case of pheochromocytoma) or hypotensive period (in the case of excessive medication).

COST-EFFECTIVENESS
OF AMBULATORY BLOOD PRESSURE MONITORING

Ambulatory blood pressure monitoring studies generally cost $100–$350 in the United States. Many insurance carriers in the United States do not reimburse for the cost of the study. However, it should be noted that the high cost of ABP monitors in the United States do not generally represent the cost of the study in other countries (where the price is generally less). Thus, there has been some controversy regarding the cost-effectiveness of ABPM. Moser has argued that if 24-h ABPM were to be performed on just 3–5 million of the hypertensives in the United States, it would add an additional $600 million to $1.75 billion dollars per year to the cost of treatment *(44)*. However, the APTH trial performed a cost–benefit analysis of ABPM versus clinical blood pressure monitoring *(37)*. They observed that the cost of medication was less for the ABP arm compared to those patients who were solely evaluated by a clinical (office) BP ($4188 versus $3390 per 100 patients treated for 1 mo). Additionally, physician fees were also reduced in the ABP arm, as those patients had to return less frequently for the monitoring of their hypertension. The authors concluded that the potential saving in the ABP group was offset by the cost of the study, rendering it equally cost-effective and more therapeutically beneficial.

Yarows and colleagues in 1994 also conducted a cost-effective study in clinical practice *(45)*. They followed two sets of patients: the treatment group that had documented hypertension on an ABPM and were given appropriate antihypertensive therapy (*n* = 192) and a diagnostic group that was documented to be hypertensive in the physician's office and was off antihypertensive therapy (*n* = 131). The diagnostic group had a 24-h ABPM conducted and the prevalence of WCH in this group was determined to be 34% (using a 24-h mean diastolic pressure of 85 mmHg) *(46)*. The authors ascertained the average yearly cost of antihypertensive medications for the 192 hypertensive subjects to be $578.40 (range: $94.90–$4361.75). They concluded that in the diagnostic group, the fee for the ABPM ($188) would be offset by the savings for 1 yr of antihypertensive therapy (if no medications were used for the WCH patients).

REFERENCES

1. Prisant LM. Ambulatory blood pressure monitoring in the diagnosis of hypertension. Cardiol Clin 1995;13:479–490.
2. Synder F, Hobson JA, Morrison DF, et al. Changes in respirations, heart rate, and systolic pressure in human sleep. J Appl Physiol 1964;19:417–422.
3. Kario K, Matsua T, Kobayashi H, et al. Nocturnal fall of blood pressure and silent cerebrovascular damage in elderly hypertensive patients: advanced silent cerebrovascular damage in extreme dippers. Hypertension 1996;27:130–135.
4. O'Brien E, Scheridan J, O'Malley K. Dippers and nondippers [letter]. Lancet 1988;2:397.
5. Pickering TG. The clinical significance of diurnal blood pressure variation: dippers and nondippers. Circulation 1990;81:700–702.
6. Hany S, Baumgart P, Frielingsdorf F, Vetter H, Vetter W. Circadian blood pressure variability in secondary and essential hypertension. J Hypertens 1987;5(Suppl 5):487–489.
7. Ohkubo T, Imai Y, Tsuji I, Nagai K, Watanabe N, Minami N, et al. Relation between nocturnal decline in blood pressure and mortality. Am J Hypertens 1997;10:1201–1207.
8. Mancia G, Bertinieri G, Grassi G, et al. Effects of blood pressure measurement by the doctor on patient's blood pressure and heart rate. Lancet 1983;2:695–697.

9. Devereux RB, Pickering TG. Ambulatory blood pressure in assessing the cardiac impact and prognosis of hypertension. In: O'Brien E, O'Malley K, eds. Blood Pressure Measurement. Handbook of Hypertension, vol 14. Elsevier, Amsterdam, 1991, pp. 261–285.
10. Lui JE, Roman MJ, Pini R, Schwartz JE, Pickering T, Devereux RB. Cardiac and arterial organ damage in adults with elevated ambulatory and normal office blood pressures. Ann Intern Med 1999;131:564–572.
11. White WB, Schulman P, McCabe EJ, Nardone MB. Clinical Validation of the Accutracker, a novel ambulatory blood pressure monitor using R-wave gating for korotkoff sounds. J Clin Hypertens 1987;3:500–509.
12. Anis Anwar Y, Giacco S, McCabe EJ, Tendler BE, White WB. Evaluation of the efficacy of the Omron HEM-737 Intellisense in adults according to the recommendations of the association for the advancement of medical instrumentation (AAMI). Blood Pressure Monit 1998; 3(4):261–265.
13. White WB, Lund-Johansen P, McCabe EJ, Omvik P. Assessment of four ambulatory blood pressure monitors and measurements by clinicians versus intraarterial blood pressure at rest and during exercise. Am J Cardiol 1990;65:60–66.
14. Devereux RB, Pickering TG, Harshfield GA, Kleinert HD, Denby L, Clark L, et al. Left ventricular hypertrophy in patients with hypertension: importance of blood pressure response to regularly recurring stress. Circulation 1983;3:470–476.
15. American National Standard for Electronic or Automated Sphygmomanometers. ANSI/AAMI SP10-1987. Association for the Advancement of Medical Instrumentation, Arlington, VA, 1987.
16. O'Brien E, Petrie J, Littler W, De Sweit M, Padfield PL, O'Malley K, et al. The British Hypertension Society protocol for the evaluation of automated and semiautomated blood pressure measuring devices with special reference to ambulatory systems. J Hypertens 1990;8:607–619.
17. White WB, Berson AS, Robbins C, Jamieson MJ, Prisant M, Roccella E, et al. National standard for measurement of resting and ambulatory blood pressures with automated sphygmomanometers. Hypertension 1993;21:504–509.
18. O'Brien E, Petrie J, Littler W, de Swiet M, Padfield PL, Altman DG, et al. The British Hypertension Society protocol for the evaluation of blood pressure measuring devices. J Hypertens 1993;11(Suppl 2):S43–S62.
19. O'Brien E, Atkins N, Staessen J. State of the market. A review of ambulatory blood pressure monitoring devices. Hypertension 1995;26:835–842.
20. Pickering T, for the American Society of Hypertension Ad Hoc Panel. Recommendations for the use of home (self) and ambulatory blood pressure monitoring. Am J Hypertens 1996;9(1):1-11.
21. Parati G, Pomidossi G, Albini F, Malaspina D, Mancia G. Relationship of 24-hour blood pressure mean and variability to severity of target organ damage in hypertension. J Hypertens 1987;5:93–98
22. Frattola A, Parati G, Cuspidi C, Albini F, Mancia G. Prognostic value of 24-hour blood pressure variability. J Hypertens 1993;11:1133-1137.
23. White WB, Dey HM, Schulman P. Assessment of the daily blood pressure load as a determinant of cardiac function in patients with mild to moderate hypertension. Am Heart J 1989;118: 782–795.
24. White WB. Accuracy and analysis of ambulatory blood pressure monitoring data. Clin Cardiol 1992;15:II-10–II-13.
25. James GD, Pickering TG, Yee LS, Harshfield GA, Riva S, Laragh JH. The reproducibility of average ambulatory, home and clinic pressure. Hypertension 1988;11:545–549
26. Fotherby MD, Potter JF. Reproducibility of ambulatory and clinic blood pressure measurements in elderly hypertensive subjects. J Hypertens 1993;1:573–579.
27. Staessen JA, Thijs L, Clement D, Davidson C, Fagard R, Lehtonen A, et al. Ambulatory blood pressure decreases on long-term placebo in older patients with isolated systolic hypertension. J Hypertens 1994;12:1035-1039.

28. Palatini P, Mormino P, Canali C, Santonastaso M, De Vento G, Zanata G, et al. Factors affecting ambulatory blood pressure reproducibility. Results of the HARVEST trial. Hypertension 1994;23:211–216.
29. Mansoor GA, McCabe EJ, White WB. Long-term reproducibility of ambulatory blood pressure. J Hypertens 1994;12:703–708.
30. Mochizuki Y, Okutani M, Donfeng Y, Iwasaki H, Takusagawa M, Kohno I, et al. Limited reproducibility of circadian variation in blood pressure dippers and nondippers. Am J Hypertens 1998;11:403–409.
31. Tamura K, Ishii H, Mukaiyama S, Halberg F. Clinical significance of ABPM monitoring for 48h rather than 24h. The Statistician 1990;39:301–306.
32. The Sixth Report of the Joint National Committee on Prevention, Detection, Evaluation and Treatment of High Blood Pressure. Arch Intern Med 1997;157:2413–2446.
33. Sheps SG, Pickering TG, White WB, Weber MA, Clement DL, Krakoff LR, et al. American College of Cariology position statement; ambulatory blood pressure monitoring. J Am Coll Cardiol 1994;23:1511-1513.
34. Pickering TG, James GD, Boddie C, Harshfield GA, Blank S, Laragh JH. How common is white coat hypertension? JAMA 1988;259:225–228.
35. Verdecchia P, Porcellati C, Schillaci G, Borgioni C, Ciucci A, Battistelli M, et al. Ambulatory blood pressure: an independent predictor of prognosis in essential hypertension. Hypertension 1994;24:793–801.
36. Verdecchia P, Schillaci G, Borgioni C, Ciucci A, Porcellati C. White coat hypertension. Lancet 1996;348:1444–1445.
37. Palatini P, Mormino P, Santonastaso M, Mos L, Dal Follo M, Zanata G, et al. Target-organ damage in stage I hypertensive subjects with white coat and sustained hypertension. Hypertension 1998;31(Part 1):57–63.
38. Staessen JA, Byttebier G, Buntinx F, Celis H, O'Brien ET, Fagard R, et al. Antihypertensive treatment based on conventional or ambulatory blood pressure measurement. JAMA 1997;278:1065-1072.
39. Gifford RW Jr. Resistant hypertension: introduction and definitions. Hypertension 1988;11:II65–II66.
40. Mezzetti A, Pierdomenico SD, Costantimi F, Romano F, Bucci A, Gioacchino MD, et al. White-coat resistant hypertension. Am J Hypertens 1997;10:1302–1307.
41. Redon J, Campos C, Narciso ML, Rodicio JL, Pascual JM, Ruilope LM. Prognostic value of ambulatory blood pressure monitoring in refractory hypertension: a prospective study. Hypertension 1998;31:712–718.
42. Gosse P, Ansoborlo P, Lemetayer P, Clementy J. Left ventricular mass is better correlated with arising blood pressure than with office or occasional blood pressure. Am J Hypertens 1997;10:505–510.
43. Kuwajima I, Mitani K, Miyao M, Suzuki Y, Kuramoto K, Ozawa T. Cardiac implications of the morning surge in blood pressure in elderly hypertensive patients: relation to arising time. Am J Hypertens 1995;8:29–33.
44. Moser M. Hypertension can be teated effectively without increasing the cost of care. J Hum Hypertens 1996;10(Suppl 2):S33–S38.
45. Yarows SA, Khoury S, Sowers JR. Cost-effectiveness of 24-hour ambulatory blood pressure monitoring in evaluation and treatment of essential hypertension. Am J Hypertens 1994;7:464–468.
46. Khoury S, Yarows SA, O'Brien TK, Sowers JR. Ambulatory blood pressure monitoring in a nonacademic setting—effects of age and sex. Am J Hypertens 1992;5:616–623.

II

Concepts in the Circadian Variation of Cardiovascular Disease

5

Circadian Rhythm and Environmental Determinants of Blood Pressure Regulation in Normal and Hypertensive Conditions

Francesco Portaluppi, MD
and Michael H. Smolensky, PHD

CONTENTS

From: *Contemporary Cardiology:*
Blood Pressure Monitoring in Cardiovascular Medicine and Therapeutics
Edited by: W. B. White © Humana Press Inc., Totowa, NJ

INTRODUCTION

Modern medicine emphasizes the concept of homeostasis, constancy of the *intern milieu*. Accordingly, it is assumed that biological functions and processes are relatively stable during the 24 h and other time periods and that the exacerbation of disease and risk of severe clinical events are of equal probability each hour of the day and night, day of month, and month of year. Also, it is taken for granted that the kinetics and effects of medications are independent of the time of day when they are ingested, inhaled, injected, or infused. The concept of homeostasis as proposed by Claude Bernard in France in the 19th century and elaborated upon by Walter Cannon in the United States early in the 20th century was deduced from studies performed primarily during the daytime. In their eras, the assessment of biological parameters repeatedly at more than a single time of day was not generally feasible. The laboratory techniques of yesteryear necessitated the withdrawal of very large volumes of blood to determine the concentration of hormones and other constituents. Moreover, instrumentation enabling around-the-clock measurement of physiologic variables had not yet been invented. Today, modern laboratory methods require sometimes minute amounts of blood, and ambulatory devices facilitate the monitoring of a variety of variables, such as activity, body temperature, blood pressure, heart rate, and brain activity, continuously throughout the 24 h. The findings of investigations employing this technology invariably reveal that biological functions and processes are anything but constant. Rather, they document a prominent genetically based time structure consisting of rhythms with periods as short as a second or less to as long as a year *(1–3)*. The majority of practitioners and even academic investigators know very little about biological rhythms. This chapter first discusses the fundamental properties of biological rhythms and biological timekeeping. It provides an in-depth discussion of the role of circadian (24-h) rhythms in blood pressure (BP) regulation and day–night patterns in common cardiovascular (CV) diseases.

MEDICAL CHRONOBIOLOGY:
BASIC CONCEPTS AND PRINCIPLES

A biological rhythm is a self-sustaining oscillation that is defined by a set of specific attributes—period, amplitude, and phasing. The *period* is the duration of time required to complete a single repetition of the rhythm. If the period is close or equal to 24 h, it is termed a circadian rhythm. Ultradian rhythms have periods shorter than 20 h, and infradian rhythms have periods greater than 28 h. The temporal patterns of electrical impulses of the brain and heart are illustrative examples of rhythms of very short period, and menstrual and seasonal patterns are familiar examples of rhythms with long periods.

Amplitude is a measure of the predictable-in-time variability in biological function resulting specifically from rhythmicity. The amplitude of circadian rhythms varies between biological functions and processes and also between individuals, reflecting differences in genetics, age, and health status. The amplitude of the circadian rhythm in heart rate (HR) and BP is relatively small, whereas that in serum epinephrine and cortisol concentration is quite large *(2,3)*.

Phase or *stage* refers to the timing of the peak or trough of a rhythm relative to a designated time-scale—24 h, menstrual cycle, or year. The staging of the circadian rhythm in plasma cortisol in diurnally active persons is defined by the occurrence of a prominent peak in the morning around the time of activity onset and trough during nighttime sleep.

Rhythmicity constitutes a fundamental property of all living matter—cells, tissues, and organs. Biological rhythms are thought to be the result of the evolution of life-forms in an environment that changed in a predictable manner over specific time domains—the day, month, and year. Therefore, rhythmicity is envisioned to be adaptive and advantageous to survival *(4,5)*. Humans inherit unique mechanisms that account for biological periodicities *(6)*. Biological rhythms are coordinated by so-called "pacemaker clocks" that operate at various levels of organization, with the suprachiasmatic nuclei (SCN) located within the hypothalamus being most dominant *(7,8)*. The inherited period of human circadian clocks is not precisely 24 h; in most persons it is slightly longer. Environmental time cues act as "synchronizers" of inherited clocks. Synchronizers are periodic environmental signals used by organisms to calibrate the period of pacemaker biological clocks to 24 h *(9,10)*. The most important environmental synchronizers are the timing of sunrise and sunset, duration of the daily photoperiod, and the alternation of nighttime sleep with daily activity. Information regarding the environmental light–dark cycle is conveyed via the retina to the SCN via the rentino-hypothalamic neural tract. The environmental light–dark synchronizer signals also are responsible for adjusting the phasing of the body's circadian rhythms following alteration of the sleep–activity routine resulting from adhering to rotating shift-work schedules or rapid transmeridian displacement by air travel. Under these conditions, the temporal relationship of the peaks and troughs of the body's circadian rhythms become disrupted (desynchronized) from normal, resulting in a transient deficit of biological and cognitive efficiency until resynchronization is re-established *(11)*. Desynchronization of the biological time structure gives rise to the well-known symptoms of jet lag, a common complaint of travelers to overseas destinations *(12)*. The majority of persons adhere to a fairly regular activity–rest routine. The occurrence of the peaks and troughs of circadian rhythms is quite predictable in these persons from one day to the next. In contrast, the staging of 24-h rhythms in those adhering to inconsistent rest–activity routines (e.g., in persons employed in occupations mandating rotating shift work) is less predictable.

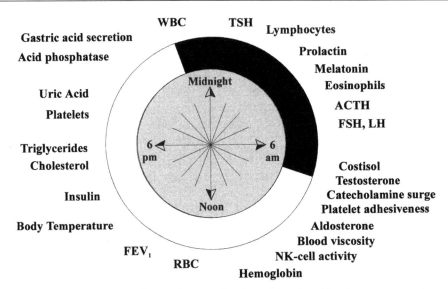

Fig. 1. Clock-like illustration of the organization of the circadian time structure shown by the average peak time of selected rhythms in clinically healthy subjects. The peak of each rhythm is depicted relative to the sleep (2230 to 0630)–wake (0630 to 2230) routine of the studied subjects. Reproduced from ref. *13*.

THE CIRCADIAN TIME STRUCTURE

The results of numerous studies help define the temporal organization of human beings *(2,3)*. One means of illustrating the circadian time structure is to depict the peak time of the body's 24-h rhythms in a clocklike diagram such as the one pictured in Fig. 1 *(13)*. In this figure, the sleep (from approx 10:30 PM to approx 6:30 AM)–wake cycle of the persons from whom the data were derived is shown on the outer rim of the clock, and the peak time of each selected variable is identified with reference to it. The peak of the rhythms in basal gastric acid secretion, white blood cell (WBC) count, and thyroid stimulating hormone (TSH) occurs during the initial hours of nighttime sleep. The crest in the rhythms of blood lymphocyte and eosinophil numbers and the blood concentration of melatonin and prolactin, plus adrenocorticotropic (ACTH), follicle-stimulating hormones (FSH), and luteinizing hormones (LH) occurs later during nighttime sleep. The cortisol rhythm peaks in the morning, and the rhythms of aldosterone, testosterone, platelet aggregation, blood viscosity, natural killer cell activity, and hemoglobin concentration crest in the morning. The spirometric parameters of lung function (the one-second forced expiratory volume [FEV_1] and peak expiratory flow rate [PEFR]) and body temperature peak in the afternoon. Insulin level is greatest late in the afternoon, and the serum concentration of cholesterol and triglycerides crests early in the evening. The peak in platelet number and serum uric acid concentration occurs later at night.

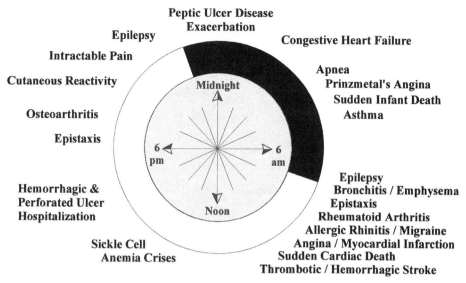

Fig. 2. Circadian rhythms in the exacerbation of chronic medical conditions and occurrence of morbid and mortal events in diurnally active persons. Shown are the approximate times relative to the diurnal activity–nocturnal sleep routine when the symptoms of common medical conditions typically are worse or when severe morbid and mortal events most likely occur. Reproduced from ref. 13.

CIRCADIAN RHYTHMS
IN OCCURRENCE AND SEVERITY OF DISEASE

The physiology and biochemistry of human beings undergo regular and dramatic variation during the course of the day and night. Thus, it is not surprising that the symptom intensity of many chronic medical conditions and the risk of life-threatening medical emergencies exhibit rather precise and predictable timings during the 24 h (Fig. 2). Those familiar with cardiovascular medicine are well aware of the circadian rhythms of angina pectoris *(14,15)*, acute myocardial infarction *(16)*, sudden cardiac death *(17)*, and thrombotic and hemorrhagic stroke *(18)*. However, numerous other medical conditions exhibit circadian rhythms in their occurrence or symptom intensity. The symptoms of peptic ulcer disease *(19)*, acute pulmonary edema *(20)*, and congestive heart failure *(21)* are most severe during the night. Asthma attacks are 100-fold or more frequent and of greater severity during the night than day *(22–24)*. The risk of death from asthma and sudden infant death syndrome (SIDS) is also greatest during the early morning hours *(24–28)*. The symptoms of allergic rhinitis *(29,30)* and the inflammation, stiffness, and pain of rheumatoid arthritis *(31)* are most intense in the morning. Migraine headache *(32)*, ventricular arrhythmia *(33–35)*, fatal pulmonary embolism, and hypertensive crises *(36)*, among other cardiac conditions *(37)* are of greatest risk during the initial hours of diurnal activity. The mood of depressed patients is typically poorest in the morning and best in the afternoon and evening *(38)*. The symptoms of osteoarthritis tend to be most bothersome in the late afternoon and evening *(39)* and the risk of perforated and bleeding ulcer *(40–42)* is greatest in the late afternoon. Certain types of seizure disorders occur more frequently at the time of the transitions between sleep and wakefulness, at night and in the morning *(43)*. Rhythmic alterations in biological function and disease status also are clearly evident over other time periods, such as the week, menstrual cycle, and year *(2,44–46)*.

TEMPORAL CONTROL OF CARDIOVASCULAR FUNCTION

Investigation of the temporal structure of the sources and mechanisms of cardiovascular rhythms is a logical and necessary step in understanding the chronobiology of BP and ischemic heart disease. Temporal variation in the CV system physiology and pathophysiology arises from day–night patterns in physical and mental activity and stress associated with the diurnal activity–nocturnal sleep cycle, plus the phase relationships of a variety of endogenous circadian rhythms that affect vascular and cardiac status and function.

The 24-h sleep–wake cycle, itself, is controlled by a large number of rhythms involving sensory, motor, autonomic, hormonal, and cerebral processes. Many changes that occur during sleep are actually independent of it *(47)*. The sleep–wake cycle results from the alternating dominance in time of mutually inhibitory interactions between arousal and activating systems, on the one hand (cholinergic, serotonergic, and histaminergic nuclear groups of the rostral pons, midbrain, and posterior hypothalamus, cholinergic neurons in the basal forebrain), and hypnogenic or deactivating systems, on the other (medial preoptic–anterior hypothalamic region and adjacent basal forebrain, medial thalamus, medulla). Circadian changes in autonomic nervous system activity play an important mechanistic role in the control of the sleep–wake cycle, and they also mediate the impact of sleep and wakefulness on CV function *per se*. For example, serotonin, arginine vasopressin, vasoactive intestinal peptide, somatotropin, insulin, and steroid hormones and their metabolites are involved in sleep induction at night, whereas corticotropin-releasing factor (CRF), adrenocorticotropin hormone (ACTH), thyrotropin-releasing hormone (TRH), endogenous opioids, and prostaglandin E_2 are involved in arousal in the morning. The cyclic 24-h pattern of these constituents is surely reflected in the phasic oscillations in CV function. Most biologically active substances (hormones, peptides, and neurotransmitters among others) exhibit significant circadian variability that is superimposed on feedback control systems. A distinctive day–night secretory pattern is thus exhibited by each. Whereas the secretion of these substances is typically episodic (i.e., manifesting high-frequency pulses), the occurrence of the secretory episodes is "gated" by mechanisms that are coupled either to sleep itself or to an endogenous pacemaker clock.

NEUROENDOCRINE INTEGRATION OF CIRCADIAN RHYTHMS AND THEIR EFFECTS ON CARDIOVASCULAR FUNCTION

The mechanisms of biological timekeeping involve a variety of neuro-humoral components that affect CV function and rhythms. For this reason, it is worthwhile to review the mechanisms of biological timekeeping. Autonomic and, in general, monoaminergic systems are responsible for integrating the mechanisms and systems of biological timekeeping. The temporal organization of these systems exhibits complex interactions with the pineal gland, from which the hormone melatonin emanates, and the SCN (the major pacemaker generator of endogenous circadian rhythms). The SCN is a self-sustaining oscillator whose period approximates 1 d. Three key components form the basis for biologic time-measuring and timekeeping mechanisms: endogenous oscillators, photoreceptor cells synchronized by the light–dark cycle, and neuroendocrine/neuronal effectors.

The first neuronal effectors are the pinealocytes. The main neuroendocrine effector, melatonin, is produced by pinealocytes of the pineal gland only during environmental darkness, with a surge during the second part of the night *(48–54)*. Melatonin is not stored after its synthesis; rather, it is released into the general circulation immediately after its formation *(55)*. Thus, it spreads important neuroendocrine information as to the onset, offset, and duration of darkness to the entire biology of vertebrate organisms. In mammals, photoreceptor cells in the retina convey information about the environmental light and dark cycle throughout the 24 h to the SCN and, thereafter, to the pineal gland via neural signals, thereby regulating the circadian rhythm of melatonin synthesis *(56,57)*. The SCN receives modulatory input from the periventricular nucleus of the thalamus *(58)*. Its norepinephrine content exhibits significant circadian rhythmicity, with the peak occurring at the beginning of the light period *(59)*. Also, 24-h variation in endogenous tyrosine hydroxylase and dopamine β-hydroxylase activity, and thus catecholamine and dopamine synthesis, is demonstrated by the pineal gland *(60,61)*. Monoamines (serotonin, histamine, norepinephrine, and dopamine) play a modulatory role in regulating the neurotransmission of signals via the retino-hypothalamic pathway to the SCN *(62)*. In fact, this neurotransmission is the result of a complex chain whose last ring is sympathetic innervation originating from the superior cervical ganglion.

Adrenergic agonists stimulate melatonin production in the pineal gland late, but not early, during the nighttime, although this effect requires the priming of darkness during the appropriate circadian phase of treatment *(63)*. The cAMP-dependent signal transduction pathway serves as a relay to stimulate melatonin synthesis *(64)*, and rhythmic adrenergic signals are essential to elucidate circadian fluctuation in cAMP-induced transcription *(65)*. At night, postganglionic fibers originating from the superior cervical ganglia release norepinephrine *(60, 66)*. Norepinephrine regulates melatonin synthesis through β-adrenergic receptors *(65,67)* by mechanisms acting distal to the SCN that generate the melatonin rhythm. Hence, it seems to be involved in the regulation of melatonin output by the SCN, but it is not implicated in the regulation of the pacemaker by light *(68)*.

Altogether, the results of numerous studies suggest that sympathetic and, in general, monoaminergic mechanisms are involved in the modulation of endogenous biological clocks and rhythms. This implies that physical and emotional stimuli that drive autonomic activation may also influence the expression of endogenous circadian rhythms. The opposite is also true. The pineal gland mediates the circadian rhythm of catecholamine secretion from the adrenal medulla, as reflected by the disrupted temporal pattern of nucleolar diameters in adrenomedullary chromaffin cells after pinealectomy *(69)*. In rats, melatonin inhibits dopamine release from the hypothalamus, but its effect is dependent on the circadian time of its administration; inhibition is greatest at 0500 h and nil at 1500 h *(70)*. A functional pineal gland (i.e., a gland that synthesizes and releases melatonin) is necessary for the expression and modulation of the circadian rhythmicity in acetylcholine-induced contraction of the prostatic portion of the rat vas deferens *(71)*. Such a contraction results from the release of norepinephrine and ATP from sympathetic nerve terminals. Melatonin directly modulates norepinephrine and serotonin synthesis through hypothalamic (mediobasal hypothalamus) and extrahypothalamic (amygdala and the pontine brain stem) pathways *(72)*. Finally, food intake and lighting conditions interact as controllers of the sympathetic nervous system and these interactions are modulated by the ventromedial hypothalamus *(73)*. However, hypothalamic (paraventricular nucleus) norepinephrine, together with neuropeptide Y and galanin, can control the total amount and the macronutrient selection of food intake at different stages of the circadian cycle *(74)*. It is of interest that experiments on rats demonstrate that lesions of the SCN abolish circadian BP, HR, and food-intake rhythms *(75)*.

In conclusion, the interactions between feedback responses to occasional environmental stimuli and endogenous circadian rhythms on monoaminergic systems have two different effects: Changes induced by external stimuli on monoaminergic neurotransmitter synthesis release chemical mediators, resulting in immediate biological responses, and inherent activity in autonomic activity modulates endogenous rhythms. These effects are both superimposed upon and modulated by rhythms that are endogenously generated by biological pacemaker clocks. Feedback responses to environmental stimuli serve to synchronize endogenous rhythms of the CV system; however, under certain circumstances, their expression may be masked. Overall, the immediate adaptation of CV function to the demands of the environment is modulated by the circadian-time-dependent responsiveness of biological oscillators. It is becoming increasingly evident, as discussed later in this chapter, that knowledge of the temporal organization of these neuro-humoral mechanisms as well as CV system function is essential for the complete understanding of circadian BP rhythms.

RHYTHMIC ORGANIZATION OF THE AUTONOMIC NERVOUS SYSTEM AND BIOGENIC AMINES

Circadian rhythms in the functioning of the autonomic nervous system are well known; sympathetic tone is dominant during the day, and vagal tone is dominant at night (76–93). In diurnally active persons, the plasma level of norepinephrine and epinephrine is highest in the morning during the initial span of daytime activity and is lowest during nighttime sleep (94–98). Urinary catecholamine excretion also exhibits marked circadian rhythmicity of comparable phasing (99–101). These day–night patterns are present not only in persons who adhere to normal routines but also in those who assume a position of constant recumbence over a prolonged duration of time. There is a strong temporal relationship between the 24-h variations in plasma dopamine and norepinephrine/epinephrine levels, indicating a dopaminergic modulation of the circadian rhythm of sympathetic nervous system activity (102).

In rats, the turnover of central dopamine and serotonin and clearance of their acid metabolites from the brain exhibits significant 24-h oscillation; turnover rates are highest between the second half of the rest and first half of the activity span (103,104). Circadian variations are found as well in the extracellular concentration of dopamine, as verified by quantitative microdialysis (105). The norepinephrine precursor tyrosine and its flow into the brain (calculated from plasma amino acid concentrations) exhibit significant day–night fluctuation (106). Such temporal variation in biogenic amines is also seen in the median eminence and in the intermediate and posterior lobes of the pituitary gland (107, 108). Parallel fluctuations are seen in the concentration of the norepinephrine metabolites 3-methoxy-4-hydroxyphenylglycol in the hippocampus and 3,4-dihydroxyphenylglycol in the hypothalamus and occipital and parietal cortex of rat brain (109). In the hypothalamus of the mouse, the concentration of norepinephrine, dopamine, and serotonin varies as much as twofold during the 24 h. Daily alterations in parent biogenic amines are reflected by concurrent changes in their metabolites (110). Also, brainstem (but not adrenal) phenylethanolamine N-methyltransferase (the enzyme which converts norepinephrine to epinephrine) activity shows a distinct 24-h fluctuation, with a nadir at 0700 h and a peak at 1500 h (111).

The epinephrine content of the peripheral organs of mammals is derived principally from the adrenal gland, with circulating epinephrine being taken up by sympathetic nerve endings in the organs of the body. In rats, cyclic 24-h alteration in nucleolar diameters, an ultrastructural feature of cellular activation, occurs in adrenomedullary chromaffin cells with a peak late in the activity period and a minimum during rest *(69)*. The epinephrine content of peripheral organs of rats increases after electric foot-shock in a circadian-time-dependent manner *(112)*, suggesting that the concentration of epinephrine in body organs plays a role in the response of the sympathetic nervous system to daily activities and stressful conditions.

In human beings, catecholamine sulfates are biologically inactive. In normotensive recumbent subjects, their circadian pattern is opposite that of biologically active free catecholamines *(113)*. During the initial portion of the sleep span, plasma noradrenaline and adrenaline sulfates peak. Before awakening, the concentration of both free noradrenaline and adrenaline suddenly increases, whereas their sulfoconjugate counterparts decline. Thus, the nocturnal decrease in the level of biologically active catecholamines may be the consequence of the activation of an endogenous system of sulfoconjugation; conversely, deactivation of the same system late during the sleep span may contribute to the significant morning increase in the concentration of biologically active catecholamines. The genetic control of catecholamine sulfoconjugation and deconjugation is primarily accomplished by two enzymes: phenolsulfotransferase and aryl sulfatase *(113)*. Temporal modulation of the gene expression of these enzymes most likely contributes to the circadian rhythm in sympathetic activity.

Environmental factors, especially the alternation of light and darkness in conjunction with the activity–sleep cycle, significantly influence the day–night pattern of catecholamine concentration. The level of norepinephrine, but not epinephrine, is strongly affected by activity, arousal, and posture *(79)*. The circadian rhythm in the plasma norepinephrine metabolite 3-methoxy-4-hydroxyphenylglycol also is evoked by day–night differences in physical activity and posture. In contrast, the 24-h pattern in the plasma dopamine metabolites homovanillic acid and 3,4-dihydroxyphenylacetic acid is regulated by a circadian oscillator, which is unaffected by the sleep–activity cycle *(109,114)*. Indeed, the nocturnal decrease in norepinephrine is observed even in healthy volunteers kept awake for 24 h by means of a regimented routine of forced activity and food consumption every hour. These findings suggest the circadian change in norepinephrine secretion is controlled by a biological clock whose activity is apparent only when the influence of sleep, posture, and activity is removed *(115)*. Nonetheless, the evidence is convincing that the observed 24-h changes in autonomic nervous system activity and biogenic amines are not explained by a single controlling influence. Temporal patterns in external stimuli are at least as important as, if not more important than, endogenous clock mechanisms.

The day–night pattern of sympathetic tone is not simply the result of the 24-h variation in catecholamine production; it is also dependent on rhythms in receptor number. Radioligand-binding studies reveal circadian changes in the number of receptors of the rat forebrain, particularly α- and β-adrenergic, muscarinic cholinergic, and striatal dopamine receptors *(116,117)*. These rhythms are endogenous in origin, as verified by studies showing their persistence in environments devoid of time (light–dark) cues *(118,119)*, dependence on the SCN *(120)*, and independence of the sleep–wake cycle *(116,120)*. The circadian rhythm in norepinephrine-stimulated cyclic AMP production in the cerebral cortex results from 24-h rhythms in α- and β-adrenergic receptors. Circadian rhythms in the postsynaptic responsiveness of hippocampal pyramidal cells to serotonin, norepinephrine, γ-aminobutyric acid, and acetylcholine have been demonstrated in the rat brain *(121)*. Short-term exposure to constant light or darkness produces a phase shift in the serotoninergic and cholinergic rhythms, suggesting their endogenous nature and their synchronization to clock time by the light–dark cycle. The circadian pattern in responsive to serotonin and norepinephrine varies in staging between December–April and May–August in rats entrained to a 12-h light–12-hour dark cycle, suggesting seasonal modulation of these rhythms *(121)*. The day–night variation in sympathetic tone also seems to entail circadian rhythms in putative second-messenger response systems involving cyclic GMP (cGMP in all brain regions except the parietal cortex) and cyclic AMP (cAMP in piriform, temporal, occipital, cingulate, and parietal cortex, amygdala, and nucleus accumbens). The correlation between receptor number and concentration of norepinephrine and dopamine metabolites is lower than expected *(109)*. The correlation is stronger with the putative second-messenger response systems, especially cGMP. The rhythms in cGMP are parallel in staging to cyclicity in α-1-adrenergic receptor function and may act as a second messenger for that receptor *(109)*. Circadian variation in the blood-brain barrier of rats acutely subjected to adrenaline-induced hypertension has also been demonstrated with lower albumin leakage into the brain during the night than day, possibly related to reduced β-adrenoceptor sensitivity at this time *(122,123)*.

Ultradian (high-frequency) oscillations in autonomic function also have been shown to be a common property of mammalian systems. However, the ultradian organization of the autonomic nervous system activity and biogenic amines has been less studied than its circadian counterpart because of methodological difficulties; such oscillations are not readily discernible from the wider fluctuations generated by circadian rhythms and extraneous stimuli. Brainstem networks generate rhythms of sympathetic nerve discharge with a frequency of 2–6 cycles per second *(124)*. In rats, special time-series techniques like spectral analysis reveal high-frequency oscillations in norepinephrine with periods of around 40 min and 90 min. These rhythms can be synchronized by certain environmental stimuli *(125)*. In the hypothalamus of the conscious rat, the release rates of dopamine, noradrenaline, and adrenaline fluctuate according to two ultradian rhythms. Dopamine exhibits 92-min and 8-h cycles, noradrenaline exhibits 92-min and

12-h cycles, and adrenaline exhibits 99-min and 12-h cycles. The release rate of dopamine and adrenaline is similar during the light and dark periods; however, it is different for noradrenaline *(126)*. In the rabbit, the release of hypothalamic catecholamines during the rest span exhibits a cycle of approx 70 min *(127)*. In humans, plasma catecholamines also display significant ultradian variations that persist even after bilateral adrenalectomy *(128)*. An about 8-h rhythm of urinary, epinephrine excretion has also been reported in man *(129)*. In addition, endogenous 12-h pulses of receptor escape from atropine blockade with acetylcholine have been demonstrated *(130)*.

CIRCADIAN ORGANIZATION OF HUMORAL FACTORS AFFECTING THE CARDIOVASCULAR SYSTEM

Renin–Angiotensin–Aldosterone System

Circadian rhythms in prorenin, plasma renin activity (PRA), angiotensin II, and aldosterone are well documented in normotensive and hypertensive conditions. They are demonstrable even in subjects restricted to long-duration recumbence *(131–141)*. The rhythms of plasma renin and aldosterone peak in the morning, and they persist, although with reduced amplitude, even in subjects who remain awake for an entire 24 h *(142)*. However, some investigators have failed to detect circadian patterns in PRA *(143–145)*, finding, instead, ultradian oscillations of about 100-min duration. These periodicities are strongly correlated with sleep-stage patterning: PRA declining during rapid eye movement (REM) sleep and peaking during the transition between deep and light sleep stages *(144,146)*. This relationship is even preserved in narcoleptic patients with disrupted sleep organization *(147)*.

Circadian rhythms in renin, angiotensin II, and aldosterone *(96,148,149)*, but not 18-hydroxycorticosterone *(150)*, are partly dependent on dopaminergic mechanisms. The sympathetic nervous system also modulates renin–aldosterone release *(151)*. In the rat pineal gland, angiotensin-converting enzyme exhibits circadian rhythmicity in activity, with the peak occurring at the end of the daily rest span. This rhythm is under negative control by norepinephrine released from the sympathetic nerves of the pineal gland *(152)*. The endogenous circadian rhythm in PRA determines the magnitude of the response of the organism to external challenge; in this regard, the exercise-induced PRA response is markedly higher at 1600 than 0400 h *(153)*. The circadian rhythm in plasma aldosterone is predominantly modulated by the 24-h rhythm in ACTH; the renin–angiotensin and dopaminergic systems play only a minor role. ACTH, which is secreted in greatest quantity during sleep, is a potent stimulus of aldosterone secretion at night. During the day, aldosterone is regulated in addition by the renin–angiotensin system *(96,151,154,155)*.

Renal Function

Circadian rhythms of renal blood flow, glomerular filtration rate, urine volume, and urinary excretions of Na, K, and Cl are well known. These rhythms are independent of temporal patterns in posture, meal timings, sleep, and activity during the 24 h *(156–165)*. In contrast, the excretion of creatinine is constant *(166,167)*. Renal blood flow and vascular resistance and glomerular filtration rate fall at night, but the decrease of urine flow is much more pronounced than expected suggesting the existence of 24-h rhythmicity of tubular reabsorption with a nighttime peak *(157,158)*. A greater amount of sodium, potassium, and aldosterone is excreted during the day than night; in contrast, the natriuretic substance kallikrein is excreted in a fixed rate throughout the 24 h *(165)*. At night, when the balance between sodium-retaining and sodium-sparing mechanisms favors natriuresis (i.e., a decreased aldosterone/kallikrein ratio), a significant correlation is detectable between sodium and potassium excretion rates as well as BP. The correlation is masked during the waking hours by the prevalence of sodium-retaining factors *(165)*. The circadian rhythm of renal sodium and potassium handling appears to be driven by the circadian rhythm of aldosterone secretion. The contribution of sympathetic factors seems to be minor *(164)*. Dopamine may play a role in the circadian variation of water and sodium handlings, as suggested by the close temporal relationship among the circadian rhythms of urinary dopamine, sodium, and water excretion *(97)*. Atrial natriuretic peptide also plays a role, as it modulates the rhythm of urinary sodium excretion *(168)*.

In summary, the renal hemodynamics exhibits significant circadian variation, and this contributes to the 24-h variation in BP. A number of physiologic rhythms are involved, such as the ones in systemic hemodynamics, structure, and permoselectivity of the glomerular basement membrane, urinary water excretion, and autonomic nervous and renin–angiotensin systems *(169)*.

Hypothalamic–Pituitary–Adrenal System

The endogenous circadian organization of the hypothalamic–pituitary–adrenal (HPA) system is paradigmatic. Rhythms in ACTH and cortisol secretion are well known, as reviewed in the classical work of Aschoff et al. *(56)*. Moreover, the sensitivity of the adrenal cortex to endogenously produced ACTH is in itself circadian time dependent and is, in part, responsible for the enhanced secretion of cortisol in the morning in response to stressful stimuli *(170)*. Catecholamines seem to be involved in the modulation of corticotropic function and cortisol rhythmicity. A rise in rat brainstem phenylethanolamine *N*-methyltransferase, the enzyme that converts norepinephrine to epinephrine, precedes the circadian rise in plasma corticosterone by several hours *(111)*. Pharmacological destruction of the ventral noradrenergic-ascending bundle, a pathway originating from the locus coeruleus and the A_1 and A_2 medullary groups of neurons that convey most of the catecholaminergic innervation to the paraventricular nuclei, suppresses the ACTH and cortisol circadian rhythms and causes the emergence of reduced-amplitude ultradian cycles *(171)*. Serotonergic neurons also impart a regulatory effect *(172)*. Nonetheless, circadian variation in plasma corticosteroid level can develop in the presence of either marked norepinephrine or serotonin depletion in areas of the central nervous system that have been implicated in the regulation of this periodicity *(173)*. Finally, ACTH plays a major role in eliciting the 24-h rhythm of aldosterone secretion, as discussed earlier *(151,155)*.

Hypothalamic–Pituitary–Thyroid System

The activity of this neuroendocrine axis affects the functioning of the CV system at multiple levels via direct positive inotropic and cronotropic actions, stimulation of tissue metabolic rate, and positive modulation of the agonistic sensitivity of the β-adrenergic receptors of the myocardium. The plasma TSH concentration exhibits significant 24-h rhythmicity. In diurnally active persons, the TSH level begins to rise in the late afternoon and is highest after midnight; the nocturnal peak occurs independently of sleep *(56)*. In actuality, the circadian variation in TSH is derived from a series of high-frequency pulsatile secretions that are of greater magnitude and frequency during the night than day. The peak in plasma TSH coincides in time with the peak concentration of norepinephrine in the thyroid gland *(174,175)*. Moreover, pharmacological manipulations with selective agonists and antagonists confirm the sympathetic modulation of TSH rhythmicity occurs through α_2- and β-adrenoceptors *(174)*. Dopamine inhibits the amplitude of the TSH pulses; however, its level does not decrease during the night. Hence, the neuroendocrine mechanism(s) underlying the nocturnal increase in TSH secretion is not dependent on decreased dopaminergic inhibition *(176–178)*.

Opioid System

The endogenous opioid system is comprised of various species of peptides *(179)*. Many of these possess potent CV system effects. Multiple forms of opioid peptides and opioid receptors have been identified. They are present in the central nervous system (in the forebrain and hindbrain nuclei and are involved in baroregulation, sympathoadrenal activation, and several other vital autonomic functions) and in peripheral neural elements (in the autonomic ganglia, adrenal gland, heart, vascular tissue, and kidneys). A circadian rhythm exists in the content of free and cryptic met-enkephalin in the heart tissue of both normotensive and spontaneously hypertensive rats *(180)*. Plasma concentrations of β-endorphins (but not met-enkephalin) also are circadian rhythmic *(181,182)*, as is the binding of the ligand to opiate receptors *(116)*. Involvement of both the sympathetic and parasympathetic systems in the actions of these peptides on CV function is established; although, little is known to date about the mechanisms of this involvement, especially in humans. Two major difficulties slowed research in this area: marked species specificity in the anatomical and functional organization of the opioid system so that animal models are only partially representative of the human beings, and poor receptor selectivity of agonist and antagonist substances that were available initially for investigation. In man, endogenous opioids modulate central nervous system BP control and they play a role in the nocturnal decline in BP *(183,184)*. δ-Opioid receptors might play a role in the nocturnal suppression of the sympathetic nervous system and the HPA axis, considering their known inhibitory effects *(185,186)* and phase relationships of the respective circadian rhythms.

Vasoactive Peptides

Atrial natriuretic peptide (ANP) is a 28-amino-acid polypeptide that affects physiologic functions and systems involved in BP regulation. It suppresses angiotensin II, plasma renin activity, aldosterone, and catecholamine concentrations. It increases sodium excretion and plasma and urinary cGMP levels, and it shifts the renal pressure–natriuresis mechanism so that the sodium balance can occur at lower arterial pressures. Thus, ANP lowers the BP and total peripheral vascular resistance. Conspicuous or sudden elevations of ANP triggers secondary sympathetic nervous system activation that counteracts its physiological actions. A distinct brain pool of ANP also has been identified, particularly in areas that are involved in the regulation of the CV system. Interactions of both circulating and brain ANP with the autonomic nervous system are well established. A review of the studies on ANP indicates that it is principally involved in the short-term control of BP and electrolyte balance, in contrast to and in opposition of the renin–angiotensin–aldosterone system, which is primarily involved in long-term BP control *(187)*. The day–night variation in the ANP level, which amounts to roughly 10 pmol/L, is unrelated to posture. The ANP rhythm peaks between 2300 and 0400 h when in diurnally active normal and hypertensive persons, the circadian rhythms of plasma renin activity and aldosterone are near or at their lowest levels *(96,188–195)*. In rats, the temporal pattern in plasma ANP concentration is paralleled by the circadian pattern in the numerical densities of the secretory granules of myoendocrine cells *(196)* and in humans by a circadian rhythm in the plasma concentration of the second-messenger cGMP *(197)*. In chronic renal and congestive heart failure patients *(198, 199)*, the circadian rhythm of BP is altered in its phasing; the nocturnal decline in BP is blunted or even reversed. Alterations in the 24-h BP pattern are paralleled by concomitant changes in the circadian rhythm of ANP, both before and after treatment *(200)*.

The calcitonin-gene-related peptide (CGRP) is a 37-amino-acid peptide produced by tissue-specific alternative RNA processing of the calcitonin gene *(201–203)*. The wide distribution of CGRP-rich fibers and high-affinity binding sites in the central and peripheral nervous system strongly suggests that CGRP has a neuromodulator and neurotransmitter role that is not limited solely to the regulation of peripheral vascular tone and blood flow. It may also be involved in a variety of metabolic and behavioral functions *(204–206)*. CGRP-binding sites are distributed in different parts of the central and peripheral nervous system of animals and humans *(207–211)*. CGRP-containing fibers are found throughout the CV system, in the heart, and especially within the coronary arteries, sinoatrial and atrioventricular nodes, and papillary muscles *(212,213)*. The concentration of CGRP is high in the adventitia of the arteries and veins *(212)*, and perivascular CGRP fibers are found in all vascular beds. Most likely, CGRP blood levels are representative of peptide spillover with release from nerve terminals that promote vasodilatation *(214,215)*. A circadian rhythm in plasma CGRP has been demonstrated in both normotensive *(216,217)* and hypertensive persons *(218)*. In vivo and in vitro studies suggest CGRP is a potent vasodilator *(219–227)*. Injection of CGRP into the coronary system of the rat, pig, and man results in dose-related increments in coronary flow *(220,224)*. Systemic infusion of CGRP or its perfusion in the isolated rat kidney decreases vascular resistance and enhances both renal blood flow and glomerular filtration *(226)*. The mechanisms by which CGRP regulates vascular tone are unclear. It might act directly on the vascular smooth muscle in exerting a potent vasodilator effect *(228,229)* or through an interaction with endothelial cells *(204,230)*. Intravenous infusion of CGRP in pharmacological doses decreases the mean BP and total peripheral resistance in rats *(223)* and man *(219,231)* and increases the HR. A bolus injection of the peptide results in increased PRA and plasma aldosterone concentrations *(232,233)*. Plasma CGRP levels increase in healthy subjects after assuming an upright position or following low-dose infusion of angiotensin II *(234)*. Thus, the renin–angiotensin system could modulate plasma CGRP secretion either directly through a vasopressor effect on peripheral blood vessels or indirectly through neurohormonal mechanisms that modulate vascular tone and BP. In fact, acute activation of cholinergic transmission by the acetylcholinesterase inhibitor pyridostigmine bromide increases CGRP plasma levels, whereas the muscarinic receptor antagonist pirenzepine exerts no significant effect *(235)*. This implies that the cholinergic system modulates the circulating levels of CGRP in the absence of a tonic cholinergic contribution to CGRP secretion under basal physiologic conditions.

Plasma vasopressin is also circadian rhythmic *(236)*. Although this peptide is thought to influence the functioning of the CV system, there is an absence of convincing data thus far.

CIRCADIAN ORGANIZATION
OF CARDIOVASCULAR PHYSIOLOGY

Arterial BP

The circadian rhythm in BP has long been recognized both in normal and hypertensive conditions *(237–246)*. Patients with a fixed HR *(247)* and bedbound normal *(240)* and hypertensive *(139)* persons exhibit a significant nocturnal decline in BP, which remains unaltered by antihypertensive therapy *(248)*. The circadian rhythm of uncomplicated essential hypertensive patients oscillates around a higher BP level than in normotensive persons, although it exhibits the same day–night pattern. The typical circadian BP pattern of diurnally active subjects has two daytime peaks—the first around 0900 h and the second around 1900 h—a small afternoon nadir around 1500 h, and a profound nocturnal nadir around 0300 h. The amplitude of the 24-h variation is slightly greater in diastolic (DBP) than systolic (SBP) BP, ranging between 10% and 20% of the daytime mean *(249,250)*. A significant increase in BP before awakening was initially reported by Millar-Craig and associates *(242)*. This was disputed by Floras and co-workers *(251)* and Littler *(243)*, who felt it was an averaging artifact. Reanalysis of the original work, however, confirmed the initial findings *(252)*. Through the years, the prewaking rise in BP has been alternately refuted *(253,254)* and confirmed *(249,255)*. It is difficult to determine the precise time when patients awaken from nighttime sleep, and this might explain the different interpretations of BP curves. The BP varies with the sleep stage *(241)*. Deep sleep (slow-wave sleep stages 3 and 4) is associated with the lowest BP levels, whereas light sleep (slow-wave sleep stages 1 and 2 and REM sleep) is associated with higher BP levels. During the first part of the night, deep sleep prevails, and the BP declines to its lowest level. During the second part of the night, REM episodes are frequent, together with brief episodes of arousal in response to external stimuli. The findings of an intra-arterial BP study on a large group of normal subjects reveal that the early morning rise in BP commences before awakening from nighttime sleep. Thus, it is incorrect to attribute the morning rise in BP solely to arousal *(255)*. Minor differences in the circadian BP profile related to ethnicity *(256,257)* and age *(258,259)* are well known. Using a BP measuring device equipped to assess physical activity, two distinct patterns of morning rise in BP have been identified. One, characterized by a gradual rise during late sleep, is common in younger subjects. The other, characterized by a steep rise after waking from sleep perhaps reflecting pronounced response to mental stress, is common in older patients *(260)*. Pregnancy does not seem to affect the circadian BP pattern *per se (261,262)*, although a reduced nocturnal fall in BP has been reported in healthy pregnant women *(263)*.

Day–night differences in physical and mental activity are the major determinants of the 24-h variation in BP *(264–266)*. Studies of rotating and night-shift workers reveal an immediate shift of the circadian BP rhythm, demonstrating the close linkage between activity level and BP *(267–271)*. This is a classical example of how external factors are able to mask the expression of intrinsic physiologic rhythms. Even though environmental factors prominently affect BP, certain aspects of the 24-h BP pattern are thought to have a genetic component, including the shape of the 24-h profile as well as the daytime mean and peak time of SBP and DBP *(272–274)*. In rats, the lesioning of the SCN abolishes the circadian rhythm in BP and HR without affecting the sleep–wake and motor activity cycle *(275)*.

Considerable evidence indicates the sympathetic system drives the BP circadian rhythm. A circadian rhythm of baroreflex reactivity and adrenergic vascular response has been demonstrated *(276)*. Intrarterial BP studies involving a variety of antihypertensive agents indicate that the before-awakening and upon-arousal morning steep rise in BP is the result of increased α-adrenoceptor activity *(252)*. Propranolol reduces the pressor range (the difference between basal and maximum BP readings) in most patients, and an inverse relationship can be demonstrated between changes in pressor range and noradrenaline concentration *(277)*. The circadian rhythms of BP and sympathoadrenergic activity, as exemplified by plasma and urine catecholamine concentration, plasma and lymphocyte cAMP concentrations, and β-adrenoceptor density and affinity on lymphocytes, are synchronous. This is the case for normotensive persons and primary hypertension patients who exhibit a normal BP circadian profile. It is true also for patients who exhibit abnormal catecholamine secretion and a circadian BP curve *(278)*. Circadian changes in sympathoadrenal and pressor reactivity to exercise are strongly correlated *(279)*. Spectral analysis of BP and interbeat HR interval data provide markers of autonomic activity and arterial baroreflex sensitivity. Using this technique, a clear 24-h variation in sympathetic and vagal tone, although not in arterial baroreflex sensitivity, is demonstrably independent of changes in activity level and posture *(93)*. The recumbent 24-h mean arterial BP of normal and hypertensive subjects is strongly correlated with plasma and urinary norepinephrine *(96,139,280–283)* and epinephrine concentration *(284)*. However, in elderly subjects, the correlation may be lacking or may even be inverted *(95,282)*. Bromocriptine treatment depresses the 24-h mean arterial BP and reduces the strength of its relationship with plasma norepinephrine. This suggests that the circadian rhythm of sympathetic nervous system activity and BP in patients with essential hypertension is modulated by a central and/or peripheral dopaminergic mechanism *(280,285)*.

An inverse circadian relationship in the staging of the rhythms in ANP and BP has been reported both in normotensive *(193)* and hypertensive *(195)* persons. This relationship has been substantiated in normotensive individuals studied two times 5 yr apart. On both occasions, the circadian parameters of the ANP and BP rhythms (mean 24-h level, 24-h amplitude of variation, and clock times of the peak and trough) showed a significant negative correlation *(286)*. An inverse circadian correlation also has been reported between the BP and CGRP *(217,218)*.

The circadian pattern of BP also seems to be dependent on circadian rhythms of the endogenous opioid system, HPA axis, the renin–angiotensin–aldosterone system, and vasoactive peptides as discussed earlier. Evidence in favor of this view comes from the study of many diverse pathological conditions in which alterations in the circadian rhythm of these neurohumoral factors, either primary or secondary to disruption of autonomic nervous system activity, are reflected by a persistent alteration of the 24-h BP pattern. A reduced or reversed nocturnal decline in BP has been reported in patients who have orthostatic autonomic failure *(287)*, ShyDrager syndrome *(288)*, vascular dementia *(289)*, Alzheimer-type dementia *(290)*, cerebral atrophy *(291)*, cerebrovascular disease *(292–296)*, ischemic arterial disease after carotid endarterectomy *(297)*, neurogenic hypertension *(298)*, fatal familial insomnia *(299)*, diabetes *(300–305)*, catecholamine-producing tumors *(306–310)*, Cushing's syndrome *(311)*, exogenous glucocorticoid administration *(312,313)*, mineralocorticoid excess syndromes *(314–316)*, Addison's disease *(317)*, pseudohypoparathyroidism *(283)*, sleep apnea syndrome *(318)*, normotensive and hypertensive asthma *(319)*, chronic renal failure *(314,320–330)*, severe hypertension *(331)*, salt-sensitive essential hypertension *(332)*, gestational hypertension *(333)*, toxemia of pregnancy *(334,335)*, and essential hypertension with left ventricular hypertrophy *(336,337)*, and following renal *(338)*, liver *(313,339)*, and cardiac transplantation *(340–345)* related to immunosuppressive treatment, congestive heart failure *(200,346–348)*, and recombinant human erythropoietin therapy *(349)*. A circadian profile characterized by daytime hypertension and nighttime hypotension has been described in hemodynamic brain infarction associated with prolonged disturbance of the blood-brain barrier *(350)*. In these patients, the range of variation in BP between the day and sleep-time BP level was significantly increased from expected—to 20% for SBP and 23% for DBP.

Disturbances of the circadian rhythm of autonomic nervous system activity and neuro-humoral factors that play a role in central and/or peripheral BP regulation are clearly involved in the genesis of alterations in the typical 24-h BP pattern. An imbalance of sympathetic versus parasympathetic activity is the major determinant of the alterations. This is true not only in the various forms of neurogenic dysautonomias but also in diabetes and chronic renal failure, where the change in the circadian pattern is minimal *(305)* or absent *(351)* before the onset of autonomic neuropathy. In chronic heart failure, tonic activation of the sympathetic nervous system throughout the day and night is present and seems to be the major determinant of the observed changes in the BP rhythm. Experiments on rats demonstrate that the altered BP pattern of heart failure is independent of changes in locomotor activity *(352)*. An identical imbalance of the circadian rhythm of autonomic activity has been demonstrated in essential hypertensive patients who exhibit a blunted nocturnal decline in BP *(353)*. However, the absence of the nocturnal fall in BP, conventionally defined as a sleep-time decrease in BP amounting to less than 10% of the daytime mean, does not necessarily imply an obliteration of the 24-h BP rhythm. This has been demonstrated in chronic renal insufficiency *(323)*, where a significant circadian rhythm in BP of reduced amplitude and peak time shifted toward the nighttime hours is frequently found; this type of pattern also is seen in patients diagnosed with fatal familial insomnia *(299)*.

Fatal familial insomnia, a prion disease leading to selective degeneration of the anterior ventral and mediodorsal nuclei of the thalamus *(354,355)* is a rare cause of genetically determined secondary hypertension. The cardinal feature of this condition is total and sustained insomnia. Thus, this condition offers a unique opportunity to study the circadian rhythms of BP and HR, along with their hormonal correlates, without interference of the sleep–wake cycle. In this disease, a significant 24-h pattern in BP and HR is detectable months after the complete obliteration of the sleep–wake cycle *(299)*. The 24-h BP pattern is reduced in amplitude with disappearance of the normal nocturnal fall in BP. Alteration of the circadian BP pattern appears to be closely related to dysfunction of the HPA axis. In fact, serum cortisol is significantly elevated in fatal familial insomnia, whereas ACTH remains normal, strongly suggesting an abnormality in feedback suppression of ACTH. In addition, distinct nocturnal peaks are detected in the circadian rhythm of these hormones. Cortisol hypersecretion occurs during the nighttime. Thus, there is a reversal of the normal sleep-related inhibition of cortisol and ACTH secretion. Moreover, the abnormalities in glucocorticoid and BP patterns precede the development of hypertension and severe dysautonomia. Taken together, the findings from studies of fatal familial insomnia patients point to a primary role of glucocorticoids in modulating the circadian rhythm of BP. Previous studies on Cushing's syndrome *(311)* and patients treated with exogenous glucocorticoids *(312)* revealed similar findings. Catecholamines, alone, seem less important in modulating the 24-h pattern of BP, because catecholamine-producing tumors obliterate the nocturnal BP decline only when the plasma concentration of catecholamines is extremely high *(310)*.

The absence of the normal nocturnal decline in BP appears to carry a higher CV and cerebral risk by prolonging the time during which the increased BP impact is exerted on target tissues and organs. Recent data support this view; the average nighttime BP level and magnitude of the nocturnal BP fall are significantly correlated with target organ damage, either cardiac *(336,337,356–360)*, cerebral *(293,294,361)*, or renal *(328,330,362)*. A large prospective study demonstrated that CV morbidity is higher in nondipper than dipper hypertensive women *(363)*. Left ventricular structure seems more load dependent in women than men with essential hypertension, as demonstrated by higher echocardiographic indices of left ventricular hypertrophy in female but not male nondippers than dippers

(360). Sodium sensitivity may be a marker of enhanced risk of renal and CV complications, and it is of interest that sodium-sensitive essential hypertensive patients show a loss of the nocturnal fall in BP *(364)*. The rate of rise in BP at the commencement of the daily activity period also is related to CV risk. In elderly hypertensive patients, the sharp morning increase in BP after arising from night-time sleep is related to the echocardiographic parameters of hypertensive target organ damage *(365)*. If these preliminary data are confirmed, restoration of the normal circadian BP pattern should be considered a therapeutic goal in all of those conditions in which it is abnormal. However, the feasibility and means of achieving this, plus the way of conducting an evaluation of the prospective significance of such a normalization, has yet to be sufficiently addressed. Only in patients with hemodynamic brain infarction has the drug-induced normalization of the pathological circadian BP profile been pursued *(350)*. Restoration of the normal nocturnal decline in BP also has been shown to be possible in chronic renal failure with evening, as opposed to morning, once-a-day isradipine oral dosing *(366)*.

The question of whether the 24-h pattern in BP is representative of an endogenous circadian rhythm or the consequence of the cycle of daytime physical activity and nighttime sleep has long been debated. It is evident that the lack of activity cannot be the sole explanation for the 24-h pattern of BP. The BP rhythm has a clear genetic basis that is driven by a variety of neuro-humoral constituents that exhibit intrinsic circadian rhythmicity, as discussed earlier. Moreover, the fact the BP rhythm loses or reverses its nocturnal fall in a variety of pathological conditions in which sleep and activity show only minor change constitutes additional evidence for an endogenous component.

Heart Rate

The circadian rhythm of the HR closely parallels that of BP in normal conditions. The 24-h profile (defined in terms of the daytime mean, amplitude, and peak time) has a strong genetic basis *(266)*. The circadian rhythm of HR is intrinsic and driven by fluctuations in autonomic nervous system activity. In all medical conditions that cause loss or reversal of the nocturnal fall in BP, nocturnal bradycardia is at least partially preserved. This indicates that the modulating influence of both variables is only partially coincident. This notion is further supported by the findings of a study on rats made hypertensive by transgenic implantation of the mouse salivary gland renin gene (TGR[mRen-2]27) *(367)*. The HR and BP circadian rhythms in these animals are out of phase by 12 h. Sleep appears to account for only a small amount of the entire nocturnal decline in HR. This is demonstrated by the persistence of the nocturnal bradycardia for months after total sleep deprivation in fatal familial insomnia patients *(299)*. Rhythms in autonomic function play a major role. In fact, the progressive alteration of the 24-h pattern in HR and catecholamines found in fatal familial insomnia closely parallels the clinical and other signs of progressive sympathetic overactivity and they are reflected in strikingly similar profiles throughout the different stages of the disease *(299)*. Because bradycardia during sleep is more the result of parasympathetic activation than sympathetic withdrawal, its preservation in fatal familial insomnia patients who have preserved parasympathetic activity is not unexpected. Inhibition of fetal and maternal adrenal glands modifies the fetal HR rhythm, suggesting adrenal involvement *(368)*. The nocturnal fall in HR is an important physiological phenomenon. In monkeys, its prevention by atrial pacing results in rapidly progressing heart failure resulting from sustained elevated left ventricular workload *(369)*. This finding suggests that alteration of the normal nighttime bradycardia could be regarded as an undesirable side effect of pharmacological treatment, although the prognostic and therapeutic implications of such are not established.

Electrical Properties of the Heart

Atrial and ventricular rates exhibit clear circadian variability, with peaks during the day and troughs during the night *(370–372)*. These patterns are already present during fetal life *(373,374)*. A circadian rhythm is also demonstrated in sinus node and AV nodal function, myocardial refractoriness, Q-T interval duration, and R- and T-wave voltage *(80,246,375–381)*. The day–night variation in the Q-T interval, which is more pronounced in normally innervated than transplanted hearts *(80,382)*, is related to the temporal variation in autonomic tone and circulating catecholamine concentration. The circadian-rhythm-dependent refractoriness of normal cardiac tissue and accessory pathways exerts protection at night against electrical induction of reciprocating tachycardia in addition to transient arrhythmia in the evening. In fact, day–night variation in ventricular arrhythmias has been demonstrated; there is significant reduction during sleep and no association with physical activity *(383–388)*. In patients with left-sided Kent bundles, nocturnal protection against electrical induction of reciprocating tachycardia is associated with prolongation of atrial, atrioventricular nodal, ventricular, and Kent bundle refractoriness *(389)*. Ventricular premature beats are more commonly induced by hypoglycemia during wakefulness than sleep *(390)*. The HR *(391)* and left ventricular function *(392)* are major determinants of the 24-h pattern in ventricular premature depolarization in certain subsets of patients. Only in patients with premature beats that are HR dependent and left ventricular ejection fraction greater than 0.30 is circadian rhythmicity demonstrable. Circadian periodicity is demonstrated also in the occurrence of bradyarrhythmias *(393)* and the ventricular response to atrial fibrillation *(394)*.

The possible influence of the circadian rhythm of BP on HR in heart patients has been studied with unclear results. A strong correlation between the incidence of ventricular extrasystoles and BP and HR was detected in patients with left ventricular hypertrophy, whereas in the absence of hypertrophy, supraventricular extrasystoles were higher in incidence during peaks of BP and HR *(395)*. In another study, an independent positive correlation between BP and ectopic beats was detected in 8 of 12 subjects, whereas the HR was a nonsignificant negative factor for ectopic beats *(396)*. Taken together, the findings of the various studies suggest a primary role of neural activity in modulating the electrical disturbances underlying ventricular ectopy, even though at least one study found no significant circadian variation in any electrophysiologic measure of ventricular electrical instability *(397)*.

Cardiovascular Hemodynamics

Knowledge of circadian rhythms in CV hemodynamics is far from complete. The nocturnal decline in BP should be related to decreased cardiac output and peripheral vascular resistance, or both. Except for the results of one study *(239)*, the nocturnal decrease in cardiac output has been found to parallel the nighttime decline in BP *(398–403)*. It should be noted, however, that the data of most studies are limited. The weight of the instrumentation used to assess subjects may have artificially limited the level of physical activity during the day, resulting in an underestimation of the true difference in hemodynamic parameters over the 24 h. Moreover, it is extremely difficult to reliably estimate cardiac output at night without interrupting sleep. Impedance cardiography *(399,402)* is useful, but its reliability is questioned. Using the pulse contour algorithm of Wesseling et al. *(404)* applied to beat-to-beat intra-arterial BP recordings, Veerman and colleagues *(403)* avoided most of the limitations of earlier studies. They documented a 9 mmHg nocturnal decrease in mean arterial BP, an 18-bpm drop in HR, a 7% fall in stroke volume, and a 29% decline in cardiac output from daytime values. They also observed a 22% increase in total peripheral resistance. The latter finding is at odds with that of an earlier study showing a 36% reduction in peripheral resistance during the night in healthy volunteers confined to bed *(405)*. Moreover, it is opposite to what is assumed to take place based on the well-documented decrease in sympathetic activity and enhancement of vagal tone during sleep *(76–93)*. Studies on primates also found total peripheral resistance to be increased during the night *(406,407)*. The physiological basis for this unexpected finding may be the decreased requirement for blood flow and oxygen nocturnally by resting skeletal muscles. In fact, a circadian pattern in oxygen consumption has been demonstrated *(408)*. A decreased peripheral requirement for oxygen and blood flow may result in increased peripheral resistance through the induction of vasoconstriction by autoregulatory mechanisms. However, the relatively sparse data on temporal changes of tissue blood flow do not support this hypothesis. Total (cutaneous, subcutaneous, and muscle) arterial blood flow in patients whose legs were fitted with an orthopedic device was 28% higher during the night than day *(405)*. The same day–night difference in subcutaneous blood flow also was substantiated in healthy individuals *(409)*. Renal blood flow is markedly reduced at night *(377)*; however, leg *(405)* and cerebral *(410)* blood flow is increased. Variation in the nature of the day–night pattern of blood flow in different regions of the body suggests cardiac output is redistributed and decreased in sleep. In the sleeping rat, a decrease in the effective circulating blood volume is reported to be a consequence of the translocation of blood to the periphery secondary to reduced venous tone *(411)*. Venous tone declines during sleep in humans as well *(398)*. In addition, central venous pressure declines *(412)* and hematocrit increases *(413)* during the night as a result of an absolute decrease in blood volume resulting from water loss, secondary to expiration, insensible perspiration, and urine formation. The only explanation that accounts for all the reported findings is a generalized reduction in vascular tone induced by sympathetic withdrawal or parasympathetic activation with preferential vasodilation in the extremities and relatively less marked dilation in other tissues and organs, such as the kidneys. In the morning, the distribution of cardiac output favors the kidneys at the expense of the extremities.

The arterial vessels adapt well to the hemodynamic changes that occur at night. In fact, nocturnal vasodilation subsequent to changes in autonomic activation results in increased arterial diameter. The reduced BP during the night could compromise the buffering function of the large arteries that act to transform the systolic flow jet from the heart into a more continuous flow for tissue perfusion. However, distension of both the elastic common carotid artery and the muscular brachial artery was shown to decrease at night, leaving vascular compliance unchanged *(414)*. In conclusion, the circadian patterns of arterial diameter and tension are inversely related, so that circadian changes in elastic properties have little effect on the buffering function of the large arteries of the body over the 24 h *(414)*.

Changes in pulmonary arterial pressure during wakefulness and sleep have been reported in healthy men. Arterial pressure is elevated moderately by 2–4 mmHg during non-REM and REM sleep relative to the daytime level *(415)*. A similar day–night variation in pulmonary artery diastolic pressure has been observed in patients with coronary artery disease; it is higher between midnight and 0600 h than during the day *(416,417)*.

The circadian rhythm in autonomic nervous system activity seems to be the major determinant of the circadian changes in circulation. Consistent with this view is the demonstration of a circadian rhythm of α-sympathetic vasoconstrictor activity in the forearm; it is enhanced in the morning and reduced in the evening *(418)*. In resting humans, the evidence is compelling that changes in plasma norepinephrine during the daytime hours are positively correlated with changes in peripheral vascular resistance but negatively correlated with changes in cardiac output *(419)*. Unfortunately, the referenced study was limited to daytime assessments that were done only for a limited duration of 5 h. There has yet to be a direct investigation of these relationships at night.

Circadian-rhythm-dependent differences in the reactivity of the coronary arteries have been demonstrated in response to adrenergic and parasympathetic stimuli, as well as physical exercise *(420,421)*. Normal, but not atherosclerotic, coronary arteries maintain basal tone throughout the day. In fact, no circadian differences in coronary blood flow or vasodilatory response to a 2-mg intra-coronary infusion of nifedipine was seen in normal conditions. In atherosclerotic coronary arteries, however, a decreased extent of drug-induced vasodilation was substantiated in the afternoon without change in blood flow *(422)*. This reflects an increase in the tone of atherosclerotic coronary vessels in the morning result-ing from endothelial dysfunction that results in a failure to limit the constrictor response associated with the morning increase in sympathetic outflow and cir-culating catecholamines.

Amplification by serotonin of other mediators (e.g., epinephrine and/or ADP) influences coronary blood flow significantly *(423)*. Even pineal melatonin pro-duction and secretion has been shown to directly affect the 24-h variation in cardiac function, namely day–night changes in the Ca^{2+}- and Mg^{2+}-dependent ATPase activity in the sarcolemma of heart tissue *(424)*. Other potential rhyth-mic factors may contribute to the circadian changes in CV hemodynamics; these include cyclic 24-h differences in the endogenous opioid and plasma renin–angiotensin–aldosterone systems, hypothalamic–pituitary neuro-hormonal axes, and vasoactive peptides, as is the case for BP.

Venous hemodynamics also undergo a significant circadian change *(425)*. Using an air plethysmography method, significant changes in venous valvular function (venous filling index) were detected indicating progressive insuffi-ciency in the late afternoon relative to the early morning, whereas calf muscle pump function and ambulatory venous pressures remained constant. The study concluded that changes in venous hemodynamic occur as a consequence of daily activity and valvular dysfunction. A circadian variation in portal pressure has also been reported. It progressively declines during the afternoon and evening and rises during the night to a peak around 0900 h *(426)*.

In conclusion, it appears that peripheral vascular resistance, arterial and pulmo-nary BP, portal pressure, HR, myocardial contractility, oxygen demand, and, most probably, cardiac output are circadian rhythmic. All of them peak in the morning. These 24-h changes are thought to be a consequence of the circadian rhythm in autonomic function and activity plus the abrupt rise in sympathetic outflow and circulating catecholamines coincident with the commencement of daytime activity in the morning. Neuro-humoral modulations as well as anatomo-pathological changes may differentially intervene in various disease states. The large hemodynamic changes that occur over the 24 h seem relevant to the therapy of BP disturbances, particularly hypertension. Almost nothing is known about the temporal pattern of systemic hemodynamics in hypertensive states of dif-ferent origin. Antihypertensive medications may need to be selected for their differential effects on hemodynamic mechanisms to achieve efficient control of BP throughout both day and night.

Blood Coagulation and Fibrinolysis

The day–night difference in sympathetic activation and glucocorticoid secretion causes blood cells to move between different body compartments. This helps explain the significant increase in both myeloid progenitor cell and polymorphonuclear leukocyte numbers in normal subjects between 0800 to 1500 h *(427)*. Circadian rhythms have been demonstrated in the aggregation of white blood cells and various activity markers of free radicals (thiobarbituric acid reactive substances, plasma thiols, and red cell lysate thiols *[428]*), and these may contribute to the 24-h temporal pattern of thrombotic events.

Platelet aggregation in response to adenosine diphosphate, epinephrine, arachidonic acid, and collagen displays a bimodal daily variation with peaks in the morning and afternoon. However, platelet adhesion exhibits a peak only in the morning *(429)*. Plasma levels of β-thromboglobulin and platelet factor 4 (indices of in vivo platelet activation) are lowest in supine subjects at rest between 0700 and 0800 h. They increase during daytime activity, peaking around 1500 h *(430,431)*. Thrombin–antithrombin III complexes and D-dimers (indices of activation of coagulation) do not exhibit 24-h variation *(431)*. Promotion of nitric oxide production decreases platelet aggregation and seems to eliminate cyclic variations in blood flow of stenosed and endothelium-injured arteries of mongrel dogs, whereas reduction in nitric oxide formation enhances platelet aggregation and induces cyclic variations in flow *(432)*.

A circadian rhythm of fibrinolysis is well established *(433–439)*. In diurnally active persons, total fibrinolytic activity is maximal around 1800 h and least around 0300 h. This circadian pattern is dependent on two enzymes, tissue-type plasminogen activator (t-PA) and plasminogen activator inhibitor type 1 (PAI-1), the latter being a fast and irreversible inhibitor of the former. The staging of the rhythm in t-PA activity is the same as that in fibrinolysis, although it is roughly 12 h out of phase with the rhythm of PAI-1. Plasma levels of t-PA and PAI-1 appear to exhibit gender differences; they are lower and have an earlier peak in women than in men *(440)*. The plasma concentration of other components of the fibrinolytic system have not been demonstrated to be circadian rhythmic.

A reduced-amplitude circadian fluctuation in fibrinolysis has been detected in eldery *(441,442)*, coronary artery disease *(443–445)*, and hypertriglyceridemia *(446–449)* subjects, whereas persons with extensive peripheral atherosclerosis show a loss of the physiological correlations between t-PA and PAI-1 *(450)*. Recently, evidence of a potential interaction between the renin–angiotensin system and fibrinolytic function has been reported. Infusion of angiotensin II in normotensive and hypertensive subjects results in the rapid increase in circulating levels of PAI-1, but not t-PA *(451)*.

Early Morning Hyperglycemia

The early morning increase in plasma glucose concentration and insulin requirement in diabetic patients *(452,453)* may be an exaggeration of the physiologic circadian variation in hepatic insulin sensitivity induced by antecedent changes in catecholamine and/or growth hormone secretion *(454)*. Plasma insulin, glucagon, and somatostatin exhibit ultradian rhythms *(455)*. Plasma insulin also displays a circadian rhythm with an evening peak. This rhythm is 12 h out of phase with the rhythm in pancreatic α-cell granules *(196)*. A modest rise in plasma glucose and glucose production rate is present in healthy young subjects in the early morning; however, it is absent in most healthy older subjects *(456)*. Insulin sensitivity is decreased at night in comparison to the mid-afternoon in healthy people, and in insulin-dependent diabetes mellitus (IDDM) patients; this phenomenon is exaggerated, even in those with defective counterregulation to hypoglycemia *(457)*. The "dawn phenomenon" (the morning elevation of plasma glucose concentration in diurnally active diabetics) is absent in newly diagnosed untreated non-insulin-dependent diabetes mellitus (NIDDM) patients. It appears after a year or so of dietary management and diet plus sulfonylurea treatment. This suggests the treatment and/or duration of diabetes play important roles in its pathogenesis *(458)*. In IDDM, the "dawn phenomenon" is the combination of an initial decrease in insulin requirement between approximately 2400 h and 0300 h and an increase in the insulin requirement between approximately 0500 and 0800 h. The "dawn phenomenon" is of pathogenetic importance. It results from changes in hepatic and extrahepatic insulin sensitivity that are best attributed to nocturnal growth hormone secretion and/or nocturnal increases in sympathetic nervous system activity *(459–462)*, changes in insulin clearance *(462, 463)*, and/or the physiologic early morning rise in plasma cortisol *(464)*, but not catecholamines and glucagon.

CIRCADIAN RHYTHMS
IN CARDIOVASCULAR DISEASE AND EVENTS

As discussed in previous sections of this chapter, the CV system is well organized in time during the 24 h. Almost all CV system functions, including HR, BP, blood flow, stroke volume, peripheral resistance, ECG parameters, plasma concentrations of vasoactive substances and their second messengers, blood volume and viscosity, platelet aggregability, plus thrombotic and fibrinolytic activity exhibit circadian variability. Although this chapter has emphasized circadian rhythms in BP and CV physiology and function, 7-d (circaseptan), yearly (circannual), and ultradian rhythms are known. Such rhythms in the physiological status of the CV system along with temporal patterns in the occurrence and intensity of environmental triggers of disease give rise to predictable-in-time differences in the susceptibility/resistance of persons to serious CV events. These so-called susceptibility/resistance rhythms are observed most notably as 24-h patterns in CV morbidity and mortality as discussed in this section.

Myocardial Ischemia

Untreated heart patients exhibit a circadian pattern in episodes of transient myocardial ischemia as evidenced by ST-segment depression *(14,465–473)*. A twofold or threefold increase in the number of transient ischemic episodes occurs in the morning, during the initial hours after arousal *(474)*. A second increase in the frequency of transient ischemic episodes is sometimes observed between 1800 and 2000 h *(475)*. In patients with established coronary artery disease, both symptomatic and silent episodes of ischemia were recorded in 72% of patients between midnight and 0900 h *(476)*. Episodes of myocardial ischemia occur most frequently between 0200 and 0400 h in patients with variant angina *(477)*. Moreover, angina attacks associated with ST-segment elevation occur more frequently during early morning sleep than afternoon activity *(478)*.

Myocardial Infarction

In day-active coronary heart disease patients, myocardial infarction (MI) onset is least frequent during the first part of the night, increased in the second part of the night, and most frequent between 0600 h and noon *(16,479–487)*. The peak of the day–night pattern in MI occurs in the morning, within the first few hours after awakening *(488)*. The coincidence of MI with awakening is substantiated in shift workers adhering to a reversed sleep–wake cycle *(489)*. Subgroups of patients might exhibit different temporal patterns, as suggested by the occurrence of smaller peaks in the evening *(482,484,486)* and daytime *(484,485)*. Age *(482,484)* and gender *(484)* have been found to affect the circadian pattern of MI onset, but this is not a universal finding *(486,487)*. A minor evening peak or even absence of 24-h variation in MI onset has been reported in patients with a history of smoking, diabetes *(482,484)*, CV disease, stroke *(486)*, or previous MI other than non-Q wave type *(484)*, presence of congestive heart failure, or non-Q-wave MI *(482,484,490)*. Altogether, it appears that different aggregations of multiple risk factors may culminate in different temporal patterns in MI onset.

Sudden Cardiac Death

Sudden cardiac death (SCD) occurs most commonly between 0600 and 1100 h in diurnally active persons; the second most common time is the afternoon. The occurrence of SCD is lowest during the night *(16,17,491–494)*. Again, when subgroups with different aggregations of risk factors are analyzed, different temporal patterns are suggested. Overall, deaths from fatal arrhythmias and MI show a major morning and minor afternoon peak of incidence; however, diabetic subjects as a group exhibit a peak between the afternoon and evening hours *(495,496)*.

Cerebrovascular Events

Both ischemic and hemorrhagic cerebrovascular events display marked temporal variability in their occurrence. The onset of ischemic cerebrovascular accidents is most frequent in the morning *(18,497–506)*, although two early studies reported a nocturnal peak *(507,508)*. A second less prominent evening peak has also been described by some investigators *(499,502–504)*, but no change in the temporal pattern is detectable in subgroups of cases classified according to the anatomical and pathophysiological attributes of the lesion *(506)*. The occurrence of subarachnoid and intracerebral hemorrhages has been reported to exhibit a bimodal pattern with a prevalent morning peak between 1000 h and noon *(508–511)*. A minor peak occurs between 1800 and 2000 h in subarachnoid hemorrhages, and between 1600 and 1800 h in intracerebral hemorrhages *(497,509, 510)*. In one study, no specific significant circadian pattern was detected *(503)*.

Arrhythmic Events

The ventricular response to chronic atrial fibrillation is circadian rhythmic. It is greatest at 1300 h and least at 0400 h *(394)*. Features of the temporal pattern in paroxysmal atrial fibrillation vary between studies. Some investigators report that it is higher in frequency during the daytime, with morning and evening peaks *(20,512)*; others report that it is higher in frequency at night *(513)*, with morning and early afternoon secondary peaks, or lacking circadian patterning altogether *(514)*. Paroxysmal supraventricular tachycardia exhibits a clear day–night pattern with a mid-afternoon peak in onset *(513–516)*. Ventricular ectopic beats are most common in the morning, with a second less prominent peak in the afternoon *(392,517–520)*. A temporal pattern in ventricular sustained tachycardia or fibrillation also has been described with a major morning and minor afternoon peak *(388,521–524)*. A progressive loss of the day–night variability in HR is observed in patients with increasing severity of Sick Sinus Syndrome *(525)*. In complete atrioventricular block, both atrial and ventricular rate display the typical 24-h sinusoidal pattern *(370)*.

Pathophysiological Mechanisms

The occurrence of CV events is triggered by several pathophysiological events, particularly sudden increases in BP, HR, sympathetic activity, basal vascular tone, vasoconstrictive hormones, prothrombotic tendency, platelet aggregability, plasma viscosity, and hematocrit. Each of these variables exhibits significant circadian rhythmicity with staging that is positively correlated in time with the occurrence of CV events. The BP reaches peak values in the morning, with a somewhat less prominent peak in the late afternoon or early evening. As discussed earlier, the morning rapid rise in BP may begin during sleep, before awakening *(242,249,252,255)* or after awakening *(243,251,253,254)*. It has been hypothesized that the morning rapid rise in BP exerts a powerful shearing force against the walls of the coronary vessels, causing rupture of unstable atherosclerotic plaques with significant thrombus formation at a time of the day when the staging of body rhythms favors intense thrombogensis *(526)*.

It is of interest that more than 80% of episodes of ambulatory ischemia are associated with substantial increases in HR *(527,528)*. The relative tachycardia that accompanies morning arousal results in increased myocardial oxygen demand *(529)*. The so-called double product (i.e., HR multiplied by SBP) is a representative and surrogate index of myocardial oxygen demand *(529–531)*. In the morning, the double product is 25–50% greater in hypertensive patients with demonstrated risk factors of CV disease than it is in young normotensive persons free of risk *(531–533)*. The higher morning BP in hypertensive ischemic heart disease patients has been linked to symptomatic and silent episodes of angina *(532,534)*, and it is likely to contribute to the elevated frequency of myocardial infarction in the morning. Nonetheless, ischemic events do occur during sleep, especially in people with severe coronary artery disease and vasospastic angina. Rapid-eye-movement (REM) sleep is associated with myocardial ischemia *(535,536)*. During deep non-REM sleep, HR, BP, and sympathetic-nerve activity are lower than during wakefulness *(92,241,415)*. During REM sleep when sympathetic-nerve activity even surpasses the levels of wakefulness, HR and BP achieve levels seen in the awake state. Hence, REM sleep constitutes a period of increased CV risk because of the reduction in coronary blood flow *(537)* and increase of coronary spasm *(536)*. This risk is time dependent in that REM sleep occurs preferentially during the second part of the night. The organization and duration of human sleep are strictly circadian-time dependent *(538)*. REM sleep is closely coupled to the circadian rhythm of core temperature *(539)*, which, in turn, is controlled by the biological clock or SCN *(540,541)*. The day–night pattern in the risk and occurrence of CV events, with its morning peak, is determined by the intrinsic circadian rhythmicity in REM sleep propensity, through increased levels of HR, BP, sympathetic activity, and prothrombic tendency.

Plasma norepinephrine level (94,542) and plasma renin activity *(131)* are higher in the morning hours and cause coronary vasoconstriction. Animal studies show that the resting coronary tone is highest in the morning and least at night *(543)*. The circadian rhythm in vascular basal tone takes place *(418)* in relation to an increased α-sympathetic vasoconstrictor activity during the morning hours. In addition, a lower ischemic threshold is found at this time *(534)*, suggesting that ischemia-induced coronary vascular resistance is increased then. This finding is also supported by a similar variation in postischemic forearm vascular resistance. Thus, in the morning, a low ischemic threshold presumably reflects elevated coronary vascular resistance. In addition, the circadian pattern of plasma cortisol secretion, characterized by a morning rise *(544)*, may indirectly reduce coronary blood flow by increasing the sensitivity of epicardial vessels to vasoconstrictor stimuli *(14)*.

In many cases of secondary hypertension and in a minority of patients with essential hypertension, the 24-h pattern of BP is blunted or reversed. In these nondipper patients, the physiological circadian balance between daytime sympathetic and nighttime parasympathetic prevalence is lost because of sustained sympathetic hyperactivity throughout the 24 h *(353)*. It is likely that altered circadian rhythms in vasoactive hormones contribute to the nondipping BP condition. This is especially true for cortisol *(311–313,351)*, catecholamines *(306–310)*, and mineralocorticoids *(314–317)*. The nondipper condition results in higher heart and cerebral risk than the normal dipper condition by prolonging the time over each 24-h period during which the impact of the increased BP is exerted on target organs. The absence of the nocturnal BP fall is significantly correlated with BP-induced target organ damage, both cardiac *(336,337,356–359)* and cerebral *(283,294,361)*. Moreover, CV morbidity has been shown to be higher in nondippers than dippers among women with ambulatory hypertension *(363)*.

Another major component of the day–night pattern in CV risk is imbalance between coagulation and fibrinolysis, as suggested by the presence of abnormalities in these systems in patients with myocardial angina and infarction *(545)*. A pro-coagulative tendency is demonstrated in the morning, when fibrinogen peaks are found, concurrent with low prothrombin and activated prothrombin time *(546–549)*. Platelet aggregability is higher in the morning in healthy *(542, 550)*, atherosclerotic *(551)*, and coronary artery disease *(552)* persons. Platelet activity is lower when in the supine position *(431)* and increased when upright *(430)*. Moreover, a higher aggregability of white blood cells combined with low levels of plasma scavengers, both predisposing to microcirculatory occlusion and thrombosis, are present in patients with ischemic heart disease *(428)*. Concurrent with the morning prothrombotic tendency is the marked decline in endogenous fibrinolytic activity. The circadian rhythm in fibrinolytic activity is well established *(434–436,553–555)*. The highest frequency of CV accidents takes place at the time of day when the PAI-1 level is near its peak *(554)*. Thus, in the morning, fibrinolytic activity is reduced because of the elevated level of PAI-1 and absence of t-PA *(444,445,556)*.

The prothrombotic tendency is also favored by the morning increase in plasma viscosity *(557)* and hematocrit *(558,559)*. High hematocrit and BP seem to act synergistically in increasing the risk of stroke in the morning; hypertensive persons who also have an elevated hematocrit have more than a twofold increase in risk compared to other hypertensives, and over a ninefold increase compared to normotensives *(560)*. An additional determinant of the increased morning risk of stroke is diminished vasodilator reserve at this time *(561)*. Finally, the endogenous release of dopamine, which promotes cell damage in experimentally produced cerebral ischemia *(562)*, shows a circadian rhythmicity in the central nervous system with enhanced metabolism and release in the morning *(563)*. Such a pattern benefits dopaminergic-dependent functions; however, it might contribute to the increased risk and frequency of cerebral infarction at this time *(564)*.

CONCLUSION

The biology of human beings is not constant during the 24 h, menstrual cycle, and year as inferred by the concept of homeostasis. Instead, most of life's functions vary predictably and often dramatically over these and other time periods. Circadian rhythms, in particular, are of great importance to clinical medicine in general *(13,565)* and to CV medicine in particular. In this chapter, we discussed in great detail the 24-h patterns of BP, HR, and other CV hemodynamics in normal and hypertensive states. These patterns arise from circadian rhythms in neuroendocrine and other functions plus day–night differences in physical activity, mental strain, and posture. In hypertensive patients at risk to CV events, the staging of the peak and trough of these critical circadian rhythms gives rise to an increased vulnerability to angina, myocardial infarct, sudden cardiac death, and stroke in the morning when environmental triggers of CV events tend to be most intense. Not only does the vulnerability to myocardial infarct vary during the 24 h, but so does its clinical course *(566)*. Symptom onset between 0600 h and noon is associated with greatest infarct size, whereas an onset time between midnight and 0600 h is associated with significantly lower risk of circulatory arrests from ventricular arrhythmias *(567)*. Moreover, the circadian-time-dependent occurrence of myocardial infarction is likely to affect the success of thrombolysis, which has been shown to be less in patients who have a morning onset *(568)*. Finally, the body's biological time structure can also exert significant influence on the pharmacokinetics and effects of antihypertensive and other medications used to treat hypertensive and other CV conditions. This will be discussed in depth in another chapter of this volume. Nonetheless, the prominent circadian patterns in BP, myocardial oxygen demand, coagulation, and CV events bring to fore the concept of chronotherapeutics (medications which proportion their concentration during the 24 h in synchrony with day–night differences in the biological requirement for therapy). In the United States, two verapamil chrono-therapies are now approved by the Food and Drug Administration. One is approved for the treatment of angina pectoris and both are approved for the treatment of hypertension. These chronotherapies have been shown to be effective in attenuating the rapid rise of BP in the morning and elevated level during daytime activity without inducing superdipping of BP during sleep. Nonetheless, it is not yet known whether they afford primary protection against CV morbidity and morality in the long term. The answer to this question must await the completion of the CONVINCE trial, which entails the comparison of conventional equal-interval, equal-dose, β-blocker, and diuretic therapy versus verapamil chronotherapy dosed once daily in the evening *(569)*.

REFERENCES

1. Halberg F. Chronobiology. Annu Rev Physiol 1969;31:675–725.
2. Reinberg A, Smolensky MH. Biological Rhythms and Medicine. Springer-Verlag, New York, 1983.
3. Touitou Y, Haus E, eds. Biological Rhythms in Clinical and Laboratory Medicine. Springer-Verlag, Heidelberg, 1992.
4. Pittendrigh CS. Temporal organization. Refection of a Darwinian clock-watcher. Annu Rev Physiol 1993;55:16–54.
5. Ticher A, Ashkenazi IE, Reinberg AE. Preservation of the functional advantage of human time structure. FASEB J 1995;9:269–272.
6. Lakatua D. Molecular and genetic aspects of chronobiology. In: Touitou Y, Haus E, eds. Biologic Rhythms in Clinical and Laboratory Medicine. Springer-Verlag, Heidelberg, 1992, pp. 65–77.
7. Moore RY, Silver R. Suprachiasmatic nucleus organization. Chronobiol Int 1998;15:475–488.
8. Reinberg A, Bicakova-Rocher A, Nouguier J, Gorceix A, Mechkouri M, Touitou Y, et al. Circadian rhythm period in reaction time to light signals: difference between right- and left-hand side. Brain Res Cogn Brain Res 1997;6:135–140.
9. Rea MA. Photic entrainment of circadian rhythms in rodents. Chronobiol Int 1998;15:395–424.
10. Hasting MH, Duffield GE, Smith EJD, Maywood S, Ebling FJP. Entrainment of the circadian system by nonphotic cues. Chronobiol Int 1998;15:425–445.
11. Ashkenazi IE, Reinberg AE, Motohashi Y. Interindividual differences in the flexibility of human temporal organization: pertinence to jet lag and shiftwork. Chronobiol Int 1997;14:99–114.
12. Arendt J, Deacon S. Treatment of circadian rhythm disorders—melatonin. Chronobiol Int 1987;14:185–204.
13. Smolensky MH, Martin RJ, Haus E, Reinberg A. Medical chronobiolgy with special reference to asthma. Chronobiol Int 1999;16: 539–563.
14. Rocco MB, Nabel EG, Selwyn AP. Circadian rhythms and coronary artery disease. Am J Cardiol 1987;59:13C–17C.
15. Mulcahy D, Keegan J, Cunningham D, Quyyumi A, Crean P, Park A, et al. Circadian variation of total ischemic burden and its alteration with anti-anginal agents. Lancet 1998; ii:755–759.
16. Cohen MC, Rohtla KM, Lavery CE, Muller JE, Mittleman MA. Meta-analysis of the morning excess of acute myocardial infarction and sudden cardiac death. Am J Cardiol 1997;79:1512–1516.
17. Muller JE, Ludmer PL, Willich SN, Tofler GH, Aylmer G, Klangos I, et al. Circadian variation in the frequency of sudden cardiac death. Circulation 1987;75:121–128.
18. Elliott WJ. Circadian variation in the timing of stoke onset. A meta-analysis. Stroke 1998; 29:992–996.
19. Moore JG, Halberg F. Circadian rhythm of gastric acid secretion in active duodenal ulcer: chronobiological statistical characteristics and comparison of acid secretory and plasma gastrin patterns in healthy and post-vagotomy and pyloroplasty patients. Chronobiol Int 1987;4: 101–110.
20. Cugini P, Di Palma L, Battisti P, Leone G, Materia E, Parenzi A, et al. Ultradian, circadian and infradian periodicity of some cardiovascular emergencies. Am J Cardiol 1990;66:240–243.
21. Kroetz C. Ein biologiescher 24-Studen-Rhythmus des Blutkreislaufs bei Gesundheit und bei Herzschivache zugleich ein Beitrag zur tageszeitlichen Haufung einiger akuter Kreislaufstorunge. Munch Med Wschr 1940;87:314–317.
22. Turner-Warwick M. Epidemiology of nocturnal asthma. Am J Med 1988;85(1B):6–8.

23. Dethlefsen U, Repges R. Ein neues therapieprinzip bei nachtlichen asthma. Med Klin 1985; 80:44–47.
24. Hetzel MR, Clark TJH, Branthwaite MA. Asthma: analysis of sudden deaths and ventilatory arrests in hospital. Br Med J 1977;i:808–811.
25. Cochrane GM, Clark TJH. A survey of mortality in patients between 35 and 65 years in the greater London hospitals in 1971. Thorax 1975;30:300–315.
26. Bateman JRM, Clark SW. Sudden death in asthma. Thorax 1979;34:40–44
27. Douglas NJ. Asthma at night. Clin Chest Med 1985;6:663–674.
28. Kelmanson IA. Circadian variation of the frequency of sudden infant death syndrome and of sudden death from life-threatening conditions in infants. Chronobiologia 1991;18:181–186.
29. Reinberg AE, Gervais P, Levi F, Smolensky M, Del Cerro L, Ugolini C. Circadian and circannual rhythms of allergic rhinitis: an epidemiologic study involving chronobiologic methods. J Allergy Clin Immunol 1988;81:51–62.
30. Smolensky MH, Reinberg A, Labrecque G. Twenty-four hour pattern in symptom intensity of viral and allergic rhinitis: treatment implications. J Allergy Immunol 1995;95:1084–1096.
31. Kowanko ICR, Knapp MS, Pownall R, Swannell AJ. Domiciliary self-measurement in rheumatoid arthritis and the demonstration of circadian rhythmicity. Ann Rheum Dis 1982; 41:453–455.
32. Solomon GD. Circadian rhythms and migraine. Cleveland Clin J Med 1992;59:326–329.
33. Behrens S, Ehlers C, Bruggemann T, Ziss W, Dissmann R, Galecka M, et al. Modification of the circadian pattern of ventricular tachyarrhythmias by beta-blocker therapy. Clin Cardiol 1997;20:253–257.
34. Venditti FJ Jr, John RM, Hull M, Tofler GH, Shahian DM, Martin DT. Circadian variation in defibrillation energy requirements. Circulation 1996;94:1607–1612.
35. Goldstein S, Zoble RG, Akiyama T, Cohen JD, Lancaster S, Liebson PR, et al. Relation of circadian ventricular ectopic activity to cardiac mortality. Am J Cardiol 1996;78:881–885.
36. Gallerani M, Manfredini R, Ricci L, Grandi E, Cappato R, Calo G, et al. Sudden death from pulmonary thromboembolism: chronobiological aspects. Eur Heart J 1992;13:661–665.
37. Portaluppi F, Manfredini R, Fersini C. From a static to a dynamic concept of risk: the circadian epidemiology of cardiovascular risk. Chronobiol Int 1999;16:33–50.
38. Wehr TA. Circadian rhythm disturbances in depression and mania. In: Brown FM, Graeber RC, eds. Rhythmic Aspects of Behavior. Lawrence Erlbaum Assoc., Hillsdale, NJ, 1982, pp. 399–428.
39. Bellamy N, Sothern RB, Campbell J. Rhythmic variations in pain perception in osteoarthritis of the knee. J Rheumatol 1990;17:364–372.
40. Illingsworth CFW, Scott LDW, Jamieson RA. Acute perforated peptic ulcer. Frequency and incidence in the west of Scotland. Br Med J 1944;ii:617–620.
41. Svanes C, Sothern RB, Sorbye H. Rhythmic patterns in incidence of peptic ulcer perforation over 5.5 decades in Norway. Chronobiol Int 1998;15:241–264.
42. Manfredini R, Gallerani M, Salmi R, Calo G, Pasin M, Bigoni M, et al. Circadian variation in the time of onset of acute gastrointestinal bleeding. J Emerg Med 1994;12:5–9.
43. Langdon-Down M, Brain WR. Time of day in relation to convulsion in epilepsy. Lancet 1929;May 18:1029–1032.
44. Dalton KD. The Premenstrual Syndrome. Charles C. Thomas, Springfield, IL, 1964.
45. Gallerani M, Manfredini R, Fersini C. Chronoepidemiology in human disease. Ann Ist Super Sanita 1993;29:569–579.
46. Case AM, Reid RL. Effects of the menstrual cycle on medical disorders. Arch Intern Med 1998;158:1405–1412.
47. McGinty D, Szymusiak R. Neurobiology of sleep. In: Saunders NA, Sullivan CE, eds. Sleep and Breathing, 2nd ed. Marcel Dekker, New York, 1994, pp. 1–26.

48. Arendt J, Paunier L, Sizonenko PC. Melatonin radioimmunoassay. J Clin Endocrinol Metab 1975;40:347–350.
49. Smith I, Mullen PE, Silman RE, Snedden W, Wilson BW. Absolute identification of melatonin in human plasma and cerebrospinal fluid. Nature 1976;260:716–718.
50. Vaughan GM, Pelham RW, Pang SF, Loughlin LL, Wilson KM, Sandock KL, et al. Nocturnal elevation of plasma melatonin and urinary 5-hydroxyindoleacetic acid in young men: attempts at modification by brief changes in environmental lighting and sleep and by autonomic drugs. J Clin Endocrinol Metab 1976;42:752–764.
51. Wilson BW, Snedden W, Silman RE, Smith I, Mullen P. A gas chromatography–mass spectrometry method for the quantitative analysis of melatonin in plasma and cerebrospinal fluid. Anal Biochem 1977;81:283–291.
52. Lewy AJ, Markey SP. Analysis of melatonin in human plasma by gas chromatography negative chemical ionization mass spectrometry. Science 1978;201:741–743.
53. Vaughan GM, Allen JP, Tullis W, Siler-Khodr TM, de la Pena A, Sackman JW. Overnight plasma profiles of melatonin and certain adenohypophyseal hormones in men. J Clin Endocrinol Metab 1978;47:566–571.
54. Weinberg U, D'Eletto RD, Weitzman ED, Erlich S, Hollander CS. Circulating melatonin in man: episodic secretion throughout the light–dark cycle. J Clin Endocrinol Metab 1979;48: 114–118.
55. Reiter RJ. Pineal melatonin: cell biology of its synthesis and of its physiological interactions. Endocr Rev 1991;12:151–180.
56. Aschoff J, Daan S, Groos GA. Vertebrate Circadian Systems. Springer-Verlag, Heidelberg, 1982.
57. Cassone VM. Effects of melatonin on vertebrate circadian systems. Trends Neurosci 1990;13: 457–464.
58. Krause DN, Dubocovich ML. Regulatory sites in the melatonin system of mammals. Trends Neurosci 1990;13:464–470.
59. Semba J, Toru M, Mataga N. Twenty-four hour rhythms of norepinephrine and serotonin in nucleus suprachiasmaticus, raphe nuclei, and locus coeruleus in the rat. Sleep 1984;7:211–218.
60. Craft CM, Morgan WW, Reiter RJ. 24-Hour changes in catecholamine synthesis in rat and hamster pineal glands. Neuroendocrinology 1984;38:193–198.
61. Racke K, Krupa H, Schroder H, Vollrath L. In vitro synthesis of dopamine and noradrenaline in the isolated rat pineal gland: day–night variations and effects of electrical stimulation. J Neurochem 1989;53:354–361.
62. Liou SY, Shibata S, Ueki S. Effect of monoamines on field potentials in the suprachiasmatic nucleus of slices of hypothalamus of the rat evoked by stimulation of the optic nerve. Neuropharmacology 1986;25:1009–1014.
63. Hong SM, Rollag MD, Ramirez J, Stetson MH. A single injection of adrenergic agonists enhances pineal melatonin production in Turkish hamsters. J Pineal Res 1993;14:138–144.
64. Vanecek J, Sugden D, Weller J, Klein DC. Atypical synergistic alpha 1- and beta-adrenergic regulation of adenosine 3',5'-monophosphate and guanosine 3',5'-monophosphate in rat pinealocytes. Endocrinology 1985;116:2167–2173.
65. Stehle JH, Foulkes NS, Molina CA, Simonneaux V, Pevet P, Sassone-Corsi P. Adrenergic signals direct rhythmic expression of transcriptional repressor CREM in the pineal gland. Nature 1993;365:314–320.
66. Brownstein M, Axelrod J. Pineal gland: 24-hour rhythm in norepinephrine turnover. Science 1974;184:163–165.
67. Axelrod J. The pineal gland: a neurochemical transducer. Science 1974;184:1341–1348.
68. Zatz M, Mullen DA. Norepinephrine, acting via adenylate cyclase, inhibits melatonin output but does not phase-shift the pacemaker in cultured chick pineal cells. Brain Res 1988;450: 137–143.

69. Kachi T, Banerji TK, Quay WB. Quantitative cytological analysis of functional changes in adrenomedullary chromaffin cells in normal, sham-operated, and pinealectomized rats in relation to time of day: I. Nucleolar size. J Pineal Res 1984;1:31–49.

70. Zisapel N, Egozi Y, Laudon M. Circadian variations in the inhibition of dopamine release from adult and newborn rat hypothalamus by melatonin. Neuroendocrinology 1985;40: 102–108.

71. Carneiro RC, Cipolla-Neto J, Markus RP. Diurnal variation of the rat vas deferens contraction induced by stimulation of presynaptic nicotinic receptors and pineal function. J Pharmacol Exp Ther 1991;259:614–619.

72. Alexiuk NA, Vriend JP. Extrahypothalamic effects of melatonin administration on serotonin and norepinephrine synthesis in female Syrian hamsters. J Neural Transm Gen Sect 1993;94: 43–53.

73. Yoshida T, Bray GA. Effects of food and light on norepinephrine turnover. Am J Physiol 1988;254(5 Pt 2):R821–R827.

74. Tempel DL, Leibowitz SF. Diurnal variations in the feeding responses to norepinephrine, neuropeptide Y and galanin in the PVN. Brain Res Bull 1990;25:821–825.

75. Janssen BJ, Tyssen CM, Duindam H, Rietveld WJ. Suprachiasmatic lesions eliminate 24-h blood pressure variability in rats. Physiol Behav 1994;55:307–311.

76. Cowley AW Jr, Liard JF, Guyton AC. Role of baroreceptor reflex in daily control of arterial blood pressure and other variables in dogs. Circ Res 1973;32:564–576.

77. Ewing DJ, Borsey DQ, Travis P, Bellavere F, Neilson JM, Clarke BF. Abnormalities of ambulatory 24-hour heart rate in diabetes mellitus. Diabetes 1983;32:101–105.

78. Clement DL, De Pue N, Jordaens LJ, Packet L. Adrenergic and vagal influences on blood pressure variability. Clin Exp Hypertens A 1985;7:159–166.

79. Linsell CR, Lightman SL, Mullen PE, Brown MJ, Causon RC. Circadian rhythms of epinephrine and norepinephrine in man. J Clin Endocrinol Metab 1985;60:1210–1215.

80. Bexton RS, Vallin HO, Camm AJ. Diurnal variation of the QT interval—influence of the autonomic nervous system. Br Heart J 1986;55:253–258.

81. Mancia G, Parati G, Pomidossi G, Casadei R, Di Rienzo M, Zanchetti A. Arterial baroreflexes and blood pressure and heart rate variabilities in humans. Hypertension 1986;8:147–153.

82. Kasting GA, Eckberg DL, Fritsch JM, Birkett CL. Continuous resetting of the human carotid baroreceptor-cardiac reflex. Am J Physiol 1987;252:R732–R736.

83. Parati G, Di Rienzo M, Bertinieri G, Pomidossi G, Casadei R, Groppelli A, et al. Evaluation of the baroreceptor–heart rate reflex by 24-hour intra-arterial blood pressure monitoring in humans. Hypertension 1988;12:214–222.

84. Bell LB, Dorward PK, Rudd CD. Influence of cardiac afferents on time-dependent changes in the renal sympathetic baroreflex of conscious rabbits. Clin Exp Pharmacol Physiol 1990; 17:545–555.

85. Furlan R, Guzzetti S, Crivellaro W, Dassi S, Tinelli M, Baselli G, et al. Continuous 24-hour assessment of the neural regulation of systemic arterial pressure and RR variabilities in ambulant subjects. Circulation 1990;81:537–547.

86. Hayano J, Sakakibara Y, Yamada M, Kamiya T, Fujinami T, Yokoyama K, et al. Diurnal variations in vagal and sympathetic cardiac control. Am J Physiol.1990;258:H642–H646.

87. Kamath MV, Fallen EL. Diurnal variations of neurocardiac rhythms in acute myocardial infarction. Am J Cardiol 1991;68:155–160.

88. Goldsmith RL, Bigger JT, Steinman RC, Fleiss JL. Comparison of 24-hour parasympathetic activity in endurance-trained and untrained young men. J Am Coll Cardiol 1992;20:552–558.

89. Molgaard H, Christensen PD, Sorensen KE, Christensen CK, Mogensen CE. Association of 24-h cardiac parasympathetic activity and degree of nephropathy in IDDM patients. Diabetes 1992;41:812–817.

90. Detollenaere MS, Duprez DA, De Buyzere ML, Vandekerckhove HJ, De Backer GG, Clement DL. 24 Hour ambulatory blood pressure variability and cardiac parasympathetic function 2 and 6 weeks after acute myocardial infarction. Clin Auton Res 1993;3:255–259.

91. Hartikainen J, Tarkiainen I, Tahvanainen K, Mantysaari M, Lansimies E, Pyorala K. Circadian variation of cardiac autonomic regulation during 24-h bed rest. Clin Physiol 1993;13: 185–196.

92. Somers VK, Dyken ME, Mark AL, Abboud FM. Sympathetic-nerve activity during sleep in normal subjects. N Engl J Med 1993;328:303–307.

93. van de Borne P, Nguyen H, Biston P, Linkowski P, Degaute JP. Effects of wake and sleep stages on the 24-h autonomic control of blood pressure and heart rate in recumbent men. Am J Physiol 1994;266(2 Pt 2):H548–H554.

94. Turton MB, Deegan T. Circadian variations of plasma catecholamine, cortisol and immunoreactive insulin concentrations in supine subjects. Clin Chim Acta 1974;55:389–397.

95. Prinz PN, Halter J, Benedetti C, Raskind M. Circadian variation of plasma catecholamines in young and old men: relation to rapid eye movement and slow wave sleep. J Clin Endocrinol Metab 1979;49:300–304.

96. Richards AM, Nicholls MG, Espiner EA, Ikram H, Cullens M, Hinton D. Diurnal patterns of blood pressure, heart rate and vasoactive hormones in normal man. Clin Exp Hypertens A 1986;8:153–166.

97. Kawano Y, Kawasaki T, Kawazoe N, Abe I, Uezono K, Ueno M, et al. Circadian variations of urinary dopamine, norepinephrine, epinephrine and sodium in normotensive and hypertensive subjects. Nephron 1990;55:277–282.

98. Kawano Y, Tochikubo O, Minamisawa K, Miyajima E, Ishii M. Circadian variation of hemodynamics in patients with essential hypertension: comparison between early morning and evening. J Hypertens 1994;12:1405–1412.

99. Lakatua DJ, Haus E, Halberg F, Halberg E, Wendt HW, Sackett-Lundeen LL, et al. Circadian characteristics of urinary epinephrine and norepinephrine from healthy young women in Japan and U.S.A. Chronobiol Int 1986;3:189–195.

100. Westerink BH, ten Kate N. 24 h excretion patterns of free, conjugated and methylated catecholamines in man. J Clin Chem Clin Biochem 1986;24:513–519.

101. Lakatua DJ, Nicolau GY, Bogdan C, Plinga L, Jachimowicz A, Sackett-Lundeen L, et al. Chronobiology of catecholamine excretion in different age groups. Prog Clin Biol Res 1987; 227B:31–50.

102. Sowers JR, Vlachakis N. Circadian variation in plasma dopamine levels in man. J Endocrinol Invest 1984;7:341–345.

103. Lemmer B, Berger T. Diurnal rhythm in the central dopamine turnover in the rat. Naunyn Schmiedebergs Arch Pharmacol 1978;303:257–261.

104. Hutson PH, Sarna GS, Curzon G. Determination of daily variations of brain 5-hydroxytryptamine and dopamine turnovers and of the clearance of their acidic metabolites in conscious rats by repeated sampling of cerebrospinal fluid. J Neurochem 1984;43:291–293.

105. Smith AD, Olson RJ, Justice JBJ. Quantitative microdialysis of dopamine in the striatum: effect of circadian variation. J Neurosci Methods 1992;44:33–41.

106. Schweiger U, Warnhoff M, Pirke KM. Norepinephrine turnover in the hypothalamus of adult male rats: alteration of circadian patterns by semistarvation. J Neurochem 1985;45:706–709.

107. Scheving LE, Harrison WH, Gordon P, Pauly JE. Daily fluctuation (circadian and ultradian) in biogenic amines of the rat brain. Am J Physiol 1968;214:166–173.

108. Koulu M, Bjelogrlic N, Agren H, Saavedra JM, Potter WZ, Linnoila M. Diurnal variation in the concentrations of catecholamines and indoleamines in the median eminence and in the intermediate and posterior lobes of the pituitary gland of the male rat. Brain Res 1989;503: 246–252.

109. Kafka MS, Benedito MA, Roth RH, Steele LK, Wolfe WW, Catravas GN. Circadian rhythms in catecholamine metabolites and cyclic nucleotide production. Chronobiol Int 1986;3:101–115.

110. Huie JM, Sharma RP, Coulombe RAJ. Diurnal alterations of catecholamines, indoleamines and their metabolites in specific brain regions of the mouse. Comp Biochem Physiol C 1989; 94:575–579.

111. Turner BB, Wilens TE, Schroeder KA, Katz RJ, Carroll BJ. Comparison of brainstem and adrenal circadian patterns of epinephrine synthesis. Neuroendocrinology 1981;32:257–261.

112. Sudo A. Adrenaline in various organs of the rat: its origin, location and diurnal fluctuation. Life Sci 1987;41:2477–2484.

113. Kuchel O, Buu NT. Circadian variations of free and sulfoconjugated catecholamines in normal subjects. Endocr Res 1985;11:17–25.

114. Sack DA, James SP, Doran AR, Sherer MA, Linnoila M, Wehr TA. The diurnal variation in plasma homovanillic acid level persists but the variation in 3-methoxy–4-hydroxyphenylglycol level is abolished under constant conditions. Arch Gen Psychiatry 1988;45:162–166.

115. Candito M, Pringuey D, Jacomet Y, Souetre E, Salvati E, Ardisson JL, et al. Circadian rhythm in plasma noradrenaline of healthy sleep-deprived subjects. Chronobiol Int 1992;9: 444–447.

116. Wirz-Justice A, Tobler I, Kafka MS, Naber D, Marangos PJ, Borbely AA, et al. Sleep deprivation: effects on circadian rhythms of rat brain neurotransmitter receptors. Psychiatry Res 1981;5:67–76.

117. Lemmer B, Lang PH. Evidence for a circadian-phase-dependency in 3H-dihydroalprenolol binding and cyclic AMP content in heart ventricles of L-D synchronized rats. Pol J Pharmacol Pharm 1984;36:275–280.

118. Kafka MS, Wirz-Justice A, Naber D. Circadian and seasonal rhythms in alpha- and beta-adrenergic receptors in the rat brain. Brain Res 1981;207:409–419.

119. Mehta J, Malloy M, Lawson D, Lopez L. Circadian variation in platelet alpha 2-adrenoceptor affinity in normal subjects. Am J Cardiol 1989;63:1002–1005.

120. Kafka MS, Wirz-Justice A, Naber D, Moore RY, Benedito MA. Circadian rhythms in rat brain neurotransmitter receptors. Fed Proc 1983;42:2796–2801.

121. Brunel S, de Montigny C. Diurnal rhythms in the responsiveness of hippocampal pyramidal neurons to serotonin, norepinephrine, gamma-aminobutyric acid and acetylcholine. Brain Res Bull 1987;18:205–212.

122. Johansson BB, Martinsson L. The blood-brain barrier in adrenaline-induced hypertension. Circadian variations and modification by beta-adrenoreceptor antagonists. Acta Neurol Scand 1980;62:96–102.

123. Mato M, Ookawara S, Tooyama K, Ishizaki T. Chronobiological studies on the blood-brain barrier. Experientia 1981;37:1013–1015.

124. Gebber GL, Barman SM. Rhythmogenesis in the sympathetic nervous system. Fed Proc 1980;39:2526–2530.

125. Tapp WN, Levin BE, Natelson BH. Ultradian rhythm of plasma norepinephrine in rats. Endocrinology 1981;109:1781–1783.

126. Dietl H, Prast H, Philippu A. Pulsatile release of catecholamines in the hypothalamus of conscious rats. Naunyn Schmiedebergs Arch Pharmacol 1993;347:28–33.

127. Robinson RL, Dietl H, Bald M, Kraus A, Philippu A. Effects of short-lasting and long-lasting blood pressure changes on the release of endogenous catecholamines in the hypothalamus of the conscious, freely moving rabbit. Naunyn Schmiedebergs Arch Pharmacol 1983; 322:203–209.

128. Takiyyuddin MA, Neumann HP, Cervenka JH, Kennedy B, Dinh TQ, Ziegler MG, et al. Ultradian variations of chromogranin A in humans. Am J Physiol 1991;261(4 Pt 2): R939–R944.

129. Simpson HW, Bartter FC, Halberg F, Gill JR, Delea C, Gullner HG, et al. A circaoctohoran rhythm of urine epinephrine excretion in man. Prog Clin Biol Res 1990;341A:157–160.

130. Rounds HD. A cholinergic receptor 12-hour interval-timer displaying "circa" periodicities. Comp Biochem Physiol C 1984;77:59–63.

131. Gordon RD, Wolfe LK, Island DP, Liddle GW. A diurnal rhythm in plasma renin activity in man. J Clin Invest 1966;45:1587–1592.

132. Katz FH, Romfh P, Smith JA. Episodic secretion of aldosterone in supine man; relationship to cortisol. J Clin Endocrinol Metab 1972;35:178–181.

133. Armbruster H, Vetter W, Beckerhoff R, Nussberger J, Vetter H, Siegenthaler W. Diurnal variations of plasma aldosterone in supine man: relationship to plasma renin activity and plasma cortisol. Acta Endocrinol (Copenh) 1975;80:95–103.

134. Katz FH, Romfh P, Smith JA. Diurnal variation of plasma aldosterone, cortisol and renin activity in supine man. J Clin Endocrinol Metab 1975;40:125–134.

135. Modlinger RS, Sharif-Zadeh K, Ertel NH, Gutkin M. The circadian rhythm of renin. J Clin Endocrinol Metab 1976;43:1276–1282.

136. Beilin LJ, Deacon J, Michael CA, Vandongen R, Lalor CM, Barden AE, et al. Circadian rhythms of blood pressure and pressor hormones in normal and hypertensive pregnancy. Clin Exp Pharmacol Physiol 1982;9:321–326.

137. Freeman RH, Davis JO, Williams GM, Seymour AA. Circadian changes in plasma renin activity and plasma aldosterone concentration in one-kidney hypertensive rats. Proc Soc Exp Biol Med 1982;169:86–89.

138. Liebau H, Manitius J. Diurnal and daily variations of PRA, plasma catecholamines and blood pressure in normotensive and hypertensive man. Contrib Nephrol 1982;30:57–63.

139. Tuck ML, Stern N, Sowers JR. Enhanced 24-hour norepinephrine and renin secretion in young patients with essential hypertension: relation with the circadian pattern of arterial blood pressure. Am J Cardiol 1985;55:112–115.

140. Shiraki K, Konda N, Sagawa S, Claybaugh JR, Hong SK. Cardiorenal–endocrine responses to head-out immersion at night. J Appl Physiol 1986;60:176–183.

141. Kool MJ, Wijnen JA, Derkx FH, Struijker Boudier HA, Van Bortel LM. Diurnal variation in prorenin in relation to other humoral factors and hemodynamics. Am J Hypertens 1994;7:723–730.

142. Stumpe KO, Kolloch R, Vetter H, Gramann W, Kruck F, Ressel C, et al. Acute and long-term studies of the mechanisms of action of beta-blocking drugs in lowering blood pressure. Am J Med 1976;60:853–865.

143. Mullen PE, James VH, Lightman SL, Linsell C, Peart WS. A relationship between plasma renin activity and the rapid eye movement phase of sleep in man. J Clin Endocrinol Metab 1980;50:466–469.

144. Lightman SL, James VH, Linsell C, Mullen PE, Peart WS, Sever PS. Studies of diurnal changes in plasma renin activity, and plasma noradrenaline, aldosterone and cortisol concentrations in man. Clin Endocrinol (Oxf) 1981;14:213–223.

145. Brandenberger G, Follenius M, Muzet A, Ehrhart J, Schieber JP. Ultradian oscillations in plasma renin activity: their relationships to meals and sleep stages. J Clin Endocrinol Metab 1985;61:280–284.

146. Brandenberger G, Follenius M, Simon C, Ehrhart J, Libert JP. Nocturnal oscillations in plasma renin activity and REM–NREM sleep cycles in humans: a common regulatory mechanism? Sleep 1988;11:242–250.

147. Schulz H, Brandenberger G, Gudewill S, Hasse D, Kiss E, Lohr K, et al. Plasma renin activity and sleep–wake structure of narcoleptic patients and control subjects under continuous bedrest. Sleep 1992;15:423–429.

148. Vagnucci AH, McDonald RH Jr, Drash AL, Wong AK. Intradiem changes of plasma aldosterone, cortisol, corticosterone and growth hormone in sodium restriction. J Clin Endocrinol Metab 1974;38:761–776.

149. Sowers JR, Stern N, Nyby MD, Jasberg KA. Dopaminergic regulation of circadian rhythms of blood pressure, renin and aldosterone in essential hypertension. Cardiovasc Res 1982;16: 317–323.

150. Sowers JR, Beck FW. Dopaminergic regulation of 18-hydroxycorticosterone and aldosterone secretion in man. Acta Endocrinol (Copenh) 1983;102:258–264.

151. Nicholls MG, Espiner EA, Ikram H, Maslowski AH, Hamilton EJ, Bones PJ. Hormone and blood pressure relationships in primary aldosteronism. Clin Exp Hypertens A 1984;6: 1441–1458.

152. Nahmod VE, Balda MS, Pirola CJ, Finkielman S, Gejman PV, Cardinali DP. Circadian rhythm and neural regulation of rat pineal angiotensin converting enzyme. Brain Res 1982; 236:216–220.

153. Stephenson LA, Kolka MA, Francesconi R, Gonzalez RR. Circadian variations in plasma renin activity, catecholamines and aldosterone during exercise in women. Eur J Appl Physiol 1989;58:756–764.

154. Takeda R, Miyamori I, Ikeda M, Koshida H, Takeda Y, Yasuhara S, et al. Circadian rhythm of plasma aldosterone and time dependent alterations of aldosterone regulators. J Steroid Biochem 1984;20:321–323.

155. Follenius M, Krauth MO, Saini J, Brandenberger G. Effect of awakening on aldosterone. J Endocrinol Invest 1992;15:475–478.

156. Mills JN. Diurnal rhythm in urine flow. J Physiol 1950;113:528–536.

157. Sirota JH, Baldwin DW, Villareal H. Diurnal variations of renal function in man. J Clin Invest 1950;29:187–192.

158. Stanbury SW, Thompson AE. Diurnal variations in electrolyte excretion. Clin Sci 1951;10: 267–293.

159. Wesson LG. Electrolyte excretion in relation to diurnal cycles of renal function. Medicine 1964;43:547–592.

160. Moore-Ede MC, Herd JA. Renal electrolyte circadian rhythms: independence from feeding and activity patterns. Am J Physiol 1977;232:F128–F135.

161. Moore-Ede MC, Meguid MM, Fitzpatrick GF, Boyden CM, Ball MR. Circadian variation in response to potassium infusion. Clin Pharmacol Ther 1978;23:218–227.

162. Kawasaki T, Ueno M, Uezono K, Kawano Y, Abe I, Kawazoe N, et al. The renin–angiotensin–aldosterone system and circadian rhythm of urine variables in normotensive and hypertensive subjects. Jpn Circ J 1984;48:168–172.

163. de Leeuw PW, van Leeuwen SJ, Birkenhager WH. Effect of sleep on blood pressure and its correlates. Clin Exp Hypertens A 1985;7:179–186.

164. Trevisani F, Bernardi M, De Palma R, Pancione L, Capani F, Baraldini M, et al. Circadian variation in renal sodium and potassium handling in cirrhosis. The role of aldosterone, cortisol, sympathoadrenergic tone, and intratubular factors. Gastroenterology 1989;96:1187–1198.

165. Staessen JA, Birkenhager W, Bulpitt CJ, Fagard R, Fletcher AE, Lijnen P, et al. The relationship between blood pressure and sodium and potassium excretion during the day and at night. J Hypertens 1993;11:443–447.

166. Kirkland JL, Lye M, Levy DW, Banerjee AK. Patterns of urine flow and electrolyte excretion in healthy elderly people. Br Med J (Clin Res Ed) 1983;287:1665–1667.

167. Dyer AR, Stamler R, Grimm R, Stamler J, Berman R, Gosch FC, et al. Do hypertensive patients have a different diurnal pattern of electrolyte excretion? Hypertension 1987;10: 417–424.

168. Janssen WM, de Zeeuw D, van der Hem GK, de Jong PE. Atrial natriuretic factor influences renal diurnal rhythm in essential hypertension. Hypertension 1992;20:80–84.

169. Pons M, Cambar J, Waterhouse JM. Renal hemodynamic mechanisms of blood pressure rhythms. Ann NY Acad Sci 1996;783:95–112.

170. Engeland WC, Byrnes GJ, Gann DS. The pituitary–adrenocortical response to hemorrhage depends on the time of day. Endocrinology 1982;110:1856–1860.
171. Szafarczyk A, Alonso G, Ixart G, Malaval F, Assenmacher I. Diurnal-stimulated and stress-induced ACTH release in rats is mediated by ventral noradrenergic bundle. Am J Physiol 1985;249:E219–E226.
172. Johnson RF, Randall W. Mediation of the photoperiodic effect on grooming reflexes by glucocorticoid hormones and serotonin. Behav Neurosci 1983;97:195–209.
173. Krieger DT. Effect of intraventricular neonatal 6-OH dopamine or 5,6-dihydroxytryptamine administration on the circadian periodicity of plasma corticosteroid levels in the rat. Neuroendocrinology 1975;17:62–74.
174. Jaffer A, Russell VA, Taljaard JJ. Noradrenergic and dopaminergic modulation of thyrotropin secretion in the rat. Brain Res 1987;404:267–272.
175. Barontini M, Romeo HE, Armando I, Cardinali DP. 24 Hour changes in catecholamine content of rat thyroid and submaxillary glands. J Neural Transm 1988;71:189–194.
176. Scanlon MF, Weetman AP, Lewis M, Pourmand M, Rodriguez-Arnao MD, Weightman DR, et al. Dopaminergic modulation of circadian thyrotropin rhythms and thyroid hormone levels in euthyroid subjects. J Clin Endocrinol Metab 1980;51:1251–1256.
177. Perez-Lopez FR, Gonzalez-Moreno CM, Abos MD, Andonegui JA, Corvo RH. Pituitary response to a dopamine antagonist at different times of the day in normal women. Acta Endocrinol (Copenh) 1982;100:481–485.
178. Rossmanith WG, Mortola JF, Laughlin GA, Yen SS. Dopaminergic control of circadian and pulsatile pituitary thyrotropin release in women. J Clin Endocrinol Metab 1988;67:560–564.
179. Negri M, Lotti G, Grossman A. Clinical Perspectives of Opioid Peptide Production. Wiley, London, 1992.
180. Dumont M, Ouellette M, Brakier-Gingras L, Lemaire S. Circadian regulation of the biosynthesis of cardiac met-enkephalin and precursors in normotensive and spontaneously hypertensive rats. Life Sci 1991;48:1895–1902.
181. Shanks MF, Clement-Jones V, Linsell CJ, Mullen PE, Rees LH, Besser GM. A study of 24-hour profiles of plasma met-enkephalin in man. Brain Res 1981;212:403–409.
182. McIntosh TK. Prolonged disruption of plasma beta-endorphin dynamics after trauma in the nonhuman primate. Endocrinology 1987;120:1734–1741.
183. Laubie M, Schmitt H, Vincent M, Remond G. Central cardiovascular effects of morphinomimetic peptides in dogs. Eur J Pharmacol 1977;46:67–71.
184. Rubin P, Blaschke TF, Guilleminault C. Effect of naloxone, a specific opioid inhibitor, on blood pressure fall during sleep. Circulation 1981;63:117–121.
185. degli Uberti EC, Salvadori S, Trasforini G, Margutti A, Ambrosio MR, Rossi R, et al. Effect of deltorphin on pituitary-adrenal response to insulin-induced hypoglycemia and ovine corticotropin-releasing hormone in healthy man. J Clin Endocrinol Metab 1992;75:370–374.
186. degli Uberti EC, Ambrosio MR, Vergnani L, Portaluppi F, Bondanelli M, Trasforini G, et al. Stress-induced activation of sympathetic nervous system is attenuated by the selective δ-opioid receptor agonist deltorphin in healthy man. J Clin Endocrinol Metab 1993;77:1490–1494.
187. Portaluppi F, Vergnani L, degli Uberti EC. Atrial natriuretic peptide and circadian blood pressure regulation: clues from a chronobiological approach. Chronobiol Int 1993;10:176–189.
188. Donckier J, Anderson JV, Yeo T, Bloom SR. Diurnal rhythm in the plasma concentration of atrial natriuretic peptide [Letter]. N Engl J Med 1986;315:710–711.
189. Winters CJ, Sallman AL, Vesely DL. Circadian rhythm of prohormone atrial natriuretic peptides 1–30, 31–67 and 99–126 in man. Chronobiol Int 1988;5:403–409.
190. Colantonio D, Pasqualetti P, Casale R, Natali G. Is atrial natriuretic peptide important in the circadian rhythm of arterial blood pressure? [Letter]. Am J Cardiol 1989;63:1166.

191. McCance DR, Roberts G, Sheridan B, McKnight JA, Leslie H, Merrett JD, et al. Variations in the plasma concentration of atrial natriuretic factor across 24 hours. Acta Endocrinol (Copenh) 1989;120:266–270.

192. Miyamoto S, Shimokawa H, Sumioki H, Nakano H. Physiologic role of endogenous human atrial natriuretic peptide in preeclamptic pregnancies. Am J Obstet Gynecol 1989;160:155–159.

193. Portaluppi F, Montanari L, Bagni B, degli Uberti E, Trasforini G, Margutti A. Circadian rhythms of atrial natriuretic peptide, blood pressure and heart rate in normal subjects. Cardiology 1989;76:428–432.

194. Sumioki H, Shimokawa H, Miyamoto S, Uezono K, Utsunomiya T, Nakano H. Circadian variations of plasma atrial natriuretic peptide in four types of hypertensive disorder during pregnancy. Br J Obstet Gynaecol 1989;96:922–927.

195. Portaluppi F, Bagni B, degli Uberti E, Montanari L, Cavallini R, Trasforini G, et al. Circadian rhythms of atrial natriuretic peptide, renin, aldosterone, cortisol, blood pressure and heart rate in normal and hypertensive subjects. J Hypertens 1990;8:85–95.

196. Watanabe M, Uchiyama Y. Twenty-four hour variations in subcellular structures of rat pancreatic islet B-, A- and D-cells, and of portal plasma glucose and insulin levels. Cell Tissue Res 1988;253:337–345.

197. Weil J, Strom TM, Heim JM, Lang RE, Schindler M, Haufe M, et al. Influence of diurnal rhythm, posture and right atrial size on plasma atrial natriuretic peptide levels. Z Kardiol 1988;77(Suppl 2):36–40.

198. Portaluppi F, Montanari L, Vergnani L, Tarroni G, Cavallini AR, Gilli P, et al. Loss of nocturnal increase in plasma concentration of atrial natriuretic peptide in hypertensive chronic renal failure. Cardiology 1992;80:312–323.

199. Portaluppi F, Montanari L, Ferlini M, Vergnani L, D'Ambrosi A, Cavallini AR, et al. Consistent changes in the circadian rhythms of blood pressure and atrial natriuretic peptide in congestive heart failure. Chronobiol Int 1991;8:432–439.

200. Portaluppi F, Montanari L, Ferlini M, Vergnani L, Bagni B, Degli Uberti EC. Differences in blood pressure regulation of congestive heart failure, before and after treatment, correlate with changes in the circulating pattern of atrial natriuretic peptide. Eur Heart J 1992;13:990–996.

201. Amara SG, Jonas V, Rosenfeld MG, Ong ES, Evans RM. Alternative RNA processing in calcitonin gene expression generates mRNAs encoding different polypeptide products. Nature 1982;298:240–244.

202. Rosenfeld MG, Amara SG, Evans RM. Alternative RNA processing: determining neuronal phenotype. Science 1984;225:1315–1320.

203. Kawai Y, Takami K, Shiosaka S, Emson PC, Hillyard CJ, Girgis S, et al. Topographic localization of calcitonin gene-related peptide in the rat brain: an immunohistochemical analysis. Neuroscience 1985;15:747–763.

204. Brain SD, Williams TJ, Tippins JR, Morris HR, MacIntyre I. Calcitonin gene-related peptide is a potent vasodilator. Nature 1985;313:54–56.

205. Girgis SI, Macdonald DW, Stevenson JC, Bevis PJ, Lynch C, Wimalawansa SJ, et al. Calcitonin gene-related peptide: potent vasodilator and major product of calcitonin gene. Lancet 1985;2:14–16.

206. Goodman EC, Iversen LL. Calcitonin gene-related peptide: novel neuropeptide. Life Sci 1986;38:2169–2178.

207. Tschopp FA, Tobler PH, Fischer JA. Calcitonin gene-related peptide in the human thyroid, pituitary and brain. Mol Cell Endocrinol 1984;36:53–57.

208. Skofitsch G, Jacobowitz DM. Autoradiographic distribution of ^{125}I calcitonin gene-related peptide binding sites in the rat central nervous system. Peptides 1985;6:975–986.

209. Skofitsch G, Jacobowitz DM. Quantitative distribution of calcitonin gene-related peptide in the rat central nervous system. Peptides 1985;6:1069–1073.

210. Skofitsch G, Jacobowitz DM. Calcitonin gene-related peptide: detailed immunohistochemical distribution in the central nervous system. Peptides 1985;6:721–745.
211. Tschopp FA, Henke H, Petermann JB, Tobler PH, Janzer R, Hokfelt T, et al. Calcitonin gene-related peptide and its binding sites in the human central nervous system and pituitary. Proc Natl Acad Sci USA 1985;82:248–252.
212. Mulderry PK, Ghatei MA, Rodrigo J, Allen JM, Rosenfeld MG, Polak JM, et al. Calcitonin gene-related peptide in cardiovascular tissues of the rat. Neuroscience 1985;14: 947–54.
213. Wimalawansa SJ, MacIntyre I. Calcitonin gene-related peptide and its specific binding sites in the cardiovascular system of rat. Int J Cardiol 1988;20:29–37.
214. Uddman R, Edvinsson L, Ekblad E, Hakanson R, Sundler F. Calcitonin gene-related peptide (CGRP): perivascular distribution and vasodilatory effects. Regul Pept 1986;15:1–23.
215. Bendtsen F, Schifter S, Henriksen JH. Increased circulating calcitonin gene-related peptide (CGRP) in cirrhosis. J Hepatol 1991;12:118–123.
216. De los Santos ET, Mazzaferri EL. Calcitonin gene-related peptide: 24-hour profile and responses to volume contraction and expansion in normal men. J Clin Endocrinol Metab 1991;72:1031–1035.
217. Trasforini G, Margutti A, Portaluppi F, Menegatti M, Ambrosio MR, Bagni B, et al. Circadian profile of plasma calcitonin gene-related peptide in healthy man. J Clin Endocrinol Metab 1991;73:945–951.
218. Portaluppi F, Trasforini G, Margutti A, Vergnani L, Ambrosio MR, Rossi R, et al. Circadian rhythm of calcitonin gene-related peptide in uncomplicated essential hypertension. J Hypertens 1992;10:1227–1234.
219. Gennari C, Fischer JA. Cardiovascular action of calcitonin gene-related peptide in humans. Calcif Tissue Int 1985;37:581–584.
220. McEwan J, Larkin S, Davies G, Chierchia S, Brown M, Stevenson J, et al. Calcitonin gene-related peptide: a potent dilator of human epicardial coronary arteries. Circulation 1986;74: 1243–1247.
221. Struthers AD, Brown MJ, Macdonald DW, Beacham JL, Stevenson JC, Morris HR, et al. Human calcitonin gene related peptide: a potent endogenous vasodilator in man. Clin Sci 1986;70:389–393.
222. Tippins JR. CGRP: a novel neuropeptide from the calcitonin gene is the most potent vasodilator known. J Hypertens 1986;4(Suppl 5):S102–S105.
223. DiPette DJ, Schwarzenberger K, Kerr N, Holland OB. Systemic and regional hemodynamic effects of calcitonin gene-related peptide. Hypertension 1987;9:III142–III146.
224. Ezra D, Laurindo FR, Goldstein DS, Goldstein RE, Feuerstein G. Calcitonin gene-related peptide: a potent modulator of coronary flow. Eur J Pharmacol 1987;137:101–105.
225. Lappe RW, Slivjak MJ, Todt JA, Wendt RL. Hemodynamic effects of calcitonin gene-related peptide in conscious rats. Regul Pept 1987;19:307–312.
226. Kurtz A, Muff R, Fischer JA. Calcitonin gene products and the kidney. Klin Wochenschr 1989;67:870–875.
227. Wang BC, Bie P, Leadley RJJ, Goetz KL. Cardiovascular effects of calcitonin gene-related peptide in conscious dogs. Am J Physiol 1989;257(4 Pt 2):R726–R731.
228. Edvinsson L, Fredholm BB, Hamel E, Jansen I, Verrecchia C. Perivascular peptides relax cerebral arteries concomitant with stimulation of cyclic adenosine monophosphate accumulation or release of an endothelium-derived relaxing factor in the cat. Neurosci Lett 1985;58: 213–217.
229. Shoji T, Ishihara H, Ishikawa T, Saito A, Goto K. Vasodilating effects of human and rat calcitonin gene-related peptides in isolated porcine coronary arteries. Naunyn Schmiedebergs Arch Pharmacol 1987;336:438–444.

230. Kubota M, Moseley JM, Butera L, Dusting GJ, MacDonald PS, Martin TJ. Calcitonin gene-related peptide stimulates cyclic AMP formation in rat aortic smooth muscle cells. Biochem Biophys Res Commun 1985;132:88–94.

231. Gennari C, Nami R, Agnusdei D, Bianchini C, Pavese G. Acute cardiovascular and renal effects of human calcitonin gene-related peptide. Am J Hypertens 1989;2(2 Pt 2):45S–49S.

232. Itabashi A, Kashiwabara H, Shibuya M, Tanaka K, Masaoka H, Katayama S, et al. The interaction of calcitonin gene-related peptide with angiotensin II on blood pressure and renin release. J Hypertens 1988;6(Suppl):S418–S420.

233. Kurtz A, Muff R, Born W, Lundberg JM, Millberg BI, Gnadinger MP, et al. Calcitonin gene-related peptide is a stimulator of renin secretion. J Clin Invest 1988;82:538–543.

234. Portaluppi F, Vergnani L, Margutti A, Ambrosio MR, Bondanelli M, Trasforini G, et al. Modulatory effect of the renin-angiotensin system on the plasma levels of calcitonin gene-related peptide in normal man. J Clin Endocrinol Metab 1993;77:816–820.

235. Trasforini G, Margutti A, Vergnani L, Ambrosio MR, Valentini A, Rossi R, et al. Evidence that enhancement of cholinergic tone increases basal plasma levels of calcitonin gene-related peptide in normal man. J Clin Endocrinol Metab 1994;78:763–766.

236. Katz FH, Smith JA, Lock JP, Loeffel DE. Plasma vasopressin variation and renin activity in normal active humans. Horm Res 1979;10:289–302.

237. Hill L. On rest, sleep and work and the concomitant changes in the circulation of the blood. Lancet 1898;1:282–285.

238. Snyder F, Hobson A, Morrison DF, Goldfrank F. Changes in respiration, heart rate and systolic blood pressure in human sleep. J Appl Physiol 1964;19:417–422.

239. Bristow JD, Honour AJ, Pickering TG, Sleight P. Cardiovascular and respiratory changes during sleep in normal and hypertensive subjects. Cardiovasc Res 1969;3:476–485.

240. Reinberg A, Ghata J, Halberg F, Gervais P, Abulker C, Dupont J, et al. Rythmes circadiens du pouls, de la pression arterielle, des excretions urinaires en 17-hydroxycorticosteroides catecholamines et potassium chez l'homme adulte sain, actif et au repos. Ann Endocrinol (Paris) 1970;31:277–287.

241. Coccagna G, Mantovani M, Brignani F, Manzini A, Lugaresi E. Laboratory note. Arterial pressure changes during spontaneous sleep in man. Electroencephalogr Clin Neurophysiol 1971;31:277–281.

242. Millar-Craig MW, Bishop CN, Raftery EB. Circadian variation of blood-pressure. Lancet 1978;1:795–797.

243. Littler WA. Sleep and blood pressure: further observations. Am Heart J 1979;97:35–37.

244. Halberg F, Halberg E, Halberg J, Halberg F. Chronobiologic assessment of human blood pressure variation in health and disease. In: Weber MA, Drayer JIM, eds. Ambulatory Blood Pressure Monitoring. Springer Verlag, New York, 1984, pp. 137–156.

245. Portaluppi F, Smolensky MH. Time-dependent structure and control of arterial blood pressure. Ann NY Acad Sci 1996:vol 783.

246. Smolensky MH, Tatar SE, Bergman SA, Losman JG, Barnard, CN, Dasco CC, et al. Circadian rhythmic aspects of cardiovascular function. Chronobiologia 1977;3:333–371.

247. Davies AB, Gould BA, Cashman PM, Raftery EB. Circadian rhythm of blood pressure in patients dependent on ventricular demand pacemakers. Br Heart J 1984;52:93–98.

248. Raftery EB, Millar-Craig MW, Mann S, Balasubramanian V. Effects of treatment on circadian rhythms of blood pressure. Biotelem Patient Monit 1981;8:113–120.

249. Degaute JP, van de Borne P, Linkowski P, Van Cauter E. Quantitative analysis of the 24-hour blood pressure and heart rate patterns in young men. Hypertension 1991;18:199–210.

250. Middeke M, Schrader J. Nocturnal blood pressure in normotensive subjects and those with white coat, primary, and secondary hypertension. Br Med J 1994;308:630–632.

251. Floras JS, Jones JV, Johnston JA, Brooks DE, Hassan MO, Sleight P. Arousal and the circadian rhythm of blood pressure. Clin Sci Mol Med 1978;4(Suppl 1):S395–S397.

252. Gould BA, Raftery EB. Twenty-four-hour blood pressure control: an intraarterial review. Chronobiol Int 1991;8:495–505.
253. Athanassiadis D, Draper GJ, Honour AJ, Cranston WI. Variability of automatic blood pressure measurements over 24 hour periods. Clin Sci 1969;36:147–156.
254. Mancia G, Ferrari A, Gregorini L, Parati G, Pomidossi G, Bertinieri G, et al. Blood pressure and heart rate variabilities in normotensive and hypertensive human beings. Circ Res 1983; 53:96–104.
255. Broadhurst P, Brigden G, Dasgupta P, Lahiri A, Raftery EB. Ambulatory intra-arterial blood pressure in normal subjects. Am Heart J 1990;120:160–166.
256. Chaturvedi N, McKeigue PM, Marmot MG. Resting and ambulatory blood pressure differences in Afro-Caribbeans and Europeans. Hypertension 1993;22:90–96.
257. Gretler DD, Fumo MT, Nelson KS, Murphy MB. Ethnic differences in circadian hemodynamic profile. Am J Hypertens 1994;7:7–14.
258. Imai Y, Munakata M, Hashimoto J, Minami N, Sakuma H, Watanabe N, et al. Age-specific characteristics of nocturnal blood pressure in a general population in a community of northern Japan. Am. J Hypertens 1993;6(6 Pt 2):179S–183S.
259. Minamisawa K, Tochikubo O, Ishii M. Systemic hemodynamics during sleep in young or middle-aged and elderly patients with essential hypertension. Hypertension 1994;23:167–173.
260. Suzuki Y, Kuwajima I, Mitani K, Kuramoto K. The relation of morning rise in blood pressure to pressure response to exercise and mental stress. Jpn J Geriat 1993;30:841–848.
261. Contard S, Chanudet X, Coisne D, Battistella P, Marichal JF, Pitiot M, et al. Ambulatory monitoring of blood pressure in normal pregnancy. Am J Hypertens 1993;6:880–884.
262. Halligan A, O'Brien E, O'Malley K, Mee F, Atkins N, Conroy R, et al. Twenty-four-hour ambulatory blood pressure measurement in a primigravid population. J Hypertens 1993;11: 869–873.
263. Seligman SA. Diurnal blood pressure variation in pregnancy. J Obstet Gynaecol Br Commonwlth 1971;78:417–422.
264. Clark LA, Denby L, Pregibon D, Harshfield GA, Pickering TG, Blank S, et al. A quantitative analysis of the effects of activity and time of day on the diurnal variations of blood pressure. J Chronic Dis 1987;40:671–681.
265. James GD, Pickering TG. The influence of behavioral factors on the daily variation of blood pressure. Am J Hypertens 1993;6(6 Pt 2):170S–173S.
266. Degaute JP, Van Cauter E, van de Borne P, Linkowski P. Twenty-four-hour blood pressure and heart rate profiles in humans. A twin study. Hypertension 1994;23:244–253.
267. Sundberg S, Kohvakka A, Gordin A. Rapid reversal of circadian blood pressure rhythm in shift workers. J Hypertens 1988;6:393–396.
268. Baumgart P, Walger P, Fuchs G, Dorst KG, Vetter H, Rahn KH. Twenty-four-hour blood pressure is not dependent on endogenous circadian rhythm. J Hypertens 1989;7:331–334.
269. Chau NP, Mallion JM, de Gaudemaris R, Ruche E, Siche JP, Pelen O, et al. Twenty-four-hour ambulatory blood pressure in shift workers. Circulation 1989;80:341–347.
270. Pieper C, Warren K, Pickering TG. A comparison of ambulatory blood pressure and heart rate at home and work on work and non-work days. J Hypertens 1993;11:177–183.
271. Goto T, Yokoyama K, Araki T, Miura T, Saitoh H, Saitoh M, et al. Identical blood pressure levels and slower heart rates among nurses during night work and day work. J Hum Hypertens 1994;8:11–14.
272. Ravogli A, Trazzi S, Villani A, Mutti E, Cuspidi C, Sampieri L, et al. Early 24-hour blood pressure elevation in normotensive subjects with parental hypertension. Hypertension 1990; 16:491–497.
273. van Hooft IM, Grobbee DE, Waal-Manning HJ, Hofman A. Hemodynamic characteristics of the early phase of primary hypertension. The Dutch Hypertension and Offspring Study. Circulation 1993;87:1100–1106.

274. Somes GW, Harshfield GA, Alpert BS, Goble MM, Schieken RM. Genetic influences on ambulatory blood pressure patterns. The Medical College of Virginia Twin Study. Am. J Hypertens 1995;8:474–478.

275. Witte K, Schnecko A, Buijs R, Lemmer B. Circadian rhythms in blood pressure and heart rate in SCN-lesioned and unlesioned transgenic hypertensive rats. Biol Rhythm Res 1995; 26:458–459 (abstract).

276. Hossmann V, Fitzgerald GA, Dollery CT. Circadian rhythm of baroreflex reactivity and adrenergic vascular response. Cardiovasc Res 1980;14:125–129.

277. de Leeuw PW, Falke HE, Kho TL, Vandongen R, Wester A, Birkenhager WH. Effects of beta-adrenergic blockade on diurnal variability of blood pressure and plasma noradrenaline levels. Acta Med Scand 1977;202:389–392.

278. Middeke M. Synchronizität von zirkadianer Blutdruckrhythmik und sympatho-adrenerger Aktivität. Z Kardiol 1992;81(Suppl 2):55–58.

279. Hickey MS, Costill DL, Vukovich MD, Kryzmenski K, Widrick JJ. Time of day effects on sympathoadrenal and pressor reactivity to exercise in healthy men. Eur J Appl Physiol 1993; 67:159–163.

280. Sowers JR. Dopaminergic control of circadian norepinephrine levels in patients with essential hypertension. J Clin Endocrinol Metab 1981;53:1133–1137.

281. Bernardi M, Trevisani F, De Palma R, Ligabue A, Capani F, Baraldini M, et al. Chronobiological evaluation of sympathoadrenergic function in cirrhosis. Relationship with arterial pressure and heart rate. Gastroenterology 1987;93:1178–1186.

282. Thompson ME, Nicolau GY, Lakatua DJ, Sackett-Lundeen L, Plinga L, Bogdan C, et al. Endocrine factors of blood pressure regulation in different age groups. Prog Clin Biol Res 1987;227B:79–95.

283. Brickman AS, Stern N, Sowers JR. Circadian variations of catecholamines and blood pressure in patients with pseudohypoparathyroidism and hypertension. Chronobiologia 1990; 17:37–44.

284. Stern N, Beahm E, McGinty D, Eggena P, Littner M, Nyby M, et al. Dissociation of 24-hour catecholamine levels from blood pressure in older men. Hypertension 1985;7:1023–1029.

285. Sowers JR, Nyby M, Jasberg K. Dopaminergic control of prolactin and blood pressure: altered control in essential hypertension. Hypertension 1982;4:431–437.

286. Sothern RB, Vesely DL, Kanabrocki EL, Hermida RC, Bremner FW, Third JLHC, et al. Temporal (circadian) and functional relationship between atrial natriuretic peptides and blood pressure. Chronobiol Int 1994;12:106–120.

287. Mann S, Altman DG, Raftery EB, Bannister R. Circadian variation of blood pressure in autonomic failure. Circulation 1983;68:477–483.

288. Martinelli P, Coccagna G, Rizzuto N, Lugaresi E. Changes in systemic arterial pressure during sleep in Shy–Drager syndrome. Sleep 1981;4:139–146.

289. Tohgi H, Chiba K, Kimura M. Twenty-four-hour variation of blood pressure in vascular dementia of the Binswanger type. Stroke 1991;22:603–608.

290. Otsuka A, Mikami H, Katahira K, Nakamoto Y, Minamitani K, Imaoka M, et al. Absence of nocturnal fall in blood pressure in elderly persons with Alzheimer-type dementia. J Am Geriatr Soc 1990;38:973–978.

291. Tominaga M, Tsuchihashi T, Kinoshita H, Abe I, Fujishima M. Disparate circadian variations of blood pressure and body temperature in bedridden elderly patients with cerebral atrophy. Am J Hypertens 1995;8:773–781.

292. Stoica E, Enulescu O. Inability to deactivate sympathetic nervous system in brainstem infarct patients. J Neurol Sci 1983;58:223–234.

293. Shimada K, Kawamoto A, Matsubayashi K, Ozawa T. Silent cerebrovascular disease in the elderly. Correlation with ambulatory pressure. Hypertension 1990;16:692–699.

294. Shimada K, Kawamoto A, Matsubayashi K, Nishinaga M, Kimura S, Ozawa T. Diurnal blood pressure variations and silent cerebrovascular damage in elderly patients with hypertension. J Hypertens 1992;10:875–878.

295. Matsumura K, Abe I, Fukuhara M, Kobayashi K, Sadoshima S, Hasuo K, et al. Attenuation of nocturnal BP fall in essential hypertensives with cerebral infarction [Letter]. J Hum Hypertens 1993;7:309–310.

296. Sander D, Klingelhöfer J. Changes of circadian blood pressure patterns after hemodynamic and thromboembolic brain infarction. Stroke 1994;25:1730–1737.

297. Asmar RG, Julia PL, Mascarel VL, Fabiani JN, Benetos A, Safar ME. Ambulatory blood pressure profile after carotid endarterectomy in patients with ischaemic arterial disease. J Hypertens 1994;12:697–702.

298. Franklin SS, Sowers JR, Batzdorf U. Relationship between arterial blood pressure and plasma norepinephrine levels in a patient with neurogenic hypertension. Am J Med 1986;81: 1105–1107.

299. Portaluppi F, Cortelli P, Avoni P, Vergnani L, Contin E, Maltoni P, et al. Diurnal blood pressure variation and hormonal correlates in fatal familial insomnia. Hypertension 1994;23: 569–576.

300. Hornung RS, Mahler RF, Raftery EB. Ambulatory blood pressure and heart rate in diabetic patients: an assessment of autonomic function. Diabet Med 1989;6:579–585.

301. Wiegmann TB, Herron KG, Chonko AM, Mac Dougall ML, Moore WV. Recognition of hypertension and abnormal blood pressure burden with ambulatory blood pressure recordings in type I diabetes mellitus. Diabetes 1990;39:1556–1560.

302. Fogari R, Zoppi A, Malamani GD, Lazzari P, Destro M, Corradi L. Ambulatory blood pressure monitoring in normotensive and hypertensive type 2 diabetes. Prevalence of impaired diurnal blood pressure patterns. Am J Hypertens 1993;6:1–7.

303. Ikeda T, Matsubara T, Sato Y, Sakamoto N. Circadian blood pressure variation in diabetic patients with autonomic neuropathy. J Hypertens 1993;11:581–587.

304. Lurbe A, Redon J, Pascual JM, Tacons J, Alvarez V, Batlle DC. Altered blood pressure during sleep in normotensive subjects with type I diabetes. Hypertension 1993;21:227–235.

305. Chau NP, Bauduceau B, Chanudet X, Larroque P, Gautier D. Ambulatory blood pressure in diabetic subjects. Am J Hypertens 1994;7:487–491.

306. Isshiki T, Akatsuka N, Tsuneyoshi H, Oka H. Periodic fluctuation of blood pressure in a case of norepinephrine secreting extra-adrenal pheochromocytoma. Jpn Heart J 1986;27:437–442.

307. Imai Y, Abe K, Miura Y, Nihei M, Sasaki S, Minami N, et al. Hypertensive episodes and circadian fluctuations of blood pressure in patients with phaeochromocytoma: studies by long-term blood pressure monitoring based on a volume–oscillometric method. J Hypertens 1988;6:9–15.

308. Oishi S, Sasaki M, Ohno M, Umeda T, Sato T. Periodic fluctuation of blood pressure and its management in a patient with pheochromocytoma. Case report and review of the literature. Jpn Heart J 1988;29:389–399.

309. Dabrowska B, Feltynowski T, Wocial B, Szpak W, Januszewicz W. Effect of removal of phaeochromocytoma on diurnal variability of blood pressure, heart rhythm and excretion of catecholamines. J Hum Hypertens 1990;4:397–399.

310. Statius van Eps RG, van den Meiracker AH, Boomsma F, Man in't Veld AJ, Schalekamp MADH. Diurnal variation of blood pressure in patients with catecholamine-producing tumors. Am J Hypertens 1994;7:492–497.

311. Imai Y, Abe K, Sasaki S, Minami N, Nihei M, Munakata M, et al. Altered circadian blood pressure rhythm in patients with Cushing's syndrome. Hypertension 1988;12:11–19.

312. Imai Y, Abe K, Sasaki S, Minami N, Munakata M, Nihei M, et al. Exogenous glucocorticoid eliminates or reverses circadian blood pressure variations. J Hypertens 1989;7:113–120.

313. van de Borne P, Gelin M, Van de Stadt J, Degaute JP. Circadian rhythms of blood pressure after liver transplantation. Hypertension 1993;21:398–405.

314. Imai Y, Abe K, Sasaki S, Munakata M, Minami N, Sakuma H, et al. Circadian blood pressure variation in patients with renovascular hypertension or primary aldosteronism. Clin Exp Hypertens A 1992;14:1141–1167.

315. White WB, Malchoff C. Diurnal blood pressure variability in mineralocorticoid excess syndrome. Am J Hypertens 1992;5:414–418.

316. Veglio F, Pinna G, Melchio R, Rabbia F, Molino P, Torchio C, et al. Twenty-four-hour power spectral analysis by maximum entropy method of blood pressure in primary hyperaldosteronism. Blood Pressure 1993;2:189–196.

317. Fallo F, Fanelli G, Cipolla A, Betterle C, Boscaro M, Sonino N. 24-Hour blood pressure profile in Addison's disease. Am J Hypertens 1994;7:1105–1109.

318. Tilkian AG, Guilleminault C, Schroeder JS, Lehrman KL, Simmons FB, Dement WC. Hemodynamics in sleep-induced apnea. Studies during wakefulness and sleep. Ann Intern Med 1976;85:714–719.

319. Franz IW, Erb D, Tonnesmann U. Gestorte 24-Stunden-Blutdruckrhythmik bei normotensiven und hypertensiven Asthmatikern. Z Kardiol 1992;81(Suppl 2):13–16.

320. Baumgart P. Circadian rhythm of blood pressure: internal and external time triggers. Chronobiol Int 1991;8:440–450.

321. Heber ME, Lahiri A, Thompson D, Raftery EB. Baroreceptor, not left ventricular, dysfunction is the cause of hemodialysis hypotension. Clin Nephrol 1989;32:79–86.

322. Middeke M, Mika E, Schreiber MA, Beck B, Wächter B, Holzgreve H. Ambulante indirekte Blutdrucklangzeitmessung bei primärer und sekundärer Hypertonie. Klin Wochenschr 1989; 67:713–716.

323. Portaluppi F, Montanari L, Ferlini M, Gilli P. Altered circadian rhythms of blood pressure and heart rate in non-hemodialysis chronic renal failure. Chronobiol Int 1990;7:321–327.

324. Middeke M, Kluglich M, Holzgreve H. Circadian blood pressure rhythm in primary and secondary hypertension. Chronobiol Int 1991;8:451–459.

325. Portaluppi F, Montanari L, Massari M, Di Chiara V, Capanna M. Loss of nocturnal decline of blood pressure in hypertension due to chronic renal failure. Am J Hypertens 1991;4: 20–26.

326. Rosansky SJ. Nocturnal hypertension in patients receiving chronic hemodialysis [Letter]. Ann Intern Med 1991;114:96.

327. Hayashi T, Shoji T, Kitamura E, Okada N, Nakanishi I, Tsubakihara Y. Circadian blood pressure pattern in the patients with chronic glomerulonephritis. Nippon Jinzo Gakkai Shi 1993;35:233–237.

328. Timio M, Lolli S, Verdura C, Monarca C, Merante F, Guerrini E. Circadian blood pressure changes in patients with chronic renal insufficiency: a prospective study. Renal Failure 1993;15:231–237.

329. Torffvit O, Agardh CD. Day and night variation in ambulatory blood pressure in type 1 diabetes mellitus with nephropathy and autonomic neuropathy. J Intern Med 1993;233:131–137.

330. Del Rosso G, Amoroso L, Santoferrara A, Fiederling B, Di Liberato L, Albertazzi A. Impaired blood pressure nocturnal decline and target organ damage in chronic renal failure. J Hypertens 1994;12(Suppl 3):S15 (abstract).

331. Shaw DB, Knapp MS, Davies DH. Variations in blood pressure in hypertensives during sleep. Lancet 1963;1:797–798.

332. de la Sierra A, del Mar Lluch M, Coca A, Aguilera MT, Sánchez M, Sierra C, et al. Assessment of salt sensitivity in essential hypertension by 24-h ambulatory blood pressure monitoring. Am J Hypertens 1995;8:970–977.

333. Olofsson P. Characteristics of a reversed circadian blood pressure rhythm in pregnant women with hypertension. J Hum Hypertens 1995;9:565–570.

334. Redman CW, Beilin LJ, Bonnar J. Reversed diurnal blood pressure rhythm in hypertensive pregnancies. Clin Sci Mol Med 1976;3:687s–689s.

335. Beilin LJ, Deacon J, Michael CA, Vandongen R, Lalor CM, Barden AE, et al. Diurnal rhythms of blood pressure, plasma renin activity, angiotensin II and catecholamines in normotensive and hypertensive pregnancies. Clin Exp Hypertens B 1983;2:271–293.

336. Verdecchia P, Schillaci G, Guerrieri M, Gatteschi C, Benemio G, Boldrini F, et al. Circadian blood pressure changes and left ventricular hypertrophy in essential hypertension. Circulation 1990;81:528–536.

337. Kuwajima I, Suzuki Y, Shimosawa T, Kanemaru A, Hoshino S, Kuramoto K. Diminished nocturnal decline in blood pressure in elderly hypertensive patients with left ventricular hypertrophy. Am Heart J 1992;123:1307–1311.

338. Soergel M, Maisin A, Azancot-Benisty A, Loirat C. Ambulante Blutdruckmessung bei nierentransplantierten Kindern und Jugendlichen. Z Kardiol 1992;81(Suppl 2):67–70.

339. Taler SJ, Textor SC, Canzanello VJ, Wilson DJ, Wiesner RH, Krom RA. Loss of nocturnal blood pressure fall after liver transplantation during immunosuppressive therapy. Am J Hypertens 1995;8:598–605.

340. Reeves RA, Shapiro AP, Thompson ME, Johnsen AM. Loss of nocturnal decline in blood pressure after cardiac transplantation. Circulation 1986;73:401–408.

341. Dart AM, Yeoh JK, Jennings GL, Cameron JD, Esmore DS. Circadian rhythms of heart rate and blood pressure after heart transplantation. J Heart Lung Transplant 1992;11:784–792.

342. Sehested J, Thomas F, Thorn M, Schifter S, Regitz V, Sheikh S, et al. Level and diurnal variations of hormones of interest to the cardiovascular system in patients with heart transplants. Am J Cardiol 1992;69:397–402.

343. van de Borne P, Leeman M, Primo G, Degaute JP. Reappearance of a normal circadian rhythm of blood pressure after cardiac transplantation. Am J Cardiol 1992;69:794–801.

344. Idema RN, van den Meiracker AH, Balk AH, Bos E, Schalekamp MA, Man in't Veld AJ. Decreased circadian blood pressure variation up to three years after heart transplantation. Am J Cardiol 1994;73:1006–1009.

345. Idema RN, van den Meiracker AH, Balk AH, Bos E, Schalekamp MA, Man in't Veld AJ. Abnormal diurnal variation of blood pressure, cardiac output, and vascular resistance in cardiac transplant recipients. Circulation 1994;90:2797–2803.

346. Caruana MP, Lahiri A, Cashman PM, Altman DG, Raftery EB. Effects of chronic congestive heart failure secondary to coronary artery disease on the circadian rhythm of blood pressure and heart rate. Am J Cardiol 1988;62:755–759.

347. Suzuki Y, Kuwajima I, Kanemaru A, Shimosawa T, Hoshino S, Sakai M, et al. The cardiac functional reserve in elderly hypertensive patients with abnormal diurnal change in blood pressure. J Hypertens 1992;10:173–179.

348. van de Borne P, Abramowicz M, Degre S, Degaute JP. Effects of chronic congestive heart failure on 24-hour blood pressure and heart rate patterns: a hemodynamic approach. Am Heart J 1992;123:998–1004.

349. van de Borne P, Tielemans C, Vanherweghem JL, Degaute JP. Effect of recombinant human erythropoietin therapy on ambulatory blood pressure and heart rate in chronic haemodialysis patients. Nephrol Dial Transplant 1992;7:45–49.

350. Sander D, Klingelhofer J. Circadian blood pressure patterns in four cases with hemodynamic brain infarction and prolonged blood-brain barrier disturbance. Clin Neurol Neurosurg 1993;95:221–229.

351. van de Borne P, Tielemans C, Collart F, Vanherweghem JL, Degaute JP. Twenty-four-hour blood pressure and heart rate patterns in chronic hemodialysis patients. Am J Kidney Dis 1993;22:419–425.

352. Teerlink JR, Clozel JP. Hemodynamic variability and circadian rhythm in rats with heart failure: role of locomotor activity. Am J Physiol 1993;264(6 Pt 2):H2111–H2118.

353. Kohara K, Nishida W, Maguchi M, Hiwada K. Autonomic nervous function in nondipper essential hypertensive subjects. Evaluation by power spectral analysis of heart rate variability. Hypertension 1995;26:808–814.

354. Lugaresi A, Baruzzi A, Cacciari E, Cortelli P, Medori R, Montagna P, et al. Lack of vegetative and endocrine circadian rhythms in fatal familial thalamic degeneration. Clin Endocrinol 1987;26:573–580.

355. Medori R, Tritschler HJ, LeBlanc A, Villare F, Manetto V, Chen HY, et al. Fatal familial insomnia, a prion disease with a mutation at codon 178 of the prion protein gene. N Engl J Med 1992;326:444–449.

356. Kobrin I, Oigman W, Kumar A, Ventura HO, Messerli FH, Frohlich ED, et al. Diurnal variation of blood pressure in elderly patients with essential hypertension. J Am Geriatr Soc 1984;32:896–899.

357. Palatini P, Penzo M, Racioppa A, Zugno E, Guzzardi G, Anaclerio M, et al. Clinical relevance of nighttime blood pressure and of daytime blood pressure variability. Arch Intern Med 1992;152:1855–1860.

358. Rizzoni D, Muiesan ML, Montani G, Zulli R, Calebich S, Agabiti-Rosei E. Relationship between initial cardiovascular structural changes and daytime and nighttime blood pressure monitoring. Am J Hypertens 1992;5:180–186.

359. Verdecchia P, Schillaci G, Gatteschi C, Zampi I, Battistelli M, Bartoccini C, et al. Blunted nocturnal fall in blood pressure in hypertensive women with future cardiovascular morbid events. Circulation 1993;88:986–992.

360. Schmieder RE, Rockstroh JK, Aepfelbacher F, Schulze B, Messerli FH. Gender-specific cardiovascular adaptation due to circadian blood pressure variations in essential hypertension. Am J Hypertens 1995;8:1160–1166.

361. O'Brien E, Sheridan J, O'Malley K. Dippers and nondippers. Lancet 1988;2:397.

362. Bianchi S, Bigazzi R, Baldari G, Sgherri G, Campese VM. Diurnal variations of blood pressure and microalbuminuria in essential hypertension. Am J Hypertens 1994;7:23–29.

363. Verdecchia P, Porcellati C, Schillaci G, Borgioni C, Ciucci A, Battistelli M, et al. Ambulatory blood pressure. An independent predictor of prognosis in essential hypertension. Hypertension 1994;24:793–801.

364. Uzu T, Kazembe FS, Ishikawa K, Nakamura S, Inenaga T, Kimura G. High sodium sensitivity implicates nocturnal hypertension in essential hypertension. Hypertension 1996;28:139–142.

365. Kuwajima I, Mitani K, Miyao M, Suzuki Y, Kuramoto K, Ozawa T. Cardiac implications of the morning surge in blood pressure in elderly hypertensive patients: relation to arising time. Am J Hypertens 1995;8:29–33.

366. Portaluppi F, Vergnani L, Manfredini R, degli Uberti EC, Fersini C. Time-dependent effect of isradipine on the nocturnal hypertension of chronic renal failure. Am J Hypertens 1995;8:719–726.

367. Lemmer B, Mattes A, Bohm M, Ganten D. Circadian blood pressure variation in transgenic hypertensive rats. Hypertension 1993;22:97–101.

368. Arduini D, Rizzo G, Parlati E, Giorlandino C, Valensise H, Dell'Acqua S, et al. Modifications of ultradian and circadian rhythms of fetal heart rate after fetal-maternal adrenal gland suppression: a double blind study. Prenat Diagn 1986;6:409–417.

369. Talan MI, Engel BT, Chew PH. Systematic nocturnal atrial demand pacing results in high-output heart failure. J Appl Physiol 1992;72:1803–1809.

370. Christ JE, Hoff HE. An analysis of the circadian rhythmicity of atrial and ventricular rates in complete heart block. J Electrocardiol 1975;8:69–72.

371. Ashkar E. Twenty-four-hour pattern of circulation by radiotelemetry in the unrestrained dog. Am J Physiol 1979;236:R231–R236.

372. Alboni P, Codeca L, Padovan G, Tomaini D, Destro A, Margutti A, et al. Variazioni circadiane della frequenza sinusale in soggetti con nodo del seno normale e patologico. G Ital Cardiol 1981;11:1211–1218.

373. Patrick J, Campbell K, Carmichael L, Probert C. Influence of maternal heart rate and gross fetal body movements on the daily pattern of fetal heart rate near term. Am J Obstet Gynecol 1982;144:533–538.

374. Visser GH, Goodman JD, Levine DH, Dawes GS. Diurnal and other cyclic variations in human fetal heart rate near term. Am J Obstet Gynecol 1982;142:535–544.

375. Manzoli U, Sensi S, Coppola E, Schiavoni G, Domenichelli B, Lucente M, et al. Il ritmo circadiano della soglia di stimolazione miocardica. G Ital Cardiol 1978;8(Suppl 3):S158–S159.

376. Thormann J, Schlepper M, Kramer W. Diurnal changes and reproducibility of corrected sinus node recovery time. Cathet Cardiovasc Diagn 1983;9:439–451.

377. de Leonardis V, de Scalzi M, Fabiano FS, Cinelli P. A chronobiologic study on some cardiovascular parameters. J Electrocardiol 1985;18:385–394.

378. Cinca J, Moya A, Figueras J, Roma F, Rius J. Circadian variations in the electrical properties of the human heart assessed by sequential bedside electrophysiologic testing. Am Heart J 1986;112:315–321.

379. Gillis AM, Mac Lean KE, Guilleminault C. The QT interval during wake and sleep in patients with ventricular arrhythmias. Sleep 1988;11:333–339.

380. Cinca J, Moya A, Bardaji A, Rius J, Soler-Soler J. Circadian variations of electrical properties of the heart. Ann NY Acad Sci 1990;601:222–233.

381. Mitsuoka T, Ueyama C, Matsumoto Y, Hashiba K. Influences of autonomic changes on the sinus node recovery time in patients with sick sinus syndrome. Jpn Heart J 1990;31:645–660.

382. Alexopoulos D, Rynkiewicz A, Yusuf S, Johnston JA, Sleight P, Yacoub MH. Diurnal variations of QT interval after cardiac transplantation. Am J Cardiol 1988;61:482–485.

383. Lown B, Calvert AF, Armington R, Ryan M. Monitoring for serious arrhythmias and high risk of sudden death. Circulation 1975;52:189–198.

384. Sensi S, Manzoli U, Capani F, Domenichelli B, Lucente M, Schiavoni G, et al. Circadian rhythm of ventricular ectopy [Letter]. Chest 1980;77:580.

385. Canada WB, Woodward W, Lee G, De Maria A, Low R, Mason DT, et al. Circadian rhythm of hourly ventricular arrhythmia frequency in man. Angiology 1983;34:274–282.

386. Lanza GA, Lucente M, Rebuzzi AG, Spagnolo A, Dulcimascolo C, Manzoli U. Ventricular parasystole: a chronobiologic study. PACE Pacing Clin Electrophysiol 1986;9:860–867.

387. Biffi A, Cugini P, Pelliccia A, Spataro A, Caselli G, Piovano G. Studio cronobiologico dell' elettrocardiogramma dinamico in atleti sani con battiti ectopici ventricolari frequenti. G Ital Cardiol 1987;17:563–568.

388. Lucente M, Rebuzzi AG, Lanza GA, Tamburi S, Cortellessa MC, Coppola E, et al. Circadian variation of ventricular tachycardia in acute myocardial infarction. Am J Cardiol 1988;62: 670–674.

389. Cinca J, Moya A, Bardaji A, Figueras J, Rius J. Daily variability of electrically induced reciprocating tachycardia in patients with atrioventricular accessory pathways. Am Heart J 1987; 114:327–333.

390. Shimada R, Nakashima T, Nunoi K, Kohno Y, Takeshita A, Omae T. Arrhythmia during insulin-induced hypoglycemia in a diabetic patient. Arch Intern Med 1984;144:1068–1069.

391. Gillis AM, Guilleminault C, Partinen M, Connolly SJ, Winkle RA. The diurnal variability of ventricular premature depolarizations: influence of heart rate, sleep, and wakefulness. Sleep 1989;12:391–399.

392. Gillis AM, Peters RW, Mitchell LB, Duff HJ, McDonald M, Wyse DG. Effects of left ventricular dysfunction on the circadian variation of ventricular premature complexes in healed myocardial infarction. Am J Cardiol 1992;69:1009–1014.

393. Otsuka K, Sato T, Saito H, Kaba H, Otsuka K, Seto K, et al. Circadian rhythm of cardiac bradyarrhythmia episodes in rats. Chronobiologia 1985;12:11–28.
394. Raeder EA. Circadian fluctuations in ventricular response to atrial fibrillation. Am J Cardiol 1990;66:1013–1016.
395. Novo S, Barbagallo M, Abrignani MG, Alaimo G, Nardi E, Corrao S, et al. Cardiac arrhythmias as correlated with the circadian rhythm of arterial pressure in hypertensive subjects with and without left ventricular hypertrophy. Eur J Clin Pharmacol 1990;39(Suppl 1): S49–S51.
396. Sideris DA, Toumanidis ST, Anastasiou-Nana M, Zakopoulos N, Kitsiou A, Tsagarakis K, et al. The circadian profile of extrasystolic arrhythmia: its relationship to heart rate and blood pressure. Int J Cardiol 1992;34:21–31.
397. McClelland J, Halperin B, Cutler J, Kudenchuk P, Kron J, McAnulty J. Circadian variation in ventricular electrical instability associated with coronary artery disease. Am J Cardiol 1990;65:1351–1357.
398. Khatri IM, Freis ED. Hemodynamic changes during sleep. J Appl Physiol 1967;22:867–873.
399. Miller JC, Horvath SM. Cardiac output during human sleep. Aviat Space Environ Med 1976; 47:1046–1051.
400. Coote JH. Respiratory and circulatory control during sleep. J Exp Biol 1982;100:223–244.
401. Takagi N. Variability of direct arterial blood pressure in essential hypertension—relationships between the fall of blood pressure during sleep and awake resting hemodynamic parameters. Jpn Circ J 1986;50:587–594.
402. Mori H. Circadian variation of haemodynamics in patients with essential hypertension. J Hum Hypertens 1990;4:384–389.
403. Veerman DP, Imholz BPM, Wieling W, Wesseling KH, van Montfrans GA. Circadian profile of systemic hemodynamics. Hypertension 1995;26:55–59.
404. Wesseling KH, de Wit B, Weber JAP, Smith NT. A simple device for the continuous measurement of cardiac output: its model basis and experimental verification. J Appl Physiol 1983;59:16–52.
405. Casiglia E, Palatini P, Baccillieri MS, Colangeli G, Petucco S, Pessina AC. Circadian rhythm of peripheral resistance: a non-invasive 24-hour study in young normal volunteers confined to bed. High Blood Pressure 1992;1:249–255.
406. Engel BT, Talan MI. Diurnal pattern of hemodynamic performance in nonhuman primates. Am J Physiol 1987;253:R779–R785.
407. Talan MI, Engel BT. Effect of sympathetic bockade on diurnal variation of hemodynamic patterns. Am J Physiol 1989;256:R778–R785.
408. Mills JN. Human circadian rhythms. Physiol Rev 1966;46:128–171.
409. Sindrup JH, Kastrup J, Jorgensen B. Regional variations in nocturnal fluctuations in subcutaneous blood flow rate in the lower leg of man. Clin Physiol 1991;11:491–499.
410. Townsend RE, Prinz PN, Obrist WD. Human cerebral blood flow during sleep and waking. J Appl Physiol 1973;35:620–625.
411. Smith TL, Coleman TG, Stanek KA, Murphy WR. Hemodynamic monitoring for 24 h in unanesthetized rats. Am J Physiol 1987;253:H1335–H1341.
412. Engel BT, Talan MI. Diurnal variation in central venous pressure. Acta Physiol Scand 1991; 141:273–278.
413. Talan MI, Engel BT, Kawate R. Overnight increases in hematocrit: additional evidence for a nocturnal fall in plasma volume. Acta Physiol Scand 1992;144:473–476.
414. Kool MJ, Wijnen JA, Hoeks AP, Struyker-Boudier HA, Van Bortel LM. Diurnal pattern of vessel-wall properties of large arteries in healthy men. J Hypertens 1991;9(Suppl 6): S108–S109.
415. Lugaresi E, Coccagna G, Mantovani M, Lebrun R. Some periodic phenomena arising during drowsiness and sleep in man. Electroencephalogr Clin Neurophysiol 1972;32:701–705.

416. Levy RD, Cunningham D, Shapiro LM, Wright C, Mockus L, Fox KM. Diurnal variation in left ventricular function: a study of patients with myocardial ischaemia, syndrome X, and of normal controls. Br Heart J 1987;57:148–153.

417. Gibbs JS, Cunningham D, Shapiro LM, Park A, Poole-Wilson PA, Fox KM. Diurnal variation of pulmonary artery pressure in chronic heart failure. Br Heart J 1989;62:30–35.

418. Panza JA, Epstein SE, Quyyumi AA. Circadian variation in vascular tone and its relation to alpha-sympathetic vasoconstrictor activity. N Engl J Med 1991;325:986–990.

419. Kennedy B, Shannahoff-Khalsa D, Ziegler MG. Plasma norepinephrine variations correlate with peripheral vascular resistance in resting humans. Am J Physiol 1994;266(2 Pt 2): H435–H439.

420. Morris JJ Jr. Mechanisms of ischemia in coronary artery disease: spontaneous decrease in coronary blood supply. Am Heart J 1990;120:746–756, 769–772.

421. Pepine CJ. Therapeutic implications of circadian variations in myocardial ischemia and related physiologic functions. Am J Hypertens 1991;4(7 Pt 2):442S–448S.

422. Raby KE, Vita JA, Rocco MB, Yeung AC, Ganz P, Fantasia G, et al. Changing vasomotor responses of coronary arteries to nifedipine. Am Heart J 1993;126:333–338.

423. Bush LR. Effects of the serotonin antagonists, cyproheptadine, ketanserin and mianserin, on cyclic flow reductions in stenosed canine coronary arteries. J Pharmacol Exp Ther 1987;240: 674–682.

424. Chen LD, Tan DX, Reiter RJ, Yaga K, Poeggeler B, Kumar P, et al. In vivo and in vitro effects of the pineal gland and melatonin on [Ca(2+)+ Mg2+]-dependent ATPase in cardiac sarcolema. J Pineal Res 1993;14:178–183.

425. Katz, ML. Comerota AJ, Kerr RP, Caputo GC. Variability of venous-hemodynamics with daily activity. L Vasc Surg 1994;19:361–365.

426. Garcia-Pagan JC, Feu F. Castells A, Luca A, Hermida RC, Rivera F, et al. Circadian variations of portal pressure and variceal hemorrage in patients with cirrhosis. Hepatology 1994; 19:595–601.

427. Morra L, Ponassi A, Caristo G, Bruzzi P, Bonelli A, Zunino R, et al. Comparison between diurnal changes and changes induced by hydrocortisone and epinephrine in circulating myeloid progenitor cells (CFU-GM) in man. Biomed Pharmacother 1984;38:167–170.

428. Bridges AB, Fisher TC, Scott N, McLaren M, Belch JJ. Circadian rhythm of white blood cell aggregation and free radical status in healthy volunteers. Free Radical Res Commun 1992; 16:89–97.

429. Fujimura A, Ohashi K, Ebihara A. Chronopharmacological study of furosemide; (IX). Influence of continuous norepinephrine infusion. Life Sci 1992;50:449–455.

430. Brezinski DA, Tofler GH, Muller JE, Pohjola-Sintonen S, Willich SN, Schafer AI, et al. Morning increase in platelet aggregability. Association with assumption of the upright posture. Circulation 1988;78:35–40.

431. Jafri SM, Van Rollins M, Ozawa T, Mammen EF, Goldberg AD, Goldstein S. Circadian variation in platelet function in healthy volunteers. Am J Cardiol 1992;69:951–954.

432. Yao SK, Ober JC, Krishnaswami A, Ferguson JJ, Anderson HV, Golino P, et al. Endogenous nitric oxide protects against platelet aggregation and cyclic flow variations in stenosed and endothelium-injured arteries. Circulation 1992;86:1302–1309.

433. Andreotti F, Davies GJ, Hackett DR, Khan MI, De Bart AC, Aber VR, et al. Major circadian fluctuations in fibrinolytic factors and possible relevance to time of onset of myocardial infarction, sudden cardiac death and stroke. Am J Cardiol 1988;62:635–637.

434. Grimaudo V, Hauert J, Bachmann F, Kruithof EK. Diurnal variation of the fibrinolytic system. Thromb Haemost 1988;59:495–499.

435. Kluft C, Jie AF, Rijken DC, Verheijen JH. Daytime fluctuations in blood of tissue-type plasminogen activator (t-PA) and its fast-acting inhibitor (PAI–1). Thromb Haemost 1988; 59:329–332.

436. Angleton P, Chandler WL, Schmer G. Diurnal variation of tissue-type plasminogen activator and its rapid inhibitor (PAI–1). Circulation 1989;79:101–106.

437. Takada A, Takada Y, Urano T, Sakakibara K, Rydzewski A. Fluctuations of euglobulin lysis time, tissue plasminogen activator, and free and total plasminogen activator inhibitor levels in plasma in daytime. Thromb Res 1990;57:13–20.

438. Bridges AB, McLaren M, Saniabadi A, Fisher TC, Belch JJ. Circadian variation of endothelial cell function, red blood cell deformability and dehydro-thromboxane B2 in healthy volunteers. Blood Coagul Fibrinolysis 1991;2:447–452.

439. Chandler WL. A kinetic model of the circulatory regulation of tissue plasminogen activator. Thromb Haemost 1991;66:321–328.

440. Urano T, Sumiyoshi K, Nakamura M, Mori T, Takada Y, Takada A. Fluctuation of tPA and PAI–1 antigen levels in plasma: difference of their fluctuation patterns between male and female. Thromb Res 1990;60:133–139.

441. Ranby M, Bergsdorf N, Nilsson T, Mellbring G, Winblad B, Bucht G. Age dependence of tissue plasminogen activator concentrations in plasma, as studied by an improved enzyme-linked immunosorbent assay. Clin Chem 1986;32:2160–2165.

442. Motohashi F, Masui Y, Kamogawa A, Hayashi T, Miyake F, Murayama M, et al. Influence of aging and circadian fluctuation of fibrinolytic factors to the responses of these factors during venous occlusion test in healthy subjects. Rinsho Byori 1992;40:172–178.

443. Huber K, Rosc D, Resch I, Schuster E, Glogar DH, Kaindl F, et al. Circadian fluctuations of plasminogen activator inhibitor and tissue plasminogen activator levels in plasma of patients with unstable coronary artery disease and acute myocardial infarction. Thromb Haemost 1988;60:372–376.

444. Sakata K, Hoshino T, Yoshida H, Ono N, Ohtani S, Yokoyama S, et al. Circadian fluctuations of tissue plasminogen activator antigen and plasminogen activator inhibitor–1 antigens in vasospastic angina. Am Heart J 1992;124:854–860.

445. Bridges AB, McLaren M, Scott NA, Pringle TH, McNeill GP, Belch JJ. Circadian variation of tissue plasminogen activator and its inhibitor, von Willebrand factor antigen, and prostacyclin stimulating factor in men with ischaemic heart disease. Br Heart J 1993;69:121–124.

446. Cucuianu MP, Rus HG, Roman S, Marcusu C, Spinu C, Manasia M, et al. Tissue-type plasminogen activator (t-PA) and dilute blood clot lysis time in nephrotic patients. Thromb Haemost 1989;61:270–274.

447. Mussoni L, Mannucci L, Sirtori M, Camera M, Maderna P, Sironi L, et al. Hypertriglyceridemia and regulation of fibrinolytic activity. Arterioscler Thromb 1992;12:19–27.

448. Avellone G, Di Garbo V, Cordova R, Raneli G, De Simone R, Bompiani GD. Fibrinolysis in hypertriglyceridaemic subjects in response to venous occlusion. Blood Coagul Fibrinolysis 1993;4:429–433.

449. Glueck CJ, Glueck HI, Mieczkowski L, Tracy T, Speirs J, Stroop D. Familial high plasminogen activator inhibitor with hypofibrinolysis, a new pathophysiologic cause of osteonecrosis? Thromb Haemost 1993;69:460–465.

450. Cortellaro M, Cofrancesco E, Boschetti C, Mussoni L, Donati MB, Cardillo M, et al. Increased fibrin turnover and high PAI–1 activity as predictors of ischemic events in atherosclerotic patients. A case-control study. The PLAT Group. Arterioscler Thromb 1993;13:1412–1417.

451. Ridker PM, Gaboury CL, Conlin PR, Seely EW, Williams GH, Vaughan DE. Stimulation of plasminogen activator inhibitor in vivo by infusion of angiotensin II. Evidence of a potential interaction between the renin-angiotensin system and fibrinolytic function. Circulation 1993;87:1969–1973.

452. Malherbe C, De Gasparo M, De Hertogh R, Hoet JJ. Circadian variations of blood sugar and plasma insulin levels in man. Diabetologia 1969;5:397–404.

453. Geffner ME, Frank HJ, Kaplan SA, Lippe BM, Levin SR. Early-morning hyperglycemia in diabetic individuals treated with continuous subcutaneous insulin infusion. Diabetes Care 1983;6:135–139.

454. Bolli GB, De Feo P, De Cosmo S, Perriello G, Ventura MM, Calcinaro F, et al. Demonstration of a dawn phenomenon in normal human volunteers. Diabetes 1984;33:1150–1153.

455. Sirek A, Vaitkus P, Norwich KH, Sirek OV, Unger RH, Harris V. Secretory patterns of glucoregulatory hormones in prehepatic circulation of dogs. Am J Physiol 1985;249:E34–E42.

456. Rosenthal MJ, Argoud GM. Absence of the dawn glucose rise in nondiabetic men compared by age. J Gerontol 1989;44:M57–M61.

457. Garrel DR, Bajard L, Harfouche M, Tourniaire J. Decreased hypoglycemic effect of insulin at night in insulin-dependent diabetes mellitus and healthy subjects. J Clin Endocrinol Metab 1992;75:106–109.

458. Atiea JA, Vora JP, Owens DR, Luzio S, Read GF, Walker RF, et al. Non-insulin-dependent diabetic patients (NIDDMs) do not demonstrate the dawn phenomenon at presentation. Diabetes Res Clin Pract 1988;5:37–44.

459. Campbell PJ, Bolli GB, Cryer PE, Gerich JE. Sequence of events during development of the dawn phenomenon in insulin-dependent diabetes mellitus. Metabolism 1985;34:1100–1104.

460. Davidson MB, Harris MD, Ziel FH, Rosenberg CS. Suppression of sleep-induced growth hormone secretion by anticholinergic agent abolishes dawn phenomenon. Diabetes 1988;37:166–171.

461. Atiea JA, Creagh F, Page M, Owens DR, Scanlon MF, Peters JR. Early-morning hyperglycemia in IDDM. Acute effects of cholinergic blockade [see comments]. Diabetes Care 1989;12:443–448.

462. Boyle PJ, Avogaro A, Smith L, Shah SD, Cryer PE, Santiago JV. Absence of the dawn phenomenon and abnormal lipolysis in type 1 (insulin-dependent) diabetic patients with chronic growth hormone deficiency. Diabetologia 1992;35:372–379.

463. Kerner W, Navascues I, Torres AA, Pfeiffer EF. Studies on the pathogenesis of the dawn phenomenon in insulin-dependent diabetic patients. Metabolism 1984;33:458–464.

464. Atiea JA, Aslan SM, Owens DR, Luzio S. Early morning hyperglycaemia "dawn phenomenon" in non-insulin dependent diabetes mellitus (NIDDM): effects of cortisol suppression by metyrapone. Diabetes Res 1990;14:181–185.

465. Waters DD, Miller DD, Bouchard A, Bosch X, Theroux P. Circadian variation in variant angina. Am J Cardiol 1984;54:61–64.

466. Quyyumi AA, Mockus L, Wright C, Fox KM. Morphology of ambulatory ST segment changes in patients with varying severity of coronary artery disease. Investigation of the frequency of nocturnal ischaemia and coronary spasm. Br Heart J 1985;53:186–193.

467. Nademanee K, Intarachot V, Josephson MA, Singh BN. Circadian variation in occurrence of transient overt and silent myocardial ischemia in chronic stable angina and comparison with Prinzmetal angina in men. Am J Cardiol 1987;60:494–498.

468. Fox K, Mulcahy D, Keegan J, Wright C. Circadian patterns of myocardial ischemia. Am Heart J 1989;118:1084–1087.

469. Aslanian NL. Chronobiological aspects of ischemic heart disease. Prog Clin Biol Res 1990;341B:583–592.

470. Rebuzzi AG, Lanza GA, Lucente M, Tamburi S, Di Pietro M, Urso L, et al. Circadian rhythm of ischemic episodes in patients with and without previous myocardial infarction. Prog Clin Biol Res 1990;341A:419–422.

471. Rocco MB. Timing and triggers of transient myocardial ischemia. Am J Cardiol 1990;66:18G–21G.

472. Behar S, Reicher-Reiss H, Goldbourt U, Kaplinsky E. Circadian variation in pain onset in unstable angina pectoris. Am J Cardiol 1991;67:91–93.

473. Hausmann D, Lichtlen PR, Nikutta P, Wenzlaff P, Daniel WG. Circadian variation of myocardial ischemia in patients with stable coronary artery disease. Chronobiol Int 1991;8:385–398.

474. Rocco MB, Barry J, Campbell S, Nabel E, Cook EF, Goldman L, et al. Circadian variation of transient myocardial ischemia in patients with coronary artery disease. Circulation 1987;75:395–400.

475. Mulcahy D, Keegan J, Cunningham D, Quyyumi A, Crean P, Park A, et al. Circadian variation of total ischaemic burden and its alteration with anti-anginal agents. Lancet 1988;2: 755–759.

476. Araki H, Koiwaya Y, Nakagaki O, Nakamura M. Diurnal distribution of ST-segment elevation and related arrhythmias in patients with variant angina: a study by ambulatory ECG monitoring. Circulation 1983;67:995–1000.

477. Ogawa H, Yasue H, Oshima S, Okumura K, Matsuyama K, Obata K. Circadian variation of plasma fibrinopeptide A level in patients with variant angina. Circulation 1989;80:1617–1626.

478. Yasue H, Omote S, Takizawa A, Nagao M, Miwa K, Tanaka S. Circadian variation of exercise capacity in patients with Prinzmetal's variant angina: role of exercise-induced coronary arterial spasm. Circulation 1979;59:938–948.

479. Pell S, D'Alonzo CA. Acute myocardial infarction in a large industrial population: report of a 6-year study of 1,356 cases. JAMA 1963;185:831–838.

480. Muller JE, Stone PH, Turi ZG, Rutherford JD, Czeisler CA, Parker C, et al. Circadian variation in the frequency of onset of acute myocardial infarction. N Engl J Med 1985;313:1315–1322.

481. Thompson DR, Blandford RL, Sutton TW, Marchant PR. Time of onset of chest pain in acute myocardial infarction. Int J Cardiol 1985;7:139–148.

482. Hjalmarson A, Gilpin EA, Nicod P, Dittrich H, Henning H, Engler R, et al. Differing circadian patterns of symptom onset in subgroups of patients with acute myocardial infarction. Circulation 1989;80:267–275.

483. Willich SN, Linderer T, Wegscheider K, Leizorovicz A, Alamercery I, Schroder R. Increased morning incidence of myocardial infarction in the ISAM Study: absence with prior beta-adrenergic blockade. ISAM Study Group. Circulation 1989;80:853–858.

484. Gilpin EA, Hjalmarson A, Ross J. Subgroups of patients with atypical circadian patterns of symptom onset in acute myocardial infarction. Am J Cardiol 1990;66:7G–11G.

485. Hansen O, Johansson BW, Gullberg B. Circadian distribution of onset of acute myocardial infarction in subgroups from analysis of 10,791 patients treated in a single center. Am J Cardiol 1992;69:1003–1008.

486. Behar S, Halabi M, Reicher-Reiss H, Zion M, Kaplinsky E, Mandelzweig L, et al. Circadian variation and possible external triggers of onset of myocardial infarction. SPRINT Study Group. Am J Med 1993;94:395–400.

487. Gallerani M, Manfredini R, Ricci L, Goldoni C, Cocurullo A, Pareschi PL. Circadian variation in the onset of acute myocardial infarction: lack of an effect due to age and sex. J Int Med Res 1993;21:158–160.

488. Goldberg RJ, Brady P, Muller JE, Chen ZY, de Groot M, Zonneveld P, et al. Time of onset of symptoms of acute myocardial infarction. Am J Cardiol 1990;66:140–144.

489. Knutsson A. Shift work and coronary heart disease. Scand J Soc Med 1989;44(Suppl):1–36.

490. Kleiman NS, Schechtman KB, Young PM, Goodman DA, Boden WE, Pratt CM, et al. Lack of diurnal variation in the onset of non-Q wave infarction. Circulation 1990;81:548–555.

491. Willich SN, Levy D, Rocco MB, Tofler GH, Stone PH, Muller JE. Circadian variation in the incidence of sudden cardiac death in the Framingham Heart Study population. Am J Cardiol 1987;60:801–806.

492. Peters RW, Muller JE, Goldstein S, Byington R, Friedman LM. Propranolol and the morning increase in the frequency of sudden cardiac death (BHAT Study). Am J Cardiol 1989;63: 1518–1520.

493. Levine RL, Pepe PE, Fromm RE, Curka PA, Clark PA. Prospective evidence of a circadian rhythm for out-of-hospital cardiac arrests. JAMA 1992;267:2935–2937.

494. Aronow WS, Ahn C. Circadian variation of primary cardiac arrest or sudden cardiac death in patients aged 62 to 100 years (mean 82). Am J Cardiol 1993;71:1455–1456.

495. Gallerani M, Manfredini R, Ricci L, Cappato R, Grandi E, Dal Monte D, et al. Sudden death may show a circadian time of risk depending on its anatomo-clinical causes and age. Jpn Heart J 1993;34:729–739.

496. Gallerani M, Manfredini R, Graziani R, Manservigi D, Bariani L, Ricci L, et al. Sudden death in diabetic subjects: evidence for a peculiar circadian variation in occurrence. Panminerva Med 1994;36:134–137.

497. Tsementzis SA, Gill JS, Hitchcock ER, Gill SK, Beevers DG. Diurnal variation of and activity during the onset of stroke. Neurosurgery 1985;17:901–904.

498. Fersini C, Manfredini R, Manfredini F, Balboni G, Fersini G. Chronobiologic aspects of recurrent transient ischemic attack. Prog Clin Biol Res 1987;227B:167–171.

499. Marler JR, Price TR, Clark GL, Muller JE, Robertson T, Mohr JP, et al. Morning increase in onset of ischemic stroke. Stroke 1989;20:473–476.

500. Arboix A, Marti-Vilalta JL. Acute stroke and circadian rhythm [Letter]. Stroke 1990;21:826.

501. Argentino C, Toni D, Rasura M, Violi F, Sacchetti ML, Allegretta A, et al. Circadian variation in the frequency of ischemic stroke. Stroke 1990;21:387–389.

502. Marsh EE, Biller J, Adams HP, Marler JR, Hulbert JR, Love BB, et al. Circadian variation in onset of acute ischemic stroke. Arch Neurol 1990;47:1178–1180.

503. Pasqualetti P, Natali G, Casale R, Colantonio D. Epidemiological chronorisk of stroke. Acta Neurol Scand 1990;81:71–74.

504. Toni D, Argentino C, Gentile M, Sacchetti ML, Girmenia F, Millefiorini E, et al. Circadian variation in the onset of acute cerebral ischemia: ethiopathogenetic correlates in 80 patients given angiography. Chronobiol Int 1991;8:321–326.

505. Ricci S, Celani MG, Vitali R, La Rosa F, Righetti E, Duca E. Diurnal and seasonal variations in the occurrence of stroke: a community-based study. Neuroepidemiology 1992;11:59–64.

506. Gallerani M, Manfredini R, Ricci L, Cocurullo A, Goldoni C, Bigoni M, et al. Chronobiological aspects of acute cerebrovascular diseases. Acta Neurol Scand 1993;87:482–487.

507. Hossmann V. Circadian changes of blood pressure and stroke. In: Zulch KJ, ed. Cerebral Circulation and Stroke. Springer-Verlag, Heidelberg, 1971, pp. 203–208.

508. Marshall J. Diurnal variation in occurrence of strokes. Stroke 1977;8:230–231.

509. Johansson BB, Norrving B, Widner H, Wu JY, Halberg F. Stroke incidence: circadian and circaseptan (about weekly) variations in onset. Prog Clin Biol Res 1990;341A:427–436.

510. Sloan MA, Price TR, Foulkes MA, Marler JR, Mohr JP, Hier DB, et al. Circadian rhythmicity of stroke onset. Intracerebral and subarachnoid hemorrhage. Stroke 1992;23:1420–1426.

511. Gallerani M, Trappella G, Manfredini R, Pasin M, Napolitano M, Migliore A. Acute intracerebral haemorrhage: circadian and circannual patterns of onset. Acta Neurol Scand 1994; 89:280–286.

512. Kupari M, Koskinen P, Leinonen H. Double-peaking circadian variation in the occurrence of sustained supraventricular tachyarrhythmias. Am Heart J 1990;120:1364–1369.

513. Rostagno C, Taddei T, Paladini B, Modesti PA, Utari P, Bertini G. The onset of symptomatic atrial fibrillation and paroxysmal supraventricular tachycardia is characterized by different circadian rhythms. Am J Cardiol 1993;71:453–455.

514. Clair WK, Wilkinson WE, McCarthy EA, Page RL, Pritchett EL. Spontaneous occurrence of symptomatic paroxysmal atrial fibrillation and paroxysmal supraventricular tachycardia in untreated patients. Circulation 1993;87:1114–1122.

515. Irwin JM, McCarthy EA, Wilkinson WE, Pritchett EL. Circadian occurrence of symptomatic paroxysmal supraventricular tachycardia in untreated patients. Circulation 1988;77:298–300.

516. Manfredini R, Gallerani M, Portaluppi F, Salmi R, Chierici F, Fersini C. Circadian variation in the occurrence of paroxysmal supraventricular tachycardia in clinically healthy subjects. Chronobiol Int 1995;12:55–61.

517. de Leonardis V, de Scalzi M, Vergassola R, Romano S, Becucci A, Cinelli P. Circadian variations of heart rate and premature beats in healthy subjects and in patients with previous myocardial infarction. Chronobiol Int 1987;4:283–289.

518. Raeder EA, Hohnloser SH, Graboys TB, Podrid PJ, Lampert S, Lown B. Spontaneous variability and circadian distribution of ectopic activity in patients with malignant ventricular arrhythmia. J Am Coll Cardiol 1988;12:656–661.

519. Lanza GA, Cortellessa MC, Rebuzzi AG, Scabbia EV, Costalunga A, Tamburi S, et al. Reproducibility in circadian rhythm of ventricular premature complexes. Am J Cardiol 1990;66: 1099–1106.

520. Siegel D, Black DM, Seeley DG, Hulley SB. Circadian variation in ventricular arrhythmias in hypertensive men. Am J Cardiol 1992;69:344–347.

521. Twidale N, Taylor S, Heddle WF, Ayres BF, Tonkin AM. Morning increase in the time of onset of sustained ventricular tachycardia. Am J Cardiol 1989;64:1204–1206.

522. Valkama JO, Huikuri HV, Linnaluoto MK, Takkunen JT. Circadian variation of ventricular tachycardia in patients with coronary arterial disease. Int J Cardiol 1992;34:173–178.

523. Arntz HR, Willich SN, Oeff M, Bruggemann T, Stern R, Heinzmann A, et al. Circadian variation of sudden cardiac death reflects age-related variability in ventricular fibrillation. Circulation 1993;88:2284–2289.

524. Lampert R, Rosenfeld L, Batsford W, Lee F, McPherson C. Circadian variation of sustained ventricular tachycardia in patients with coronary artery disease and implantable cardioverter-defibrillators. Circulation 1994;90:241–247.

525. Alboni P, degli Uberti E, Codeca L, Padovan G, Lo Vecchio G, Margutti A, et al. Circadian variations of sinus rate in subjects with sinus node dysfunction. Chronobiologia 1982;9: 173–183.

526. Johnstone MT, Mittleman M, Tofler GH, Muller JE. The pathophysiology of the onset of morning cardiovascular events. Am J Hypertens 1996;9:22S–28S.

527. Andrews TC, Fenton T, Toyosaki N, Glasser SP, Young PM, Mac Callum G, et al. Subsets of ambulatory myocardial ischemia based on heart rate activity. Circadian distribution and response to anti-ischemic medication. The Angina and Silent Ischemia Study Group (ASIS). Circulation 1993;88:92–100.

528. Benhorin J, Banai S, Moriel M, Gavish A, Keren A, Stern S, et al. Circadian variations in ischemic threshold and their relation to the occurrence of ischemic episodes. Circulation 1993;87:808–814.

529. Hinderliter A, Miller P, Bragdon E, Ballenger M., Sheps D. Myocardial ischemia during daily activities: the importance of increased myocardial oxygen demand. J Am Coll Cardiol 1991;18:405–412.

530. Chaitman BR. Exercise stress testing. In: Braunwald E, ed. Heart Disease—A Textbook of Cardiovascular Medicine, 5th ed. WB Saunders, Philadelphia, 1997, pp. 153–176.

531. White WB, Black HR, Weber MA, Elliott WJ, Bryzinski B, Fakouhi TD. Comparison of effects of controlled-onset extended-release verapamil at bedtime and nifedipine gastrointestinal therapeutic system on arising on early morning blood pressure, heart rate and the heart-rate-blood pressure product. Am J Cardiol 1998;81;424–431.

532. Deedwania PC, Nelson JR. Pathophysiology of silent myocardial Ischemia during daily life: hemodynamic evaluation by simultaneous electrocardiographic and blood pressure monitoring. Circulation 1990;82:1296–1304.

533. Hermida RC, Fernandez JR, Smolensky M, Mojon A. Alonso I, Ayala DE. Circadian variability of double (rate-pressure) product in young normotensive healthy men and women. Chronobiol Int 2001, in press.

534. Quyyumi AA, Panza JA, Diodati JG, Lakatos E, Epstein SE. Circadian variation in ischemic threshold. A mechanism underlying the circadian variation in ischemic events. Circulation 1992;86:22–28.

535. Nowlin JB, Troyer WG, Collins WS. The association of nocturnal angina pectoris with dreaming. Ann Intern Med 1965;63:1040–1046.

536. King MJ, Zir LM, Kaltman AJ, Fox AC. Variant angina associated with angiographically demonstrated coronary artery spasm and REM sleep. Am J Med Sci 1973;265:419–422.

537. Kirby DA, Verrier RL. Differential effects of sleep stage on coronary hemodynamic function during stenosis. Physiol Behav 1989;45:1017–1020.

538. Czeisler CA, Weitzman ED, Moore-Ede MC, Zimmerman JC, Knauer RS. Human sleep: its duration and organization depend on its circadian phase. Science 1980;210:1264–1267.

539. Czeisler CA, Zimmerman JC, Ronda JM, Moore-Ede MC, Weitzman ED. Timing of REM sleep is coupled to the circadian rhythm of body temperature in man. Sleep 1980;2:329–346.

540. Aschoff J, Wever R. Human circadian rhythms: a multioscillatory system. Fed. Proc 1976;35: 2326–2332.

541. Refinetti R, Menaker M. The circadian rhythm of body temperature. Physiol Behav 1992; 51:613–637.

542. Tofler GH, Brezinski D, Schafer AI, Czeisler CA, Rutherford JD, Willich SN, et al. Concurrent morning increase in platelet aggregability and the risk of myocardial infarction and sudden cardiac death. N Engl J Med 1987;316:1514–1518.

543. Fujita M, Franklin D. Diurnal changes in coronary blood flow in conscious dogs. Circulation 1987;76:488–491.

544. Weitzman ED, Fukushima D, Nogeire C, Roffwarg H, Gallagher TF, Hellman L. Twenty-four hour pattern of the episodic secretion of cortisol in normal subjects. J Clin Endocrinol Metab 1971;33:14–22.

545. Vaziri ND, Kennedy SC, Kennedy D, Gonzales E. Coagulation, fibrinolytic, and inhibitory proteins in acute myocardial infarction and angina pectoris. Am J Med 1992;93:651–657.

546. Petralito A, Mangiafico RA, Gibiino S, Cuffari MA, Miano MF, Fiore CE. Daily modifications of plasma fibrinogen, platelets aggregation, Howell's time, PTT, TT, and antithrombin II in normal subjects and in patients with vascular disease. Chronobiologia 1982;9: 195–201.

547. Conchonnet P, Decousus H, Perpoint B. Morning hypercoagulability in man. Annu Rev Chronopharmacol 1990;7:165–168.

548. Haus E, Cusulos M, Sackett-Lundeen L, Swoyer J. Circadian variations in blood coagulation parameters, alpha-antitrypsin antigen and platelet aggregation and retention in clinically healthy subjects. Chronobiol Int 1990;7:203–216.

549. Labrecque G, Soulban G. Biological rhythms in the physiology and pharmacology of blood coagulation. Chronobiol Int 1991;8:361–372.

550. Jovicic A, Mandic S. Circadian variations of platelet aggregability and fibrinolytic activity in healthy subjects. Thromb Res 1991;62:65–74.

551. Musumeci V, Rosa S, Caruso A, Zuppi C, Zappacosta B, Tutinelli F. Abnormal diurnal changes in in-vivo platelet activation in patients with atherosclerotic diseases. Atherosclerosis 1986;60:231–236.

552. Willich SN, Sintonen SP, Bathia SS. Morning increase in platelet aggregability in patients with coronary artery disease. J Am Coll Cardiol 1988;11:204 (abstract).

553. Fearnley GR, Balmforth G, Fearnley E. Evidence of a diurnal fibrinolytic rhythm with a simple method of measuring natural fibrinolysis. Clin Sci 1957;16:645–650.

554. Huber K, Rose D, Resch I, Glogar DH, Kaindl F, Binder BR. Circadian fluctuations of plasma levels of tissue plasminogen activator antigen and plasminogen activator inhibitor activity. Fibrinolysis 1989;3:41–43.

555. Andreotti F, Kluft C. Circadian variation of fibrinolytic activity in blood. Chronobiol Int 1991;6:336–351.

556. Masuda T, Ogawa H, Miyao Y, Yu Q, Misumi I, Sakamoto T, et al. Circadian variation in fibrinolytic activity in patients with variant angina. Br Heart J 1994;71:156–161.

557. Ehrly AM, Jung G. Circadian rhythm of human blood viscosity. Biorheology 1973;10: 577–583.

558. Touitou Y, Touitou C, Bogdan A, Reinberg A, Auzeby A, Beck H, et al. Differences between young and elderly subjects in seasonal and circadian variations of total plasma proteins and blood volume as reflected by hemoglobin, hematocrit, and erythrocyte counts. Clin Chem 1986;32:801–804.

559. Kubota K, Sakurai T, Tamura J, Shirakura T. Is the circadian change in hematocrit and blood viscosity a factor triggering cerebral and myocardial infarction? [Letter]. Stroke 1987; 18:812–813.

560. Wannamethee G, Perry IJ, Shaper AG. Haematocrit, hypertension and risk of stroke. J Intern Med 1994;235:163–168.

561. Ameriso SF, Mohler JG, Suarez M, Fisher M. Morning reduction of cerebral vasomotor reactivity. Neurology 1994;44:1907–1909.

562. Globus MY, Ginsberg MD, Harik SI, Busto R, Dietrich WD. Role of dopamine in ischemic striatal injury: metabolic evidence. Neurology 1987;37:1712–1719.

563. Fahn S. Fluctuations of disability in Parkinson's disease: pathophysiological aspects. In: Marsden CD, Fahn S, eds. Movement Disorders. Buttersworth Scientific, London, 1981, pp. 123–145.

564. Struck LK, Rodnitzky RL. Periodicity of ischemic stroke. Stroke 1989;20:1590.

565. Smolensky MH, Bing ML. Chronobiology and chronotherapeutics in primary care. Patient Care, Clin Focus Summer (Suppl):1997;1–15.

566. Barash D, Silverman RA, Gennis P, Budner N, Matos M, Gallagher EJ. Circadian variation in the frequency of myocardial infarction and death associated with acute pulmonary edema. J Emerg Med 1989;7:119–121.

567. Hansen O, Johansson BW, Gullberg B. The clinical outcome of acute myocardial infarction is related to the circadian rhythm of myocardial infarction onset. Angiology 1993;44: 509–516.

568. Fujita M, Araie E, Yamanishi K, Miwa K, Kida M, Nakajima H. Circadian variation in the success rate of intracoronary thrombolysis for acute myocardial infarction. Am J Cardiol 1993;71:1369–1371.

569. Black HR, Elliott WJ, Neaton JD, Grandits G, Grambsch P, Grimm RH Jr, et al. Rationale and design for the Controlled-ONset Verapamil INvestigation of Cardiovascular Endpoints (CONVINCE) Trial. Control Clin Trials 1998;19:370–390.

6

Circadian Variation of the Blood Pressure in the Population at Large

Hilde Celis, MD *and Jan A. Staessen,* MD, PHD

INTRODUCTION

Ambulatory blood pressure (ABP) measurement has several advantages. ABP readings are obtained outside the medical environment and are free of the so-called "white coat" effect *(1,2)*, often seen when the BP is conventionally measured. Therefore, the average BP level on ABP measurement provides a better estimate of a subject's usual BP than conventional readings *(3)*. In addition, the BP is recorded during the habitual daily activities, both working and resting periods, and during episodes of emotional stress and sleep. The way in which a subject's BP is modulated throughout the day to cope with these various levels of physical and emotional activity and so forth may provide meaningful pathophysiological information *(4)*. Some investigators have also speculated that the amplitude of the diurnal BP profile is characteristic for an individual *(5)*, or that a blunted or absent nocturnal fall in BP is correlated with a worse cardiovascular

From: *Contemporary Cardiology:*
Blood Pressure Monitoring in Cardiovascular Medicine and Therapeutics
Edited by: W. B. White © Humana Press Inc., Totowa, NJ

prognosis *(4)*. These views explain the growing interest in methods to describe the diurnal BP profile and its determinants.

About 20 yr ago, Raferty and colleagues *(4a)* demonstrated that the diurnal BP rhythm is preserved during bed rest and remains present in patients with an artificial pacemaker *(4)*. However, although the autonomic nervous system and other hormonal mechanisms are probably involved in maintaining the diurnal BP profile *(4,6)*, the existence of an endogenous circadian BP rhythm remains controversial. This issue is confounded by the fact that several external factors, such as physical and mental activity, emotions, and so on influence the diurnal BP profile. However, even if the BP curve would not be modulated endogenously, it still remains possible that the response of the BP to daily activities is an important individual characteristic. Indeed, the amplitude of the BP response is potentiated or dampened by cardiovascular control mechanisms and the integration of these mechanisms may differ between individual subjects *(4)*.

OVERVIEW OF METHODS
USED TO DESCRIBE THE DIURNAL BP PROFILE

Nocturnal BP Fall and Night–Day Ratio

The nocturnal BP fall and the night–day ratio can be computed from the average BP during the day and night. The nocturnal BP fall is usually calculated by subtracting the average nighttime BP from the average daytime BP. These two measures of the difference between the high and low BP spans of the day are easy to calculate but require the definition of arbitrary daytime and nighttime periods *(4)*.

CLOCK-TIME-INDEPENDENT METHOD

The most meaningful and scientifically sound method for defining daytime and nighttime BP would be to calculate the pressures for the intervals during which the subject is awake or asleep. Daytime and nighttime are usually delineated based on the times that subjects go to bed at night and get out of bed in the morning. However, these in-bed and out-of-bed periods do not necessarily coincide with the actual periods of sleep and wakefulness. However, because it is virtually impossible to note the time at which one actually falls asleep and wakes up, the times of getting in bed for the night and getting out of bed for the day are probably the most reasonable assessments for practical purposes. A disadvantage of using the times of going to bed and rising is that the periods during which the subjects are awake during the night or take a nap during the day are not taken into account. However, whereas some authors report that the inclusion of daytime sleep in the total asleep time is of great importance, others did not find a clinically relevant difference in BP between the "real" and "conventional" asleep and awake periods *(7)*.

CLOCK-TIME-DEPENDENT METHOD

Another method consists of predefining fixed clocktimes to calculate the daytime and nighttime BP. This can be done by the "wide" or the "narrow" approach. In the wide approach, the full 24 h is covered. For example, the 1990 consensus document of the Scientific Committee *(3)* proposed the daytime to last from 0700 to 2200 h and the nighttime from 2200 to 0700 h, but other dividing times have also been used. A drawback of the wide approach is that these predefined clocktimes do not usually correspond to the waking and sleeping times and that the day and the night may contain variable proportions of the awake and asleep periods *(7)*. In the narrow approach, the morning and evening intervals during which BP increases and decreases rapidly are excluded from the analysis of the diurnal BP profile. Most often, the daytime is defined as lasting from 1000 to 2000 h and the nighttime from midnight to 0600 h, but other periods have also been proposed *(7)*. An argument used against the narrow approach is that not all available information is used for the analysis. Another disadvantage is that it is still possible that subjects go to bed or wake up outside the predefined transition periods, but subjects can be instructed to observe these time intervals so that they are up and about during the day and in bed during the night *(7)*.

Square-Wave Method

The square-wave method represents an individual 24-h BP profile by a waveform consisting of two alternating contiguous periods of constant low and high pressure. Determination of the times of transition between those two periods is performed individually using a least-square error criterion. However, when this method is applied unrestricted, one outlying pressure or a short period of a few pressures can be identified as the interval of low or high BP. This can be avoided by the implementation of restrictions (e.g., that the high-pressure period has to last at least 10 h and the low-pressure period at least 6 h). A disadvantage of this method is that it identifies periods of high and low BP, which will coincide with the day and the night in most instances, except when the diurnal pattern is reversed. Furthermore, the correspondence of the transition times with the in-bed and out-of-bed times is limited, especially for subjects with small awake–asleep differences in BP *(7,8)*.

Cumulative-Sum (cusum) Analysis

The cusum method consists of selecting a reference value, such as the mean BP over 24 h, and subtracting it from each successive BP measurement. The successive deviations of each ambulatory BP reading from the reference value are then added and plotted against time. From these cusum plots, several quantitative measures of the diurnal profile can be derived. The cusum plot height is the difference between the maximum and minimum values of the cusum plot. It reflects both the extent and the duration of the nocturnal fall in BP. The cusum-derived crest and trough BP are defined as the highest and lowest time-weighted mean BP, respectively, sustained during a period of at least 6 h. The cusum-derived alteration magnitude is calculated by subtracting the cusum-derived trough BP from the cusum-derived crest BP *(8)*. The cusum method has the advantage that there is no need to define fixed daytime and nighttime intervals. However, just like the square-wave method, the cusum method also identifies periods of high and low BP, which do not necessarily coincide with the day and the night. Furthermore, the 6-h crest period is relatively short when it is meant to represent the day, but the method allows using longer periods *(7,8)*.

Fourier Method

The most frequently used strategy for modeling the 24-h BP curve is the cosinor method, which is equivalent to a Fourier series with only one harmonic with a period of 24 h. However, this method has been criticized because of the incorrect assumption that there are exactly 12 h between the acrophase (peak) and bathyphase (trough) of the wave and that the distances of the peak and the trough to the mean value are identical. The fit of the cosinor method can be markedly improved by adding harmonics with shorter periods than 24 h (Fig. 1). The use of a Fourier model with four harmonics (cosine functions with periods of 24, 12, 8, and 6 h) has been recommended for use in all subjects because this approach standardizes the degree of smoothing of the input data. It also offers an acceptable compromise between the accuracy and the complexity of the mathematical procedures required to adequately describe the diurnal BP profile in most subjects. For each of the four harmonics and for the global Fourier curve, the amplitude and the acrophase can be computed. The amplitude is half the difference between each curve's minimum and maximum, and the acrophase is the time lag between the maximum and midnight. Initially, the application of the Fourier technique necessitated that the data points be equidistant. More recently, a weighting procedure (weighted Fourier analysis) was developed, which takes into account that the interval between successive BP readings is usually not constant. The coefficients of the weighted model are estimated using weighted linear regression analysis, with the time interval between successive readings as the weighting factor. Prior to the application of Fourier analysis, the presence of a significant diurnal rhythm should be tested against the hypothesis of pure random variation using the one-sample runs test *(4,8–10)*.

DESCRIPTION OF THE DIURNAL BP PROFILE AND ITS DETERMINANTS IN THE POPULATION

The Belgian Population Study

As part of an ongoing population survey *(5)*, the ABP was measured in 58% of the subjects of a random sample of the population of a small town. The diurnal

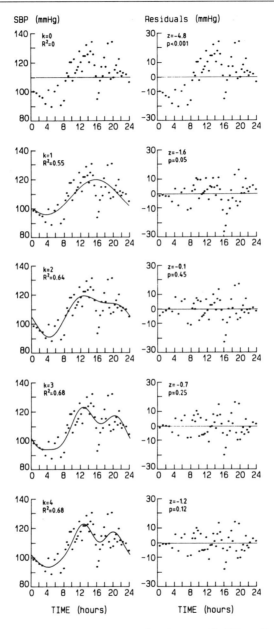

Fig. 1. A Fourier series with k harmonics was fitted to systolic BP readings with ambulatory monitoring in one subject. An increasing fit with the actually observed BP values is apparent when more harmonics are added to the model (left panels). R^2 is the percentage of the variance explained by the model. The hypothesis of pure random variation of the residual points (i.e., the difference between the observed pressure and the pressure predicted from the Fourier model [right panels]) was rejected when the probability of the Z-statistic (runs test) was less than 5%. Reproduced with permission *(9)*.

BP curve was characterized in 399 subjects (191 men) with an average (± SD) age of 49 ± 15 yr. Most of the ABP recordings were performed on weekdays (91%), and none during nighttime work. The one-sample runs test was compatible with a significant diurnal rhythm in 370 subjects (93%). For this analysis, the daytime period was defined as the interval from 1000 to 2000 h and nighttime as the interval from midnight to 0600 h. The night–day BP ratio averaged 0.87 ± 0.07 systolic and 0.81 ± 0.08 diastolic. The nocturnal BP fall was normally distributed and averaged 16 ± 9 mmHg systolic and 14 ± 7 mmHg diastolic. The amplitude of the diurnal BP curve fitted by Fourier analysis averaged 16 ± 5 mmHg systolic and 14 ± 4 mmHg diastolic. The acrophase occurred in most recordings between 0900 h and 2100 h. The acrophase in the 399 subjects combined averaged 1554 h ± 447 systolic and 1511 h ± 420 diastolic.

In a more extended sample (313 men and 317 women, age 20–88 yr) of the same population, the correlates or determinants of the diurnal BP curve were identified *(11)*. Persons on treatment with blood-pressure-lowering drugs were excluded from this analysis. Daytime was also defined as the interval from 1000 to 2000 h and nighttime from midnight to 0600 h.

Table 1 shows some calculated parameters of the diurnal BP profile (i.e., the nocturnal BP fall, the cusum-derived parameters, and the Fourier amplitudes). Tables 2 and 3 show the correlates of the parameters describing the diurnal BP curve in men and women separately.

With the exception of the cusum-derived crest and trough BPs, which were significantly higher in men than in women, the parameters derived from the diurnal BP curve were similar in men and women (Table 1). The main determinants of the crest and trough BP in men and women were age, body mass index, and pulse rate, which were mostly associated with an increase in the crest and trough BP levels. In male and female smokers the trough systolic pressure was 2–3 mmHg lower than in nonsmokers (Tables 2 and 3).

In both sexes, the nocturnal fall in systolic BP increased with the height of the conventional BP and was nearly 2 mmHg greater in male smokers than in male nonsmokers (Tables 2 and 3). The nocturnal fall in diastolic BP decreased curvilinearly with advancing age (Tables 2 and 3).

The cusum-derived circadian alteration magnitude and the cusum-derived plot height increased with a higher BP level on conventional measurement for both systolic and diastolic BP, whereas the cusum plot height of the diastolic BP was inversely correlated with age in men and women. The cusum-derived circadian alteration magnitude and the plot height of systolic BP were greater in smoking than in nonsmoking men. Similarly, the cusum-derived circadian alteration magnitude and plot height of both systolic and diastolic BP were greater in smoking than in nonsmoking women (Tables 2 and 3).

The amplitudes of the overall Fourier curve and of the first and second harmonics tended to increase in both sexes, with a higher BP level on conventional

Table 1
Parameters of the Diurnal
BP Curve in a Belgian Population Sample

	Men		Women
Number	313		317
Variance			
Sys_v (mmHg)^2	71 ± 19		69 ± 18
Dia_v (mmHg)^2	62 ± 20		63 ± 18
Nocturnal fall			
Sys_{nf}	17.8 ± 8.7		17.3 ± 8.2
Dia_{nf}	14.7 ± 6.9		15.3 ± 6.3
Cusum parameters			
Sys_c	131 ± 11	*	126 ± 11
Dia_c	82 ± 9	*	79 ± 8
Sys_t	107 ± 10	*	103 ± 10
Dia_t	61 ± 8	*	58 ± 7
Sys_{am}	24.2 ± 8.2		23.0 ± 7.4
Dia_{am}	20.4 ± 7.1		20.5 ± 6.2
Sys_{ph} (mmHg·h)	103 ± 36		98 ± 32
Dia_{ph} (mmHg·h)	87 ± 32		88 ± 27
Fourier amplitudes			
Sys_a	17.0 ± 5.0		16.3 ± 4.9
Dia_a	14.4 ± 5.0		14.2 ± 4.2
Sys_1	11.3 ± 4.8		10.8 ± 5.9
Dia_1	9.6 ± 4.2		9.6 ± 4.0
Sys_2	5.8 ± 2.9		5.9 ± 4.1
Dia_2	4.8 ± 2.7		5.0 ± 3.1
Sys_3	3.8 ± 2.1		3.6 ± 2.4
Dia_3	3.4 ± 2.2		3.1 ± 2.2
Sys_4	3.6 ± 2.1		3.6 ± 2.1
Dia_4	3.3 ± 2.1		3.2 ± 2.0

Note. Values are means ± standard deviation. $*p < 0.001$ for the difference between men and women.
Unless otherwise indicated, variables are expressed in mmHg. Sys, Dia = systolic, diastolic pressure; Sys_v, Dia_v = within subject variance of all ambulatory readings over 24 h; Sys_{nf}, Dia_{nf} = nocturnal fall in pressure; Sys_a, Dia_a = overall amplitude; Sys_c, Dia_c = cusum-derived crest pressure; Sys_t, Dia_t = cusum-derived trough pressure; Sys_{am}, Dia_{am} = cusum-derived circadian alteration magnitude; Sys_{ph}, Dia_{ph} = cusum plot height; Sys_1, Sys_2, Sys_3, Sys_4, Dia_1, Dia_2, Dia_3, Dia_4 = amplitudes of the first through fourth harmonic.
Source: From ref. *11* with permission.

measurement. The amplitude of the first harmonic of diastolic BP was inversely correlated with age in men and women, whereas the opposite was observed for the amplitude of the fourth harmonic of systolic BP. In men and women, current smokers tended to have slightly greater amplitudes of one or more of the

Table 2
Correlates of the Parameters Describing the Diurnal Blood Pressure Curve in 313 Men of a Belgian Population Sample

	R^2	INT (mmHg)	BP (mmHg)	Age (yr)	Age^2 (yr^2)	BMI (kg/m^2)	Rate (bpm)	SCa (mmol/L)	γGT (U/L)	SMK 0, 1
Blood pressure										
Sys_{24}	0.099	118.4	nc	−0.864	0.00920	0.79	ns	ns	ns	ns
Dia_{24}	0.161	42.3	nc	ns	ns	0.56	0.16	ns	3.57	ns
Sys_d	0.093	106.7	nc	ns	ns	0.78	ns	ns	ns	ns
Dia_d	0.126	48.5	nc	ns	ns	0.65	0.18	ns	ns	ns
Sys_{ni}	0.093	118.7	nc	−1.191	0.01252	0.63	ns	ns	ns	ns
Dia_{ni}	0.126	33.6	nc	0.082	ns	0.39	0.15	ns	4.35	ns
Sys_c	0.088	126.1	nc	−0.828	0.00888	0.89	ns	ns	ns	ns
Dia_c	0.108	53.1	nc	ns	ns	0.68	0.16	ns	ns	ns
Sys_t	0.090	110.0	nc	−0.865	0.00924	0.63	ns	ns	ns	−1.97
Dia_t	0.174	20.0	nc	0.598	−0.00510	0.38	0.15	ns	3.96	ns
Variance										
Sys_v	0.049	38.3	0.261	ns	ns	ns	ns	ns	ns	ns
Dia_v	—	—	—	—	—	—	—	—	—	—
Nocturnal fall										
Sys_{nf}	0.031	7.5	0.076	ns	ns	ns	ns	ns	ns	2.11
Dia_{nf}	0.030	16.8	ns	ns	−0.00084	ns	ns	ns	ns	ns
Cusum parameters										
Sys_{am}	0.047	11.4	0.097	ns	ns	ns	ns	ns	ns	2.10
Dia_{am}	0.031	15.3	0.089	ns	−0.00064	ns	ns	ns	ns	ns
Sys_{ph}	0.049	43.0	0.452	ns	ns	ns	ns	ns	ns	8.83
Dia_{ph}	0.032	65.5	0.457	−0.271	ns	ns	ns	ns	ns	ns
Fourier parameters										
Sys_a	0.046	23.2	0.054	ns	ns	ns	ns	−5.56	ns	ns
Dia_a	—	—	—	—	—	—	—	—	—	—
Sys_1	0.018	6.2	0.040	ns	ns	ns	ns	ns	ns	ns
Dia_1	0.022	10.7	ns	ns	−0.00043	ns	ns	ns	ns	ns
Sys_2	0.049	1.0	0.036	ns	ns	ns	ns	ns	ns	0.71
Dia_2	—	—	—	—	—	—	—	—	—	—
Sys_3	0.017	10.0	ns	ns	ns	ns	ns	−2.74	ns	ns
Dia_3	—	—	—	—	—	—	—	—	—	—
Sys_4	0.020	2.6	ns	0.021	ns	ns	ns	ns	ns	ns
Dia_4	—	—	—	—	—	—	—	—	—	—

Note: **Dependent variables.** Unless otherwise indicated in this footnote, the dependent variables are expressed in mmHg. Sys, Dia = systolic, diastolic pressure; Sys_{24}, Dia_{24} = 24-h ambulatory blood pressure; Sys_d, Dia_d = daytime blood pressure; Sys_{ni}, Dia_{ni} = nighttime blood pressure; Sys_c, Dia_c = cusum-derived crest pressure; Sys_t, Dia_t = cusum-derived trough pressure; Sys_v, Dia_v = within-subject variance of all ambulatory readings over 24 h (mmHg^2); Sys_{nf}, Dia_{nf} = nocturnal fall in pressure; Sys_{am}, Dia_{am} = cusum-derived circadian alteration magnitude; Sys_{ph}, Dia_{ph} = cusum plot height (mmHg·h); Sys_a, Dia_a = overall amplitude; Sys_1, Sys_2, Sys_3, Sys_4, Dia_1, Dia_2, Dia_3, Dia_4 = amplitudes of the first through fourth harmonic.

Regression model. INT = intercept. The following explanatory variables were considered: the level of blood pressure on conventional measurement at home (BP), age (linear and squared term), body mass index (BMI), pulse rate in the presence of an observer, serum total calcium (SCa), log γ-glutamyltransferase (γGT), current smoking habits (SMK, coded 0 for nonsmokers and 1 for smokers) and the urinary Na$^+$/K$^+$ ratio. All regression coefficients given in the table were significant ($p < 0.05$)—indicates that none of the correlations between the dependent and explanatory variables was significant. nc = not considered for entry into the regression model. ns = not significant.

Source: From ref. *11* with permission.

Table 3
Correlates of the Parameters Describing the Diurnal
Blood Pressure Curve in 317 Women of a Belgian Population Sample

	R^2	INT (mmHg)	BP (mmHg)	Age (yr)	Age^2 (yr^2)	BMI (kg/m^2)	Rate (bpm)	γGT (U/L)	SMK (0, 1)	$Na^+/$ K^+	Pill 0, 1
Blood pressure											
Sys_{24}	0.280	94.0	nc	−0.635	0.00873	0.56	0.13	5.93	ns	ns	4.14
Dia_{24}	0.090	50.4	nc	ns	ns	0.23	0.12	4.52	ns	ns	ns
Sys_d	0.204	88.7	nc	ns	0.00245	0.43	0.14	5.25	ns	ns	5.32
Dia_d	0.074	57.8	nc	ns	ns	0.20	0.11	3.33	ns	ns	2.55
Sys_{ni}	0.236	88.6	nc	−0.989	0.01155	0.60	0.18	6.76	ns	ns	ns
Dia_{ni}	0.119	38.0	nc	0.078	ns	ns	ns	6.75	ns	ns	ns
Sys_c	0.261	84.5	nc	ns	0.00293	0.62	0.17	5.26	ns	ns	5.29
Dia_c	0.090	58.8	nc	ns	ns	0.33	0.13	ns	ns	0.66	ns
Sys_t	0.267	82.8	nc	−0.759	0.00937	0.57	0.17	6.63	−2.91	ns	3.74
Dia_t	0.129	27.1	nc	0.587	−0.00481	ns	0.12	6.00	ns	ns	2.29
Variance											
Sys_v	0.125	19.9	0.375	ns	ns	ns	ns	ns	ns	1.55	ns
Dia_v	0.036	35.1	0.375	ns	ns	ns	ns	ns	ns	ns	ns
Nocturnal fall											
Sys_{nf}	0.047	13.7	0.107	ns	ns	−0.37	ns	ns	ns	ns	ns
Dia_{nf}	0.021	16.0	ns	ns	−0.00069	ns	ns	ns	ns	ns	ns
Cusum parameters											
Sys_{am}	0.093	5.8	0.136	ns	ns	ns	ns	ns	2.53	ns	ns
Dia_{am}	0.079	13.1	0.120	ns	ns	ns	ns	−3.71	2.09	0.50	ns
Sys_{ph}	0.070	35.7	0.488	ns	ns	ns	ns	ns	11.29	ns	ns
Dia_{ph}	0.058	61.0	0.500	−0.252	ns	ns	ns	−14.25	10.40	ns	ns
Fourier parameters											
Sys_a	0.108	3.6	0.102	ns	ns	ns	ns	ns	1.34	ns	ns
Dia_a	0.044	8.0	0.071	ns	ns	ns	ns	ns	ns	0.35	ns
Sys_1	0.023	10.2	ns	ns	ns	ns	ns	ns	1.95	ns	ns
Dia_1	0.052	7.3	0.055	−0.045	ns	ns	ns	ns	1.13	ns	ns
Sys_2	0.042	−0.5	0.054	ns	ns	ns	ns	ns	ns	ns	ns
Dia_2	0.033	0.4	0.062	ns	ns	ns	ns	ns	ns	ns	ns
Sys_3	0.051	6.6	ns	−0.173	0.00191	ns	ns	ns	0.23	ns	ns
Dia_3	—	—	—	—	—	—	—	—	—	ns	ns
Sys_4	0.056	1.1	ns	ns	0.00024	0.08	ns	ns	ns	ns	ns
Dia_4	0.016	1.7	ns	ns	0.06	ns	ns	ns	ns	ns	ns

Note: **Dependent variables.** Unless otherwise indicated in this footnote, the dependent variables are expressed in mmHg. Sys, Dia = systolic, diastolic pressure; Sys_{24}, Dia_{24} = 24-h ambulatory blood pressure; Sys_d, Dia_d = daytime blood pressure; Sys_{ni}, Dia_{ni} = nighttime blood pressure; Sys_c, Dia_c = cusum-derived crest pressure; Sys_t, Dia_t = cusum-derived trough pressure; Sys_v, Dia_v = within-subject variance of all ambulatory readings over 24 h ($mmHg^2$); Sys_{nf}, Dia_{nf} = nocturnal fall in pressure; Sys_{am}, Dia_{am} = cusum-derived circadian alteration magnitude; Sys_{ph}, Dia_{ph} = cusum plot height (mmHg·h); Sys_a, Dia_a = overall amplitude; Sys_1, Sys_2, Sys_3, Sys_4, Dia_1, Dia_2, Dia_3, Dia_4 = amplitudes of the first through fourth harmonic.

Regression model. INT = intercept. The following explanatory variables were considered: the level of blood pressure on conventional measurement at home (BP), age (linear and squared term), body mass index (BMI), pulse rate in the presence of an observer, serum total calcium (SCa), log γ-glutamyltransferase (γGT), current smoking habits (SMK, coded 0 for nonsmokers and 1 for smokers), the urinary Na^+/K^+ ratio and intake of estroprogestogens (pill, coded 0 or 1). All regression coefficients given in the table were significant ($p < 0.05$). —indicates that none of the correlations between the dependent and explanatory variables was significant. nc = not considered for entry into the regression model. ns = not significant.

Source: From ref. *11* with permission.

harmonics. In women, the amplitude of the fourth harmonic of systolic and dia-stolic BP increased with greater body mass index (Tables 2 and 3).

International Database

In an international database *(12)*, the ABP recordings of 4765 normotensive and 2555 hypertensive subjects from 10 to 99 yr of age were collected. The subjects in the database were not treated with BP-lowering drugs or corticoster-oids and were not engaging in night work at the time of the BP measurement. The study population included 3730 males and 3590 females with an average age of 48 ± 16 yr. Daytime and nighttime were defined ranging from 1000 to 2000 h and from midnight to 0600 h, respectively. In all 7320 subjects combined, the day-time BP averaged 129 ± 17 mmHg systolic and 79 ± 12 mmHg diastolic and the nighttime BP averaged 113 ± 17 mmHg systolic and 66 ± 12 mmHg diastolic.

In all subjects combined, the nocturnal BP fall averaged 17 ± 11 mmHg systo-lic and 14 ± 8 mmHg diastolic. The corresponding night–day ratios were 0.87 ± 0.08 and 0.83 ± 0.10, respectively. These means are similar to those obtained in the Belgian population study.

DETERMINANTS OF THE DIURNAL BP PROFILE

Age, Sex, and Body Mass Index. The nocturnal BP fall and the night–day ratio showed a curvilinear correlation with age (Fig. 2). These relations were compatible with a smaller nocturnal decrease in BP and higher night–day ratio in older subjects, especially those older than 70 yr of age. In the Belgian popu-lation, an inverse correlation between the nocturnal BP fall in diastolic BP and age had already been noticed and similar observations for systolic and diastolic BP have been reported in other European *(13–15)* and Asian *(16–18)* popu-lations. In general, older people spend more time in bed than younger people, but they experience reduced slow-wave sleep, more nighttime wakefulness, and increased fragmentation of sleep by awake periods. These age-related changes in the circadian sleep–wake rhythm probably explain why the highest night–day ratios were observed in older subjects.

After adjusting for age and other significant covariates (i.e., BP level on con-ventional measurement, continent of residence, and technique of ambulatory measurement), the nocturnal BP fall was greater in men than in women. The sys-tolic night–day ratio was also slightly smaller in males (Table 4).

Accounting for body mass index (available only in 5303 subjects) reduced the sex difference in the nocturnal fall of diastolic BP to a nonsignificant level (Table 4).

Normotension Versus Hypertension. A higher conventional BP was asso-ciated with a larger nocturnal BP fall, if the latter was expressed on an absolute scale (i.e., in millimeters of mercury). Furthermore, the height of the conven-tional BP correlated positively with the night–day ratio of diastolic but not sys-tolic BP. Thus, a higher conventional diastolic BP was associated with a higher

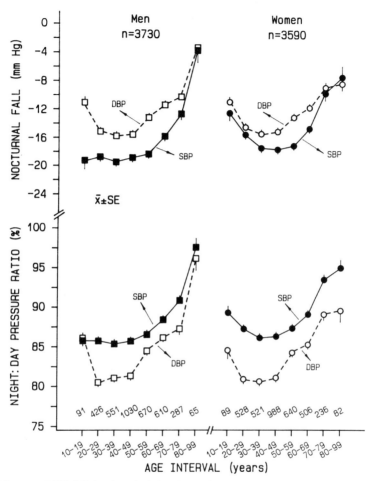

Fig. 2. Nocturnal BP fall (top) and night–day ratios (bottom) for systolic BP (filled symbols) and diastolic BP (open symbols) in 10-yr age classes in 3730 men (left) and 3590 women (right) from an international database. For each sex and age group, the number of subjects contributing to the mean (± SE) is given. Reproduced with permission from Staessen JA, et al., Nocturnal blood pressure normality: results from the Pamela Study. J Hypertens 1995;13:1377–1390. © Lippincott Williams & Wilkins.

night–day ratio (i.e., a lesser nocturnal fall in diastolic BP). Because in most subjects the etiologic diagnosis of hypertension had been established only on clinical grounds, the database may have incorporated some cases of secondary hypertension. The inclusion of such subjects may partially explain why, for diastolic BP, a weak positive correlation between the night–day ratio and the BP level on conventional measurement persisted. Indeed, such subjects usually have a considerably elevated BP, whereas their diurnal BP profile is often flattened or even inverted.

Table 4
Nocturnal BP Fall and Night–Day BP Ratio
in Various Subgroups of an International Database

| Subgroup | n | Nocturnal fall (mmHg) | | Night–Day ratio (%) | |
		SBP	DBP	SBP	DBP
Sex					
Males	3730	−16.7 ± 0.2 (A)	−12.3 ± 0.2 (A)	87.5 ± 0.2 (A)	84.8 ± 0.2 (A)
Females	3590	−15.1 ± 0.2 (B)	−11.9 ± 0.2 (B)	88.3 ± 0.2 (B)	84.9 ± 0.2 (A)
Blood pressure					
Normotension	4765	−14.8 ± 0.2 (A)	−12.0 ± 0.1 (A,C)	87.9 ± 0.1 (A)	84.2 ± 0.2 (A)
Borderline hypertension	759	−17.4 ± 0.4 (B)	−12.8 ± 0.3 (B)	87.2 ± 0.3 (B)	85.2 ± 0.4 (A)
Definite hypertension	1796	−17.8 ± 0.3 (B)	−12.3 ± 0.2 (B,C)	88.2 ± 0.2 (A)	86.9 ± 0.2 (B)
Residence					
Europe	4556	−16.7 ± 0.2 (A)	−13.5 ± 0.1 (A)	87.1 ± 0.1 (A)	83.4 ± 0.2 (A)
Asia	2213	−15.7 ± 0.3 (B)	−10.0 ± 0.2 (B)	87.9 ± 0.2 (B)	87.5 ± 0.3 (B)
Other	551	−15.3 ± 0.5 (B)	−12.9 ± 0.4 (A)	88.8 ± 0.4 (C)	83.7 ± 0.4 (A)
Recording technique					
Auscultatory	1436	−15.3 ± 0.3 (A)	−10.2 ± 0.2 (A)	88.2 ± 0.2 (A)	87.3 ± 0.3 (A)
Oscillometric	5884	−16.5 ± 0.2 (B)	−14.0 ± 0.2 (B)	87.6 ± 0.2 (B)	82.4 ± 0.2 (B)

Note: SBP indicates systolic blood pressure; DBP indicates diastolic blood pressure. Values are mean ± SE adjusted for significant covariates. Dissimilar letters indicate significant ($p \leq 0.05$) differences.

Source: From Staessen JA, et al., Nocturnal blood pressure normality: results from the Pamela Study. J Hypertens 1995;13:1377–1390. © Lippincott Williams & Wilkins.

After adjusting for significant covariates, hypertensive subjects tended to have a larger nocturnal BP fall than normotensive subjects. In addition, the night–day ratio for diastolic BP was significantly greater in subjects with definite hypertension than in the normotensive group (Table 4).

Technique of Ambulatory Recording. After adjustment for significant covariates, the nocturnal BP fall was smaller and the night–day ratios were larger in subjects whose BP had been recorded with an auscultatory rather than an oscillometric technique for ambulatory BP measurement (Table 4). In general, auscultatory and oscillometric readings have the same accuracy versus intra-arterial readings or a standard mercury manometer operated by an auscultating observer. However, the present study was not designed to identify differences between two recording techniques, and confounding or aspecific factors could therefore have been involved.

With additional adjustment for BMI in the 5303 subjects in whom it was available, the differences between both types of measurement persisted only for the nocturnal BP fall and the night–day ratio for diastolic BP. Thus, in obese arms, the obese tissue may hamper the propagation of faint Korotkoff sounds from the brachial artery to the microphone, especially at night when BP is lower.

Continent of Residence. Of the 7320 subjects, 3799 lived in northern Europe, 757 in southern Europe, 2213 in Asia, and 551 in other continents (South America, Australia, and North America). With adjustments for significant covariates applied, subjects living in northern and southern Europe showed the same nocturnal

BP fall and similar night–day ratios for systolic and diastolic BP. Therefore, they were pooled for further analysis. The night–day ratios were compatible with larger nocturnal BP falls in Europeans than in Asians (96% Japanese) (Table 4). The Asians' BP had been recorded with gas-powered recorders, which operate almost noiselessly and which are therefore assumed to interfere less with sleep quality. However, the intercontinental differences in the nocturnal BP fall could not be ascribed to the technique of ambulatory monitoring because they persisted in analyses confined to oscillometric recordings. In this international database, data handling was rigorously standardized but was uniform only within each subsample. Therefore, selective recruitment, confounding, and methodological differences could have contributed to the apparently lesser nocturnal BP fall in the Japanese. However, a lesser nocturnal BP fall has been observed in at least three independent studies in the Far East (19,20). This suggests that the higher night–day ratios in Asian populations could be real and attributable, at least in part, to genetic background, lifestyle, or both.

Nondippers Versus Dippers. Nondipping profiles were defined as showing a night–day ratio of 1 or higher because this threshold corresponds mathematically with a nighttime BP equal or higher than the daytime BP. Furthermore, nondippers were characterized as subjects showing a nondipping profile for both systolic and diastolic BP. Indeed, because the BP through the day is characterized by large variability, a few extreme values may easily shift a subject's classification, if dipping status were to be based on either systolic or diastolic pressure alone. The distinct use of both pressures may also jeopardize the internal consistency of classifications within studies, because subjects may be systolic nondippers and diastolic dippers, or vice versa. Only 3.2% (233 persons) of all subjects were nondippers. After adjustment for significant covariates, the probability of being a nondipper was significantly correlated with the linear and the quadratic term of age. The probability of being a nondipper increased 2.8 times from 30 to 60 yr, but 5.7 times from 60 to 80 yr.

After adjustments for all significant covariates, the odds of being a nondipper were the same in males and females. These odds were significantly higher in subjects with definite hypertension as opposed to normotensive subjects. Participants examined with auscultatory instead of oscillometric devices had a higher probability of being a nondipper.

The Diurnal BP Profile in Children and Adolescents

In children, ambulatory blood pressure monitoring is feasible with the application of carefully standardized and specially adapted recording techniques. Because the physiological circadian variation in children and adolescents had not yet been described in detail, Lurbe and colleagues investigated the diurnal BP curve and the nocturnal BP fall in 228 normotensive children (116 boys and 112 girls) between 6 and 16 yr (21). Normotension was defined according to the

Table 5
Characteristics of the Children

	Boys	Girls	p	Total
Number	116	112		228
Age (yr)	11 ± 3	11 ± 3		11 ± 3
Weight (kg)	43 ± 14	41 ± 12		42 ± 13
Height (cm)	145 ± 14	142 ± 14		144 ± 14
Conventional blood pressure (mmHg)				
SBP	99 ± 11	98 ± 12		99 ± 11
DBP	57 ± 9	56 ± 9		56 ± 9
Ambulatory blood pressure (mmHg)				
24-h SBP	111 ± 7	109 ± 7	0.03	110 ± 7
24-h DBP	66 ± 5	65 ± 5	0.05	66 ± 5
Daytime SBP	115 ± 8	113 ± 8	0.02	114 ± 8
Daytime DBP	71 ± 6	70 ± 6		71 ± 6
Nighttime SBP	103 ± 8	102 ± 8		102 ± 8
Nighttime DBP	57 ± 6	56 ± 6	0.05	57 ± 6

Note: Values are expressed as means ± standard deviation. SBP = systolic blood pressure; DBP = diastolic blood pressure; daytime = 0800-2200 h; night-time = 2400-0600 h. *p* indicates sex differences; only *p* levels ≤ 0.05 are reported.

Source: From Lurbe E, et al., Diurnal blood pressure curve in children and adolescents. J Hypertens **14:** 41–46. © 1996 Lippincott Williams & Wilkins.

criteria proposed by the Task Force on Blood Pressure Control in Children and none of the subjects was taking any medication. For this analysis, daytime was defined as the interval from 0800 to 2200 h and nighttime from midnight to 0600 h. The day–night ratio was calculated by dividing the average nighttime by the average daytime BP.

The main characteristics and the conventional and ambulatory BP values in both boys and girls separately are shown in Table 5 and the parameters of the diurnal BP profile are presented in Table 6. More than 80% of the children in the present analysis showed a diurnal BP rhythm that differed significantly from random variation. The systolic crest pressure was 3 mmHg higher in boys than in girls. The cusum plot height and the circadian alteration magnitude for systolic BP were also greater in boys than in girls. This observation possibly reflects the more vigorous physical activity in the male than in the female children and adolescents (Table 6).

The 24-h, daytime, and nighttime crest and trough systolic BP were positively and independently correlated with age and body weight. The 24-h, nighttime, and trough diastolic BP were positively correlated with age, but negatively with body weight (Table 7).

In most recordings, the acrophase of the overall Fourier curve with four harmonics occurred between 0900 h and 2100 h. There were no differences between

Table 6
Parameters of the Diurnal Profile in 228 Children

	Boys	Girls	p	Total
Number	116	112		228
Day–night difference				
SBP (mmHg)	12.6 ± 6.7	11.4 ± 5.7		12.0 ± 6.3
DBP (mmHg)	14.0 ± 6.1	14.4 ± 5.7		14.2 ± 5.9
Day–night ratio				
SBP (mmHg)	1.13 ± 0.07	1.11 ± 0.06		1.12 ± 0.06
DBP (mmHg)	1.25 ± 0.12	1.27 ± 0.12		1.26 ± 0.12
Fourier amplitude				
SBP (mmHg)	12.9 ± 4.4	12.1 ± 3.9		12.5 ± 4.2
DBP (mmHg)	14.0 ± 4.3	13.9 ± 3.9		14.0 ± 4.1
Acrophase				
SBP (h)	13 h 57 ± 4 h 53	13 h 31 ± 4 h 39		13 h 44 ± 4 h 46
DBP (h)	13 h 42 ± 4 h 26	13 h 00 ± 4 h 18		13 h 21 ± 4 h 22
Crest				
SBP (mmHg)	119 ± 8	116 ± 8	0.01	118 ± 8
DBP (mmHg)	75 ± 6	74 ± 6		74 ± 6
Trough				
SBP (mmHg)	101 ± 7	100 ± 8	0.05	101 ± 7
DBP (mmHg)	56 ± 6	55 ± 6		55 ± 6
Cusum plot height				
SBP (mmHg·h)	75.7 ± 28.7	68.4 ± 25.1	0.04	72.1 ± 27.2
DBP (mmHg·h)	82.0 ± 28.6	83.0 ± 25.2		82.3 ± 26.9
Circadian alteration magnitude				
SBP (mmHg)	18.0 ± 6.7	16.3 ± 5.6	0.04	17.0 ± 6.2
DBP (mmHg)	19.1 ± 6.3	19.4 ± 5.3		19.2 ± 5.8

Note: Values are expressed as means ± standard deviation. SBP = systolic blood pressure; DBP = diastolic blood pressure; daytime = 0800-2200 h; nighttime = 2400-0600 h. *p* indicates sex differences; only *p* levels ≤ 0.05 are reported.

Source: From Lurbe E, et al., Diurnal blood pressure curve in children and adolescents. J Hypertens **14**: 41–46. © 1996 Lippincott Williams & Wilkins.

boys and girls in the parameters of the overall Fourier curve. The nocturnal BP fall was normally distributed. The nocturnal BP fall as well as the day–night ratio for systolic and diastolic BP were not correlated with sex, age, body weight, and height.

INFLUENCE OF WORKING TIME
ON THE DIURNAL VARIATION OF BP

The circadian variation of BP is known to be modified by physical as well as mental activities. In contrast to other biological parameters, BP is immediately adapted to shifted phases of activity and sleep *(22)*. However, in some diseases, such as Cushing's syndrome *(23)*, BP reduction during the night is lacking and

Table 7

Correlates of the Parameters Describing the Diurnal BP Profile in 228 Children

	R^2	Intercept	Age (yr)	Weight (kg)	Sex (male = 1, female = 0)
Blood pressures (mmHg)					
24-h SBP	0.20	97.1	0.66**	0.13**	
24-h DBP	0.08	75.8	0.77***		1.37*
Daytime SBP	0.19	100.5	0.68***	0.12*	1.92*
Daytime DBP					
Nighttime SBP	0.16	89.9	0.53*	0.15**	
Nighttime DBP	0.07	53.3	0.64**	−0.11**	1.56*
Crest SBP	0.19	103.4	0.78**	0.12*	2.21*
Crest DBP					
Trough SBP	0.15	89.4	0.53*	0.13**	
Trough DBP	0.07	52.5	0.61***	−0.12**	1.46*
Cusum plot height (mmHg·h)					
SBP	0.02	68.5			7.24*
DBP					
Circadian alteration magnitude (mmHg)					
SBP	0.02	16.4			1.65*
DBP					

Note: SBP, systolic blood pressure; DBP, diastolic blood pressure. *$p < 0.05$, **$p < 0.01$, ***$p < 0.001$.

Source: From Lurbe E, et al., Diurnal blood pressure curve in children and adolescents. J Hypertens **14:** 41–46. © 1996 Lippincott Williams & Wilkins.

this suggests that activities and sleep do not necessarily induce a day and night rhythm of the BP. Some authors reported a systematic increase of BP in the early morning hours before awaking, indicating BP variations independent of activities. Others who did not find any BP increase before arousal assumed that the diurnal variations of BP were mainly the result of activities and sleep and concluded that there was no internal rhythm shaping the 24-h BP profile *(22)*.

Because physical activity is thought to influence the diurnal BP profile, the changes in working time common in some professions (e.g., shift workers) may influence the diurnal BP profile, especially when the work is performed during the night. In 1989, Baumgart and colleagues *(22)* already investigated the effects of shift work on the diurnal BP profile in 15 normotensive, healthy, physically working men who were not taking any drugs. They were working at a slowly rotating three-shift system. The ABP measurement was performed during the morning shifts and night shifts. The mean 24-h BP was identical in both shifts. There were also no differences in the BP levels in the sleeping phases or in the working phases between the two 24-h cycles. In the two shifts, the minimal and maximal hourly means over 24 h were nearly identical, indicating that the amplitudes of diurnal BP fluctuations were comparable (Fig. 3). Corresponding to the

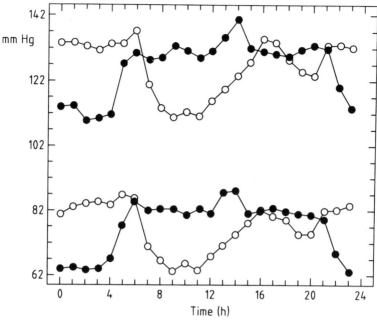

Fig. 3. Hourly means of systolic and diastolic blood pressure of shift workers during the morning (●) and night (○) shifts (*n* = 15). Reproduced from Baumgart P, et al., Twenty-four-hour blood pressure is not dependent on endogenous circadian rhythm. J Hypertens **7**: 331–334. © 1989 Lippincott Williams & Wilkins.

lag between the working periods, there was a phase difference of 8 h between the 24-h BP curves. The 24-h BP curves during the first and last day of the night shift were nearly identical. The authors concluded that the immediate adaptation of the 24-h BP curve to shifted activity and sleeping phases indicated that the diurnal BP profile is determined by activity and is largely independent of the internal circadian rhythm.

REPRODUCIBILITY OF THE DIURNAL BP PATTERN

Only few studies compared the reproducibility of various methods for the analysis of the diurnal BP profile. Usually, group reproducibility is assessed by calculating the signed difference in pressure between duplicate monitorings. The within-subject repeatability is mostly assessed by means of the repeatability coefficient. This coefficient is calculated as twice the standard deviation of the individual differences, assuming a mean difference for all subjects of zero. To allow comparisons between various measurements, the repeatability coefficient is often expressed as a percentage of nearly maximal variation (i.e., four times the standard deviation of the measurement under investigation). This index is typically around 50% for clinic BP and around 30% for the mean 24-h BP. The lower the value of the index, the better the repeatability *(7)*.

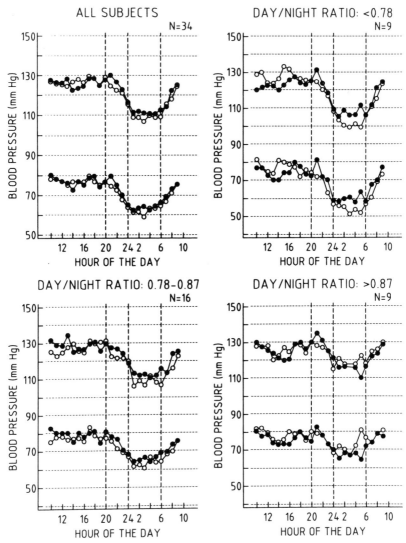

Fig. 4. The hourly means of the ABP in paired recordings performed with a median interval of 350 d in 34 subjects from a Belgian population study. Results are given for 9 strong dippers, 16 intermediate dippers, and 9 nondippers, separately, and for the 34 subjects combined. Reproduced with permission *(5)*.

In the previously mentioned Belgian population study *(5)*, 34 of the 399 participants underwent a repeat measurement of their ABP. The mean interval between the first and second ABP recording in those 34 subjects was 350 d (range: 254–430 d). There was close agreement between the paired recordings in the average 24-h, daytime, and nighttime BP and in the hourly BP means (Fig. 4). Expressed as a percentage of maximal variation, repeatability was 37% for the

24-h systolic BP and 47% for the 24-h diastolic BP. For the daytime and night-time BP levels, repeatability was comparable with that of the 24-h BP. However, repeatability tended to be substantially less for the statistical parameters describing the diurnal BP rhythm. For example, the overall amplitude of systolic and diastolic BP derived by a four-harmonic Fourier series had a repeatability coefficient equivalent to 83% of nearly maximal variation.

Of the 36 subjects who underwent a repeat ABP measurement, 9 were classified as being strong dippers (night–day ratio less than 0.78), 18 as intermediate dippers (night–day ratio between 0.78 and 0.87), and 9 as nondippers (night–day ratio greater than 0.87). In the strong dippers, the nighttime BP was significantly higher at the repeat recording than at the initial recording. This was associated with a decrease in the nocturnal BP fall and of the amplitude of the BP curve. In the nine nondippers, the nighttime BP fell at the repeat examination, but none of them had a night–day ratio of less than 0.78 and thus became a strong dipper at the repeat examination. These data suggest that, as for the conventional BP, regression to the mean is also observed for the nighttime BP, when ABP recordings are repeated in subjects selected for being a strong dipper or a nondipper. However, the alternative explanation that nondippers become accustomed to the recorder and sleep deeper at the repeat examination and that some dippers may sleep less well must also be considered.

A repeat ABP recording was also performed in a random sample of 31 of the 228 children and adolescents reported on in the above-mentioned trial by Lurbe et al. *(21)*. The median time between their repeat recordings was 123 d (range 36–273 d). Repeated measurements yielded only minor changes for the average 24-h, daytime, and nighttime BP values, thus making group means easy to reproduce. The intraindividual repeatability coefficient for the 24-h systolic and diastolic BP were 32% and 34%, respectively. However, as in adults, the reproducibility of the parameters describing the diurnal BP profile was generally lower than that of the level of the ambulatory measurements.

We can thus conclude that group means for the ABP parameters can be accurately reproduced and that in individual subjects, the agreement between paired recordings is satisfactory for the level of BP. By contrast, the parameters related to the diurnal BP rhythm are less reproducible in individual subjects. Thus, one 24-h ABP recording is not satisfactory to fully characterize an individual with respect to his/her diurnal BP profile. Increasing the number of recordings per subject or standardizing activity patterns during the recordings may increase the potential of 24-h ABP monitoring to characterize the diurnal BP profile of individual subjects *(5)*.

However, repeatability in many studies not only reflects the variability inherent to the measurement technique but also biological variability. In some studies, variability may have been inflated because of the long interval between the duplicate recordings or by seasonal and random variation in the pattern of the daily activities.

REFERENCES

1. Hoegholm A, Kristensen KS, Madsen NH, Svendsen TL. White coat hypertension diagnosed by 24-h ambulatory monitoring. Examination of 159 newly diagnosed hypertensive patients. Am J Hypertens 1992;5:64–70.
2. Pickering TG, James GD, Boddie C, Harshfield GA, Blank S, Laragh JH. How common is white coat hypertension? JAMA 1988;259:225–228.
3. The Scientific Committee. Concensus document on non-invasive ambulatory blood pressure monitoring. J Hypertens 1990;8:135–140.
4. Staessen JA, Celis H, De Cort P, Fagard R, Thijs L, Amery A. Methods for describing the diurnal blood pressure curve. J Hypertens 1991;9:S16–S18.
4a. Raferty EB. Understanding hypertension: the contribution of direct ambulatory blood pressure monitoring. In: Weber MA, Drayer JIM, eds. Ambulatory Blood Pressure Monitoring. Springer-Verlag, New York, 1983, pp. 105–116.
5. Staessen JA, Bulpitt CJ, O'Brien E, et al. The diurnal blood pressure profile. A population study. Am J Hypertens 1992;5:386–392.
6. Portaluppi F, Bagni B, degli Umberti E, et al. Circadian rhythms of atrial natriuretic peptide, renin, aldosterone, cortisol, blood pressure and heart rate in normal and hypertensive subjects. J Hypertens 1990;8:85–95.
7. Fagard RF, Staessen JA, Thijs L. Optimal definition of daytime and night-time blood pressure. Blood Pressure Monit 1997;2:315–321.
8. Thijs L, Staessen JA, Fagard R, Zachariah P, Amery A. Number of measurements required for the analysis of diurnal blood pressure profile. J Hum Hypertens 1994;8:239–244.
9. Staessen JA, Fagard R, Thijs L, Amery A. Fourier analysis of blood pressure profiles. Am J Hypertens 1993;6:184S–187S.
10. Fagard R, Staessen JA, Thijs L. Twenty-four-hour blood pressure measurements: analytic aspects. Blood Pressure Monit 1996;1:S23–S25
11. Staessen JA, Atkins N, Fagard R, et al. Correlates of the diurnal blood pressure profile in a population study. High Blood Pressure 1993;2:271–282.
12. Staessen JA, Bieniaszewski L, O'Brien E, et al. Nocturnal blood pressure fall on ambulatory monitoring in a large international database. Hypertension 1997;29:30–39.
13. Mancia G, Sega R, Bravi C, et al. Ambulatory and home blood pressure normality: results from the Pamela Study. J Hypertens 1995;13:1377–1390.
14. Wiinberg N, Hoegholm A, Christensen HR, et al. 24-h ambulatory blood pressure in 352 normal Danish subjects, related to age and gender. Am J Hypertens 1995;8:978–986.
15. Middeke M, Kluglich M. Gestorte nachtliche Blutdruckregulation by Hypertoniken im hoheren Lebensalter. Geriat Forsch 1995;3:125–132.
16. Imai Y, Munakata M, Hashimoto J, et al. Age-specific characteristics of nocturnal blood pressure in a general population in a community of Northern Japan. Am J Hypertens 1993;6:179S–183S.
17. Hayashi H, Hatano K, Tsuda M, Kanematsu K, Yoshikane M, Saito H. Relationship between circadian variation of ambulatory blood pressure and age or sex in healthy adults. Hypertens Res 1992;15:127–135.
18. Zhang W, Shi H, Wang R, et al. Reference values for the ambulatory blood pressure: results from a collaborative study. Chin J Cardiol 1995;10:325–328.
19. Imai Y, Nagai K, Sakuma M, et al. Ambulatory blood pressure of adults in Ohasama, Japan. Hypertension 1993;22:900–912.
20. Chen CH, Ting CT, Lin SJ, et al. Relation between diurnal variation of blood pressure and left ventricular mass in a Chinese population. Am J Cardiol 1995;75:1239–1243.
21. Lurbe E, Thijs L, Redon J, Alvarez V, Tacons J, Staessen JA. Diurnal blood pressure curve in children and adolescents. J Hypertens 1996;14:41–46.
22. Baumgart P, Walger P, Fuchs G, Dorst KG, Vetter H, Rahn KH. Twenty-four-hour blood pressure is not dependent on endogenous circadian rhythm. J Hypertens 1989;7:331–334.
23. Imai Y, Sasaki S, Minami N, et al. Altered circadian blood pressure rhythm in patients with Cushing's syndrome. Hypertension 1988;12:11–19.

7

Importance of Heart Rate in Determining Cardiovascular Risk

Paolo Palatini, MD

CONTENTS

INTRODUCTION

A body of evidence indicates that subjects with tachycardia are more likely to develop hypertension (1–3) and atherosclerosis in future years (4–6). However, the connection between heart rate and the cardiovascular risk has long been neglected, on the grounds that tachycardia is often associated with the traditional risk factors for atherosclerosis, such as hypertension or metabolic abnormalities (7). A high heart rate is currently considered only an epiphenomenon of a complex clinical condition rather than an independent risk factor. However, most epidemiogic studies showed that the predictive power of a fast heart rate for cardiovascular disease remains significant even when its relative risk is adjusted for all major risk factors for atherosclerosis and other confounders (4–7). In this chapter, the results of the main studies that dealt with the relation between tachycardia and cardiovascular morbidity and mortality will be summarized, and the pathogenesis of the connection between fast heart rate and cardiovascular disease will be the focus.

From: *Contemporary Cardiology:*
Blood Pressure Monitoring in Cardiovascular Medicine and Therapeutics
Edited by: W. B. White © Humana Press Inc., Totowa, NJ

EPIDEMIOLOGIC EVIDENCE

The heart rate was found to be a predictor for future development of hypertension as far back as in 1945 (8). This finding was subsequently confirmed by the Framingham study, in which the predictive power of the heart rate for future development of hypertension was similar to that of obesity (3). Several other more recent reports have confirmed those findings (1,2,9). The heart rate was found to be also a predictor of myocardial infarction (10,11) and of cardiovascular morbidity in general (5,8). A body of evidence indicates that tachycardia is also related to increased risk of cardiovascular mortality. This association was shown by Levy et al. in a survey of over 20,000 Army officers (8). Thereafter, a number of other studies confirmed this finding, showing that the resting heart rate was a powerful predictor of death from cardiovascular and noncardiovascular causes (4,5,6,12–15). The data related to sudden death were particularly impressive, especially in the Framingham study, in which a sharp upward trend in mortality was found in the men divided by quintiles of heart rate (6). Also, in the Chicago studies a strong association was found between heart rate and sudden death, but the relation was U-shaped, because of an excess of mortality also in the subjects with very low heart rates (4).

The relationship between heart rate and cardiovascular mortality persists into old age. This was shown by the Framingham (6,16) and the NHANES (5) studies performed in general populations and by two more recent studies conducted in elderly subjects (13,14). In the CASTEL study (13), the predictive power of heart rate for mortality was 1.38 for the men with a heart rate > 80 beats/minute (bpm) (top quintile) compared to those of the three intermediate quintiles, and 0.82 for the men with a heart rate < 60 bpm (bottom quintile). The relation between heart rate and mortality was particularly strong for sudden death, with an adjusted relative risk of 2.45 for the subjects in the top quintile as compared to those in the three intermediate quintiles. In the CASTEL study, no significant association between heart rate and mortality was found in the women. In another study performed on elderly men and women combined (14), a 1.14 times higher probability of developing fatal or nonfatal myocardial infarction or sudden death was found for an increment of 5 bpm of heart rate recorded over the 24 h.

In the Framingham study, the relationship of heart rate with morbidity and mortality was analyzed also within hypertensive individuals (15) followed up for 36 yr. For a heart rate increment of 40 bpm the age-adjusted and systolic-blood-pressure-adjusted relative risk for cardiovascular mortality was 1.68 in males and 1.70 in females. For sudden death, the adjusted odds ratios were 1.93 and 1.37, respectively. These relationships were still significant after adjusting for smoking, total cholesterol, and left ventricular hypertrophy.

The heart rate was found to be a strong predictor of cardiovascular mortality also in patients with myocardial infarction. This association was found in the Norwegian Timolol Multicenter Study (17) and in a study by Hjalmarson et al.

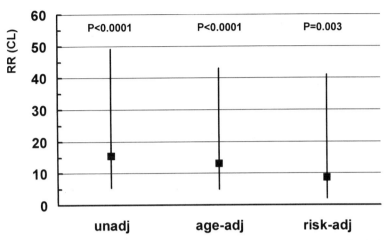

Fig. 1. Relative risks (RR) and 95% confidence limits (CL) for 1-yr mortality in 250 men divided according to whether their heart rate was < 80 bpm or ≥ 80 bpm on the seventh day after admission to the hospital for acute myocardial infarction. Unadj = unadjusted relative risk; age-adj = relative risk adjusted for age; risk-adj = relative risks adjusted for age, CK-MB peak, echocardiographic left ventricular ejection fraction, diabetes, history of hypertension, current smoking, history of angina, Killip class, thrombolysis and β-blocker therapy; *p*-values relate to the results of Cox regression analyses.

(18) in which the total mortality was 14% in the subjects with an admission heart rate < 60 bpm, 41% in the subjects with a heart rate > 90 bpm, and 48% in those with a heart rate > 110 bpm. In a subsequent study, Disegni et al. found a doubled mortality risk in postmyocardial infarction patients with a heart rate > 90 bpm compared to subjects with a heart rate < 70 bpm *(19)*. Two analyses performed in larger datasets confirmed the results of the above studies. In the GUSTO study *(20)*, a high heart rate emerged as a potent precursor of mortality, and in the GISSI-2 trial *(21)*, the predischarge heart rate was a stronger predictor of death than standard indices of risk, such as left ventricular dysfunction or ventricular arrhythmias. It is noteworthy to observe that tachycardia in postmyocardial infarction patients cannot be considered simply as a marker of heart failure, as its predictive power appeared more evident in the subjects with no or mild signs of congestive heart failure *(18,19)*. In a recent study, we found that the predictive power of heart rate for mortality in subjects with acute myocardial infarction remained significant also after adjusting for numerous confounders, including clinical and echocardiographic signs of left ventricular dysfunction (Palatini et al., unpublished observations) (Fig. 1).

PATHOGENETIC CONSIDERATIONS

The pathogenetic connection between fast heart rate and cardiovascular risk can be explained according to several different mechanisms (Fig. 2). The heart

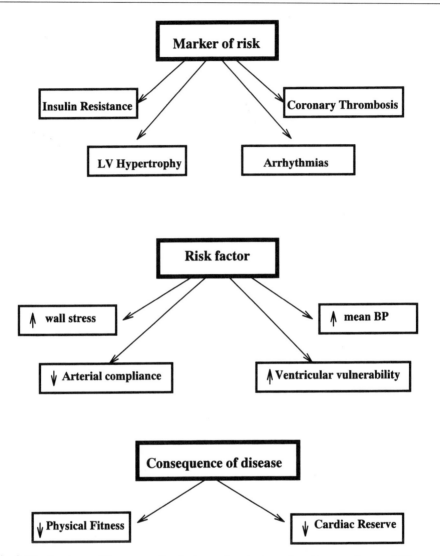

Fig. 2. Mechanisms of the connection between heart rate and cardiovascular morbidity and mortality. The heart rate can be a marker of risk or a consequence of an underlying disease, but can exert a direct action in the induction of the risk as well. LV = left ventricular; BP = blood pressure, ↑ = increased, ↓ = decreased.

rate can be considered as a marker of an underlying clinical condition related to the risk or a consequence of a latent chronic disease. However, experimental evidence suggests that a high heart rate should be regarded as a pathogenetic factor in the induction of the risk as well. In fact, tachycardia favors the occurrence of atherosclerotic lesions by increasing the arterial wall stress *(22)* and impairs arterial compliance and distensibility *(23)*. Moreover, the mean blood

Table 1
Correlation Coefficients Between Resting Heart Rate
and Other Clinical Variables in Three General and One Hypertensive Populations

Population	SBP	DBP	BMI	CT	TG	GL	INS
General							
Tecumseh	.27	.26	.11	.16	.13	NS	.19
Mirano	.22	.24	NS	.05	.08	.20*	—
Belgian	.20	.32	.13	NS	NS	.19*	.20
Hypertensive							
Harvest	.26	.10	NS	NS	NS	NS	—

SBP=systolic blood pressure; DBP = diastolic blood pressure; BMI = body mass index; CT = total cholesterol; TG = triglycerides; GL = glucose; INS = fasting insulin; NS = coefficient non significant; * = postload glucose. Data are for men only.
Data from ref. 7.

pressure has been found to be higher in subjects with faster heart rate *(24)*. This can be explained by the increase in the total time spent on systole because of the shortening of diastolic time.

The experimental evidence for a direct role of tachycardia in the induction of arterial atherosclerotic lesions was provided by studies performed in cynomolgus monkeys. Beere et al. were the first to demonstrate that reduction of heart rate by ablation of the sinoatrial node could retard the development of coronary lesions in these animals *(25)*.

Bassiouny et al. studied the effect of the product of mean heart rate and mean blood pressure (so-called hemodynamic stress) on the aorta of the monkeys *(26)* and found a striking positive relationship between the hemodynamic stress index and maximum atherosclerotic lesion thickness. Similar results were obtained by Kaplan et al., who found a significant relationship between naturally occurring differences in heart rate and atherosclerotic coronary lesions in monkeys *(27)*.

As mentioned earlier, heart rate can be considered as a marker of an abnormal clinical condition. This is suggested by the relationship found in several studies between heart rate and many risk factors for atherosclerosis *(28–30)*. In four different populations studied in the Ann Arbor laboratory, we found that the heart rate was correlated with blood pressure, degree of obesity, cholesterol, triglycerides, postload glucose, and fasting insulin (Table 1) *(31,32)*. In other words, subjects with a fast heart rate exhibited the features of the insulin-resistance syndrome. If one assumes that a fast heart rate is the marker of an abnormal autonomic control of the circulation, as demonstrated by Julius et al. *(33,34)*, it is easy to understand why subjects with tachycardia develop atherosclerosis and cardiovascular events. In fact, several studies performed in the Ann Arbor and other laboratories indicate that sympathetic overactivity can cause insulin resistance (Fig. 3). This can be obtained through acute *(35)* as well as chronic *(36)* stimulation of β-adrenergic receptors. It has been shown that chronic stimulation of

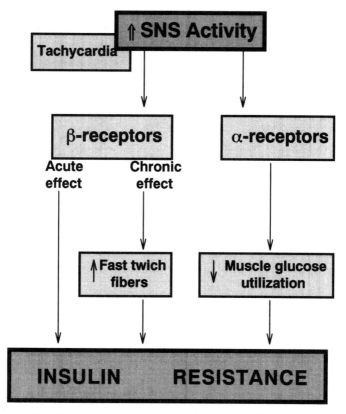

Fig. 3. Pathogenesis of the connection between tachycardia and insulin resistance. Tachycardia is a marker of the underlying sympathetic overactivity. SNS = sympathetic nervous system, ↑ = increased, ↓ = decreased.

β-receptors causes the conversion from a small to a larger proportion of insulin-resistant fast-twitch muscles *(36)*. An insulin-resistance state can be obtained also through a vasoconstriction mediated by α-adrenergic receptors, as shown by Jamerson et al. in the human forearm *(37)*. Conversely, the α-adrenergic blockade can improve insulin sensitivity in patients with hypertension *(38)*.

The connection between high heart rate and mortality can be explained also by an unrecognized underlying disease, and tachycardia can reflect poor physical fitness or loss of cardiac reserve *(4,6,13)*. In fact, an impaired left ventricular contractility may be an early clinical finding in asymptomatic hypertensive individuals, as demonstrated in the Padova *(39)* and Ann Arbor *(40)* laboratories. To rule out this possibility, in some studies the subjects who died within the first years after the baseline evaluation were eliminated *(6,13,16)*. However, in all of those studies, the heart rate–mortality association remained significant, indicating that tachycardia was not only a marker of latent left ventricular failure or of loss of vigor.

Besides causing the development of atherosclerotic lesions, a fast heart rate can also favor the occurrence of cardiovascular events, as shown by the Framingham study *(6,12,16)*. The relationship appeared weak for nonfatal cardiovascular events but was strong for fatal cardiovascular events. Moreover, as mentioned earlier, tachycardia can facilitate sudden death *(4,6,13)*. The reasons for this connection can be of a different nature. Sympathetic overactivity underlying a fast heart rate can facilitate the occurrence of coronary thrombosis through platelet activation and increased blood viscosity *(31)*. Subjects with tachycardia are more prone to ventricular arrhythmias. It is known that a heightened sympathetic tone can promote the development of left ventricular hypertrophy *(41)*, which facilitates the occurrence of arrhythmias *(42)*. Moreover, tachycardia increases oxygen consumption and ventricular vulnerability *(7,43)*. The latter mechanisms are important chiefly in subjects with acute myocardial infarction.

LOOKING FOR A THRESHOLD VALUE

The current definition of tachycardia is a heart rate > 100 bpm. Recent results obtained in our laboratory with mixture analysis suggest that this value is probably too high. In fact, in three general and one hypertensive populations, we found that the distribution of heart rate was explained by the mixture of two homogeneous subpopulations, a larger one with a "normal" heart rate and a smaller one with a "high" heart rate. The partition value between the two subpopulations was around 80–85 bpm. Furthermore, in almost all of the epidemiologic studies that showed an association between heart rate and death from cardiovascular or noncardiovascular causes, the heart-rate value above which a significant increase in risk was seen was below the 100-bpm threshold *(44)* (Table 2). On the basis of the above data we suggested that the upper normal value of heart rate should be set at 85 bpm *(44)*.

THERAPEUTIC CONSIDERATIONS

Although there is no doubt that a fast heart rate is independently related to cardiovascular and total mortality, it is not known whether the reduction of heart rate can be beneficial in prolonging life. No clinical trial has been implemented as yet in human beings with the specific purpose of studying the effect of cardiac slowing on morbidity and mortality. This issue was dealt with by Coburn et al. in mice by studying the effect of digoxin administration *(45)*. Survival increased by 29% in the digoxin-treated males and by 14% in the treated females, in comparison with two groups of untreated mice (control groups), indicating that a heart-rate reduction may confer an advantage in terms of longevity.

A beneficial effect of heart-rate reduction in retarding the development of atherosclerotic lesions was demonstrated by Kaplan et al. with β-blocker administration in cynomolgus monkeys *(46)*. After 26 mo of propranolol treatment, the

Table 2
Heart Rate Threshold Values Above Which a Significant
Increase in Mortality Was Found in Eight Epidemiologic Studies

Reference	HR threshold value		Results of the study
	Men	Women	
Levy et al., 1945 (8)	99	—	Increased 5-yr cardiovascular mortality in men.
Dyer et al., 1980 (4)	79	—	Increased 15-yr all-cause mortality in the men of the People Gas Co. study.
Dyer et al., 1980 (4)	86	—	Increased 5-yr all-cause mortality in the men of the Heart Association study.
Dyer et al., 1980 (4)	89	—	Increased 17-yr all-cause mortality in the men of the Western Electric study.
Kannel et al., 1985 (6)	87	87	Increased 26-yr sudden death mortality rate in men.
Gillum et al., 1991 (5)	84	84	Increased 10-yr all-cause mortality in black and white men and in black women.
Gillman et al., 1993 (15)	84	84	Increased 36-yr all-cause mortality in hypertensive men and women.
Palatini et al., 1999 (13)	80	84	Increased 12-yr cardiovascular mortality in elderly men.

HR = heart rate in bpm.

socially dominant animals showed a reduced development of coronary artery lesions in comparison to a group of untreated monkeys of the control group. This suggests that heart-rate reduction with β-blockers is beneficial in preventing atherosclerotic lesions, but only in animals exposed to a high environmental stress.

Most of the information on the effect of β-blockers on heart rate and morbidity and mortality in human beings comes from results obtained in post-myocardial-infarction patients. The reduction in heart rate obtained varied greatly among the trials, from 10.5% to 22.8%. β-Blocking treatment appeared beneficial in those patients in whom the heart rate was reduced by 14 bpm or more, whereas for a heart-rate reduction <8 bpm, no benefit was apparent (47). Moreover, the advantage of treatment was virtually confined to patients with a heart rate of >55 bpm.

In 26 large, placebo-controlled trials with a long-term follow-up, β-blockers proved effective primarily in reducing sudden death and death resulting from pump failure (47–51). An almost linear relationship was found between reduction in resting heart rate and decreased mortality (48,52). β-Blockers with intrinsic sympathomimetic activity, such as pindolol or practolol, showed only little effect on mortality.

Similar beneficial effects were obtained in patients with congestive heart failure (53). Carvedilol caused a marked reduction in mortality in subjects with congestive heart failure (54), but only in patients with a high heart rate (>82 bpm).

The results obtained in hypertensive subjects *(55)* were less impressive, probably the result of the untoward effects of β-blockers on high-density lipoprotein (HDL) cholesterol and triglycerides *(56)*. However, the effect of β-blockers in hypertensive patients was never examined in relation to the subjects' heart rates at baseline.

If the unsatisfactory effects of β-blockers in hypertension are the result of their unfavorable effects on plasma lipids, the use of drugs which reduce blood pressure and heart rate without altering the lipid profile appears warranted. Non-dihydropyridine-calcium antagonists *(57,58)* have been shown to be neutral on the metabolic profile and could, thus, be more effective in preventing cardiovascular mortality in hypertensive subjects with tachycardia. In addition to having a peripheral action, some of them can cross the blood-brain barrier and decrease sympathetic outflow *(58)*.

Diltiazem and verapamil have been shown to be effective in reducing the risk of cardiac events *(59–61)*, but their depressive action on cardiac inotropism makes them unsuitable for patients with acute myocardial infarction and severe left ventricular dysfunction. The new long-acting calcium antagonists that selectively block voltage-dependent T-type calcium channels *(62,63)* reduce heart rate without manifesting a depressant effect on myocardial contractility and could, thus, be indicated also for subjects with congestive heart failure *(64)*.

Centrally active antihypertensive drugs that decrease heart rate through reduction of the sympathetic discharge from the central nervous system should have a good potential for the treatment of the hypertensive patient with fast heart rate. Unfortunately, the use of clonidine, α-methyldopa, guanfacine, and guanabenz is limited by the frequent occurrence of side effects, like dry mouth, sedation, and impotence *(65)*. Moxonidine and rilmenidine are new antihypertensive agents acting on the I1-imidazoline receptors of the rostro-ventrolateral medulla of the brainstem and do not have most of the side effects encountered with the centrally acting agents *(65,66)*. Moreover, these drugs proved effective in improving the metabolic profile in the experimental animal *(67)* and also in human studies *(68)*. The goal of antihypertensive treatment should be not only to lower the blood pressure but also to reverse those functional abnormalities that often accompany the hypertensive condition. Therefore, a therapy that not only reduces blood pressure effectively but also decreases the heart rate and improves metabolic abnormalities should be sought.

REFERENCES

1. Selby JV, Friedman GD, Quesenberry CP Jr. Precursors of essential hypertension: pulmonary function, heart rate, uric acid, serum cholesterol, and other serum chemistries. Am J Epidemiol 1990;131:1017–1027.
2. Reed D, McGee D, Yano K. Biological and social correlates of blood pressure among Japanese men in Hawaii. Hypertension 1982;4:406–414.

3. Garrison RJ, Kannel WB, Stokes J III. Incidence and precursors of hypertension in young adults. Prev Med 1987;16:235–251.
4. Dyer AR, Persky V, Stamler J, et al. Heart rate as a prognostic factor for coronary heart disease and mortality: findings in three Chicago epidemiologic studies. Am J Epidemiol 1980;112: 736–749.
5. Gillum RF, Makuc DM, Feldman JJ. Pulse rate, coronary heart disease, and death: the NHANES I epidemiologic follow-up study. Am Heart J 1991;121:172–177.
6. Kannel WB, Wilson P, Blair SN. Epidemiologic assessment of the role of physical activity and fitness in development of cardiovascular disease. Am Heart J 1985;109:876–885.
7. Palatini P, Julius S. Heart rate and the cardiovascular risk. J Hypertens 1997;15:3–17.
8. Levy RL, White PD, Stroud WD, et al. Transient tachycardia: Prognostic significance alone and in association with transient hypertension. JAMA 1945;129:585–588.
9. Paffenbarger RS Jr, Thorne MC, Wing AL. Chronic disease in former college students—VIII. Characteristics in youth predisposing to hypertension in later years. Am J Epidemiol 1968;88: 25–32.
10. Schroll M, Hagerup LM. Risk factors of myocardial infarction and death in men aged 50 at entry. A ten-year prospective study from the Glostrup population studies. Dan Med Bull 1977; 24:252–255.
11. Medalie JH, Kahn HA, Neufeld HN, et al. Five-year myocardial infarction incidence—II. Association of single variables to age and birthplace. J Chronic Dis 1973;26:329–349.
12. Goldberg RJ, Larson M, Levy D. Factors associated with survival to 75 years of age in middle-aged men and women. The Framingham study. Arch Intern Med 1996;156:505–509.
13. Palatini P, Casiglia E, Julius S, et al. Heart rate: a risk factor for cardiovascular mortality in elderly men. Arch Int Med 1999;159:585–592.
14. Aronow WS, Ahn C, Mercando AD, et al. Association of average heart rate on 24-hour ambulatory electrocardiograms with incidence of new coronary events at 48-month follow-up in 1,311 patients (mean age 81 years) with heart disease and sinus rhythm. Am J Cardiol 1996;78:1175–1176.
15. Gillman MW, Kannel WB, Belanger A, et al. Influence of heart rate on mortality among persons with hypertension: The Framingham Study. Am Heart J 1993;125:1148–1154.
16. Kannel WB, Kannel C, Paffenbarger RS Jr, et al. Heart rate and cardiovascular mortality: The Framingham Study. Am Heart J 1987;113:1489–1494.
17. The Norwegian Multicenter Study Group. Timolol-induced reduction in mortality and reinfarction in patients surviving acute myocardial infarction. N Engl J Med 1981;304:801–807.
18. Hjalmarson A, Gilpin EA, Kjekshus J, et al. Influence of heart rate on mortality after acute myocardial infarction. Am J Cardiol 1990;65:547–553.
19. Disegni E, Goldbourt U, Reicher-Reiss H, et al. The predictive value of admission heart rate on mortality in patients with acute myocardial infarction. J Clin Epidemiol 1995;48: 1197–1205.
20. Lee KL, Woodlief LH, Topol EJ, et al. Predictors of 30-day mortality in the era of reperfusion for acute myocardial infarction. Results from an international trial of 41,021 patients. Circulation 1995;91:1659–1668.
21. Maggioni AP, Zuanetti G, Mantini L, et al. The predictive value of pre-discharge heart rate on 8-month mortality in 7,831 patients with acute myocardial infarction in the fibrinolytic era. Eur Heart J 1997;18(Abstract suppl):352A.
22. Gordon D, Guyton J, Karnovsky N. Intimal alterations in rat aorta induced by stressful stimuli. Lab Invest 1983;45:14–19.
23. Mangoni AA, Mircoli L, Giannattasio C, et al. Heart rate-dependence of arterial distensibility in vivo. J Hypertens 1996;14:897–901.
24. Palatini P. Exercise haemodynamics in the normotensive and the hypertensive subject. Clin Sci 1994;87:275–287.

25. Beere PA, Glagov S, Zarins CK. Retarding effect of lowered heart rate on coronary atherosclerosis. Science 1984;226:180–182.
26. Bassiouny HS, Zarins CK, Kadowaki MH, et al. Hemodynamic stress and experimental aorto-iliac atherosclerosis. J Vasc Surg 1994;19:426–434.
27. Kaplan JR, Manuck SB, Clarkson TB. The influence of heart rate on coronary artery atherosclerosis. J Cardiovasc Pharmacol 1987;10(Suppl 2):S100–S102.
28. Stamler J, Berkson DM, Dyer A, et al. Relationship of multiple variables to blood pressure—findings from four Chicago epidemiologic studies. In: Paul O, ed. Epidemiology and Control of Hypertension. Symposia Specialists, Miami, 1975, pp. 307–352.
29. Cirillo M, Laurenzi M, Trevisan M, et al. Hematocrit, blood pressure, and hypertension. The Gubbio Population Study. Hypertension 1992;20:319–326.
30. Stern MP, Morales PA, Haffner SM, et al. Hyperdynamic circulation and the insulin resistance syndrome ("Syndrome X"). Hypertension 1992;20(6):802–808.
31. Palatini P, Julius S. Association of tachycardia with morbidity and mortality: pathophysiological considerations. J Hum Hypertens 1997;11(Suppl 1):19–27.
32. Palatini P, Casiglia E, Pauletto P, et al. Relationship of tachycardia with high blood pressure and metabolic abnormalities. A study with mixture analysis in three populations. Hypertension 1997;30:1267–1273.
33. Julius S, Gudbrandsson T, Jamerson K, et al. Hypothesis. The hemodynamic link between insulin resistance and hypertension. J Hypertens 1991;9:983–986.
34. Julius S, Pascual AV, London R. Role of parasympathetic inhibition in the hyperkinetic type of borderline hypertension. Circulation 1971;44:413–418.
35. Deibert DC, DeFronzo RA. Epinephrine-induced insulin resistance in man. J Clin Invest 1980;65:717–721.
36. Zeman RJ, Ludemann R, Easton TG, et al. Slow to fast alterations in skeletal muscle fibers caused by clenbuterol, a beta-2-receptor agonist. Am J Physiol 1988;254:E726–E732.
37. Jamerson KA, Julius S, Gudbrandsson T, et al. Reflex sympathetic activation induces acute insulin resistance in the human forearm. Hypertension 1993;21(5):618–623.
38. Pollare T, Lithell H, Selinus I, et al. Application of prazosin is associated with an increase of insulin sensitivity in obese patients with hypertension. Diabetologia 1988;31:415–420.
39. Palatini P, Visentin PA, Mormino P, et al. Left ventricular performance in the early stages of systemic hypertension. Am J Cardiol 1998;81:418–423.
40. Julius S. Altered cardiac responsiveness and regulation in the normal cardiac output type of borderline hypertension. Circ Res 1975;36–37(Suppl I):I-199–I-207.
41. Julius S, Li Y, Brant D, et al. Neurogenic pressor episodes fail to cause hypertension, but do induce cardiac hypertrophy. Hypertension 1989;13:422–429.
42. Palatini P, Maraglino G, Accurso V, et al. Impaired left ventricular filling in hypertensive left ventricular hypertrophy as a marker of the presence of an arrhytmogenic substrate. Br Heart J 1995;73:258–262.
43. Palatini P. Heart rate as a cardiovascular risk factor. Eur Heart J 1999;20(Suppl B):B3–B9.
44. Palatini P. Need for a revision of the normal limits of resting heart rate. Hypertension 1999;33:622–625.
45. Coburn AF, Grey RM, Rivera SM. Observations on the relation of heart rate, life span, weight and mineralization in the digoxin-treated A/J mouse. Johns Hopkins Med J 1971;128:169–193.
46. Kaplan JR, Manuck SB, Adams MR, et al. Inhibition of coronary atherosclerosis by propranolol in behaviorally predisposed monkeys fed an atherogenic diet. Circulation 1987;76:1364–1372.
47. Kjekshus JK. Importance of heart rate in determining beta-blocker efficacy in acute and long-term acute myocardial infarction intervention trials. Am J Cardiol 1986;57:43F–49F.
48. Teo KK, Yusuf S, Furberg CD. Effects of prophylactic antiarrhythmic drug therapy in acute myocardial infarction: an overview of results from randomized controlled trials. JAMA 1993;270:1589–1595.

49. The Goteborg Metoprolol Trial in Acute Myocardial Infarction. Am J Cardiol 1984;53: 10D–50D.
50. The International Collaborative Study Group. Reduction of infarct size with the early use of timolol in acute myocardial infarction. N Engl J Med 1984;310:9–15.
51. Taylor SH, Silke B, Ebbutt A, et al. A long-term prevention study with oxprenolol in coronary heart disease. N Engl J Med 1982;307:1293–1301.
52. Kjekshus JK. Comments on beta-blockers: heart rate reduction, a mechanism of action. Eur Heart J 1985;6(Suppl A):29–30.
53. MRC Working Party. Medical Research Council trial of treatment of hypertension in older adults: principal results. Br Med J 1992;304:405–412.
54. Lehtonen A. Effect of beta blockers on blood lipid profile. Am Heart J 1985;109:1192–1198.
55. Eichorn EJ, Bristow MR. Medical therapy can improve the biological properties of the chronically failing heart. Circulation 1996;94:2285–2296.
56. Packer M, Bristow MR, Cohn JN, for the U.S. Carvedilol Heart Failure Study Group. The effect of Carvedilol on morbidity and mortality in patients with chronic heart failure. N Engl J Med 1996;334:1349–1355.
57. Stadler P, Leonardi L, Riesen W, et al. Cardiovascular effects of verapamil in essential hypertension. Clin Pharmacol Ther 1987;42:85–92.
58. Kailasam MT, Parmer RJ, Cervenka JH, et al. Divergent effects of dihydropyridine and phenylalkylamine calcium channel antagonist classes on autonomic function in human hypertension. Hypertension 1995;26:143–149.
59. The Danish Study Group on Verapamil in Myocardial Infarction. Effect of verapamil on mortality and major events after acute myocardial infarction. The Danish Verapamil Infarction Trial II (DAVIT-II). Am J Cardiol 1990;66:779–785.
60. Alderman MH, Cohen H, Rogué R, et al. Effect of long-acting and short-acting calcium antagonists on cardiovascular outcomes in hypertensive patients. Lancet 1997;349:594–598.
61. The Multicenter Diltiazem Postinfarction Trial Research Group. The effect of diltiazem on mortality and reinfarction after myocardial infarction. N Engl J Med 1988;319:385–392.
62. Luscher TF, Clozel JP, Noll G. Pharmacology of the calcium antagonist mibefradil. J Hypertens 1997;15(Suppl 3):S11–S18.
63. Kung CF, Tschudi MR, Noll G, et al. Differential effects of the calcium antagonist mibefradil in epicardial and intramyocardial coronary arteries. J Cardiovasc Pharmacol 1995;26:312–318.
64. Clozel J, Ertel EA, Ertel SI. Discovery and main pharmacological properties of mibefradil (Ro 40-5967), the first selective T-type calcium channel blocker. J Hypertens 1997;15(Suppl 5): S17–S25.
65. Van Zwieten PA. Centrally acting antihypertensives: a renaissance of interest. Mechanisms and haemodynamics. J Hypertens 1997;15(Suppl 1):S3–S8.
66. Ernsberger P, Koletsky RJ, Collins LA, et al. Sympathetic nervous system in salt-sensitive and obese hypertension: amelioration of multiple abnormalities by a central sympatholitic agent. Cardiovasc Drugs Ther 1996;10:275–282.
67. Rosen P, Ohly P, Gleichmann H. Experimental benefit of moxonidine on glucose metabolism and insulin secretion in the fructose-fed rat. J Hypertens 1997;15(Suppl 1):S31 S38.
68. Ernsberger P, Friedman JE, Koletsky RJ. The I1-Imidazoline receptor: from binding site to therapeutic target in cardiovascular disease. J Hypertens 1997;15(Suppl 1):S9–S23.

8 Sodium, Potassium, the Sympathetic Nervous System, and the Renin–Angiotensin System

Impact on the Circadian Variability in Blood Pressure

Domenic A. Sica, MD and Dawn K. Wilson, PHD

CONTENTS

INTRODUCTION

Under the usual circumstances of everyday life, the phasing of human circadian clocks and rhythms is set, or synchronized, by the sleep-in-darkness–activity-in-light, 24-h routine. These time cues greatly influence the intrinsic diurnal rhythm for blood pressure (BP). As an example of this, when shift workers are assigned to night duty, they ordinarily adhere to a different sleep–activity routine than do day workers. Because of this, the timing of their peak and trough BP differs, with reference to external clocktime, if compared to daytime active

From: *Contemporary Cardiology:*
Blood Pressure Monitoring in Cardiovascular Medicine and Therapeutics
Edited by: W. B. White © Humana Press Inc., Totowa, NJ

individuals. The biologic time structure of man is an inherited characteristic for a number of parameters, such as BP. Its normal expression, however, may be influenced by either environmental/nutritional factors or an individual's normal or pathophysiologically acquired neuro-humoral status. When normal phase relationships change between circadian bioperiodicities, BP patterns may alter radically and unpredictably. The purpose of this review is to characterize the neuro-humoral and nutritional determinants of the ambulatory blood pressure (ABP) profile in normotensive and hypertensive patients. In particular, this review focuses on the sympathetic nervous system (SNS), the renin–angiotensin–aldosterone (RAA) axis, and the role of dietary sodium (Na^+) and potassium (K^+) in shaping circadian BP patterns.

AMBULATORY BLOOD PRESSURE MONITORING AS A TOOL

Ambulatory BP monitoring is a recently developed methodology, capable of identifying and systematically evaluating factors responsible for individual differences in BP responses in the natural environment. This approach provides a means for studying an individual in a standardized fashion as he or she responds to the physical and psychological demands of a typical 24-h day. Prior research employing ABP monitoring indicates that most people display low-amplitude diurnal variations in BP, with higher pressures during waking hours and lower pressures during sleep *(1,2)*. In most normotensive subjects, average BP values decline by approx 15% during sleep *(3–5)*. In hypertensive subjects, the circadian rhythm is generally preserved, although the 24-h BP profile shifts to higher around-the-clock values *(6)*.

Ambulatory BP patterns are rarely static with considerable day-to-day variability in how nocturnal BP patterns express themselves *(7)*. It has proven tempting to assign causality to a particular dietary or neuro-humoral change in how nocturnal BP changes occur. Unfortunately, it is the rare circumstance where a specific neuro-humoral or dietary pattern is exclusively responsible for a particular nocturnal BP pattern, such as nondipping (minimal drop in nocturnal BP). Rather, factors typically coalesce with different weightings assigned to individual factors in order to arrive at a final explanation for a specific BP pattern. Comments found in this chapter should be viewed accordingly.

ELECTROLYTES AND CIRCADIAN RHYTHMS

The established associations between BP and electrolytes are for the most part most reliable when based on data from urinary excretion and/or a validated self-report of nutrient intake *(7–9)*. Urinary excretion and/or dietary recall parameters are the preferred correlates to BP, as it is widely held that they more realistically

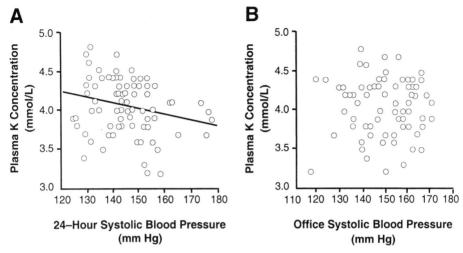

Fig. 1. Relation between plasma K⁺ and 24-h systolic blood pressure (**A**: $r = 0.336$, $p < 0.01$) or office systolic blood pressure (**B**: $r = -0.018$, $p = \text{NS}$) in 82 patients with essential hypertension. Adapted with permission of Elsevier Science from ref. *(13)*. Copyright 1997 by American Journal of Hypertension Ltd.

depict the true state of electrolyte balance. Interpreting the relationship between a plasma electrolyte, such as K⁺, and BP is inherently difficult because nutritional intake is one of only many factors known to influence plasma K⁺ values. Such factors include a circadian rhythm for plasma K⁺ (average peak → trough difference ≈ 0.60 mEq/L with lowest values at night) *(10)* and a tendency for K⁺ to migrate intracellularly, when β_2-adrenergic receptors are stimulated *(11)*.

Accordingly, very few reports have even attempted to characterize the relationship between plasma K⁺ and ABP patterns in hypertensive patients *(12,13)*. Goto et al. found significant negative correlations between daytime plasma K⁺ concentration and 24-h systolic and diastolic BP levels in patients with essential hypertension *(13)*. Plasma K⁺ also inversely correlated with both daytime and nighttime systolic and diastolic BP levels. In these studies, there was no correlation between office BP readings and plasma K⁺ concentration. No doubt, any such relationship was obscured by the inherent variability of office BP measurements (Fig. 1).

If the plasma K⁺ value in any way equates with intake, these results are consistent with prior epidemiologic studies, which have found a negative correlation between K⁺ intake and BP levels *(12)*. Goto et al. have further suggested that decreased extracellular K⁺ promotes vasoconstriction in hypertensive patients by either enhancing SNS activity or by increasing the Na⁺ content of vascular smooth muscle cells *(13)*. Additional research is needed to better understand the relative contribution of plasma electrolytes to circadian variability in BP.

NEURO-HUMORAL PATTERNS
AND CIRCADIAN BLOOD PRESSURE RHYTHMS

Atrial Natriuretic Peptide

As a prominent regulatory arm of volume homeostasis in man, the natriuretic peptides are intimately involved in the regulation of BP. Atrial natriuretic peptide (ANP) release is primarily regulated by atrial pressure though a number of other factors, such as age and level of renal and/or cardiac function, that can arbitrate the final plasma concentration for ANP. ANP can be viewed as the "mirror image" of the RAA axis in that it inhibits the release of renin and aldosterone while opposing the actions of angiotensin II and aldosterone through effects on vascular tone, cells growth, and renal sodium reabsorption. When ANP is administered to animals or humans, the BP acutely drops, a process, which is particularly prominent when the RAA is activated. For these reasons, a relationship between the time structure of ANP, other neurohormones, and 24-h BP patterns has been sought.

It has been observed that single-point-in-time morning ANP levels may have either no relationship to 24-h BP *(14)* or may separate isolated clinic hypertension (wherein ANP levels are typically normal) from sustained hypertension (wherein plasma ANP levels are increased) in elderly hypertensives *(15)*. Methodologic considerations are important to the interpretation of circadian ANP patterns. For example, Chiang et al. observed the absence of any circadian rhythm for ANP (and thus no relationship to diurnal BP change) in a group of 14 healthy volunteers in whom ANP was sampled every 3 h for 24 h *(16)*.

In other studies in which subjects were synchronized to the light–dark cycle and were given a controlled diet, a variable acrophase for ANP was found. Portaluppi et al. originally noted an acrophase for ANP to occur at around 4:00 AM. In these studies, BP and heart rate (HR) rhythms appeared to be in antiphase with the ANP rhythm, with the peak of BP and HR more or less coinciding with the trough for ANP rhythm. This pattern of response suggested a relationship between ANP levels and BP and HR *(17)*. Alternatively, Cugini et al. noted an acrophase timing for ANP at about 5:00 PM in young clinically healthy subjects and no circadian pattern for ANP in elderly subjects, although mean blood levels of ANP were noticeably higher in the elderly cohort *(18)*. There is no obvious explanation for these obviously different findings. Additional studies will be required to clarify the time pattern of ANP levels.

Plasma Renin Activity

Gordon et al. originally described a diurnal rhythm for plasma renin activity (PRA) that was independent of posture and dietary influences *(19)*, a finding subsequently corroborated by a number of other investigators *(17,20–22)*. From these observations emerged the concept of a circadian rhythm in PRA, with a nadir in the afternoon and a nocturnal increase culminating in the early morning hours, despite the occasional study having failed to demonstrate any significant variation in PRA with the time of day *(23–25)*. What remained to be determined was to define the relative role of endogenous circadian rhythmicity and the sleep–wake cycle on 24-h PRA variations because sleep can make substantial contributions to the overall variations in PRA and thereby mask the characteristics of an endogenous rhythm *(26)*.

A strong relationship exists between nocturnal oscillations in PRA and internal sleep structure *(24,27)*. Non-rapid-eye-movement (NREM) is invariably linked to increasing PRA levels, with PRA decreasing during rapid-eye-movement (REM) sleep. In normal man, modifying the renal renin content modulates only the amplitude of the nocturnal oscillations without altering their relationship to the stage of sleep *(28)*, and in the case of sleep disorders, such as sleep apnea, the PRA profiles reflect all facets of the sleep structure disturbance *(29)*. Brandenberger et al. have recently shown, using an acute shift in the normal sleep time, that increased renin release was associated with sleep whatever time it occurs, an observation atypical of an intrinsic circadian rhythm (Fig. 2) *(26)*. This group further observed that internal sleep architecture had an important modulatory role on the characteristics of the PRA oscillations and, consequently, on the 24-h pattern. When NREM–REM sleep cycles are disturbed, as is the case with the fragmented sleep of obstructive sleep apnea, there is insufficient time for PRA to increase significantly; consequently, in poor sleepers, PRA values may not vary to any significant degree throughout a 24-h time span. This may provide an explanation for the occasional study wherein PRA values fail to increase during sleep *(23–25,30)*.

Although several studies have examined the 24-h cycle of PRA, few have seen fit to examine the relationship between PRA and ABP patterns, and those that have, fail to provide a consistent picture. For example, Watson found significant positive correlations between PRA and variability in daytime BP readings after adjusting for age *(31)*. Chau et al. *(32)*, however, reported negative correlations between upright PRA and 24-h mean BP readings. Harshfield and colleagues *(33)* examined the relationship between renin–sodium profiles and ABP patterns in healthy children. The subjects were classified as low, intermediate, or high renin, inferred from the relationship between PRA and Na⁺ excretion. The subjects classified as high renin had elevated systolic and diastolic BP readings while asleep more so than did subjects in the low-renin category. These studies suggest that the relationship between the level of RAA system activity and ambulatory BP patterns is complex, with Na⁺ sensitivity and/or Na⁺ intake emerging as important co-variables in this relationship.

In addition, the 24-h pattern for PRA oppose that for BP, which tends to fall in the first few hours of sleep and to rise thereafter. Superimposed on these tendencies, periodic changes in BP occur that coincide with the presence of NREM

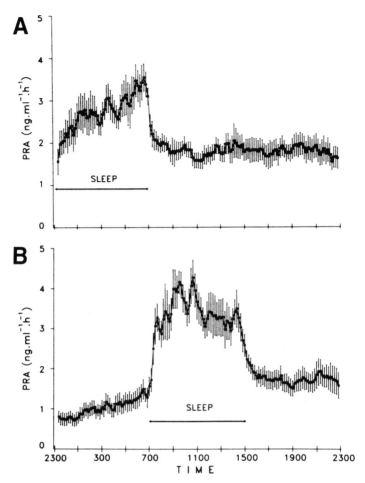

Fig. 2. Effects of an 8-h delay of the sleep–wake cycle on the 24-h plasma renin activity profiles in 10 subjects: (**A**) normal nocturnal sleep from 2300 to 0700 h and (**B**) daytime sleep from 0700 to 1500 h after a night of sleep deprivation. Values are expressed as means ± SEM. Adapted from *(26)* by permission of Lippincott Williams & Wilkins.

sleep cycles *(34)*. Such changes are characterized by slight decreases in the mean BP levels during slow-wave sleep and small increases in mean BP levels during REM sleep, during which there is a marked increase in PRA pulse activity. It is unclear as to the relationship of PRA pulse activity to these observed oscillations in nocturnal BP.

Angiotensin-Converting Enzyme Inhibitors

A failure to establish clear relationships between nocturnal RAA axis activity and BP patterns may be a function of various sensitivities to external influences

Table 1
Chronopharmacology of ACE inhibitors

Authors (ref.)	Drug/dose (mg)	Subject No. Study design	Timing (h)	Single/ multiple dose	Observations
Weisser et al. (35)	Enalapril/10	8 Normals	0800 2000	Yes/no	T_{max} ↑ with 2000 h dose
Palatini et al. (36)	Quinapril/20	18 Hypertensives, double-blind/ crossover	0800 2200	No/yes	Evening dose maintained efficacy for 24 h; morning dose lost efficacy during nighttime and early morning
Palatini et al. (37)	Benazepril/10	10 Hypertensives, single blind/ crossover	0900 2100	Yes/no	Morning had more sustained 24-h effect than did evening dose
Witte et al. (38)	Enalapril/10	8 Hypertensives, double blind/ crossover	0700 1900	Yes/yes	Evening dose maintained efficacy for 24 h; morning dose lost efficacy between 0200 and 0700 h
Morgan et al. (39)	Perindopril/4	20 Hypertensives, crossover	0900 2100	No/yes	Evening dose maintained efficacy for 24 h; morning dose lost efficacy after 18 h

and/or the interactions of other rhythms, which could obscure PRA cycles during the waking periods. One way to evaluate the importance of nocturnal PRA is to determine the nature of the vasodepressor response subsequent to administration of ACE inhibitors. Several studies have attempted such an evaluation (Table 1).

Possible circadian changes in the pharmacokinetics and effect on serum angiotensin-converting enzyme (ACE) activity of the ACE inhibitor enalapril were first evaluated in the studies of Weisser et al. (35), with several subsequent studies having been reported since that time (Table 1). Weisser et al. (35) noted that the mean serum concentration–time profiles of enalapril and its active metabolite enalaprilat were comparable whether enalapril was ingested at 0800 or 2000 h. Administration of enalapril at 2000 h did not markedly influence the bioavailability of enalapril as estimated by time to maximum concentration (T_{max}), maximum drug concentration (C_{max}), or area under the curve (AUC_{0-24}) for the active enalapril metabolite, enalaprilat. The only observed difference was an increase in T_{max} for enalapril after its evening administration (1.3 ± 0.5 [0800 h]) vs 2.4 ± 1.4 (2000 h [$p < 0.05$]), a phenomenon that has been observed with a number of other drugs.

Palatini et al. subsequently examined the relationship between daytime (0800 h) and nighttime (2200 h) administration of quinapril following 4 wk of dosing (36). The 24-h BP profiles obtained by ABP monitoring showed a more sustained antihypertensive action with the evening administration (2200 h) of quinapril compared with its morning administration (0800 h). There was a partial loss of effectiveness for quinapril during the nighttime and early morning hours when it was administered in the morning. In addition, measurement of ACE activity showed that evening administration of quinapril caused a less pronounced but more sustained decline of plasma ACE. In this regard, 24 h after the last dose of quinapril, the residual ACE inhibition was greater (62%) with evening dosing than was the case with morning dosing (40%). These authors concluded that evening administration of quinapril was preferable because it provided a more homogeneous pattern of 24-h BP control, which, in part, may have related to an extended inhibition of the ACE enzyme *(36)*.

Palatini et al. also evaluated the influence of timing of benazepril administration on 24-h intra-arterial BP measurements. In contradistinction to their previous studies with quinapril, they noted that a single 10-mg dose of benazepril administered at 0900 h more effectively covered the 24-h dosing interval than did an identical dose administered at 2100 h *(37)*. Although the single-dose nature of these studies make their interpretation difficult, they do suggest that ACE inhibitor pharmacokinetics are relevant to the circadian variability in response to an ACE inhibitor.

Witte et al. *(38)* evaluated the cardiovascular effects and pharmacokinetics of once-daily enalapril (10 mg) after either a single dose or following its chronic administration. Chronic therapy (with dosing at 0700 h) significantly reduced BP during the day but lost effectiveness between 2 and 7 AM of the succeeding day. Chronic dosing at 1900 h significantly exaggerated the nocturnal dip in BP. BP values slowly increased throughout the next day with the evening dosing regimen, with no effect on elevated afternoon values. Peak concentrations of enalaprilat were found at 3.5 h (morning) and 5.6 h (evening) after drug administration. The time-to-peak drug effect was shorter after morning dosing (7.4 ± 4.3 h [diastolic]) than evening dosing (12.1 ± 3.7 h [diastolic]). Differences in the response to enalapril could not be attributed to timewise changes in pharmacokinetics or to a different time-course of ACE inhibition. It is more likely that circadian changes in the sensitivity of the RAA system play an important role in defining timewise differences in response to an ACE inhibitor.

In a final study, Morgan et al. examined the BP response following the administration of perindopril either in the morning (0900 h) or in the evening (2100 h). It was noted in these studies that the early morning rise in BP was reduced more with the evening administration of perindopril. However, the 2100 h dose regimen did not reduce BP over 24 h, whereas the 0900 h dose achieved better BP control. These studies concluded that the time-related response profile obtained with an ACE inhibitor is unique and that chronobiology has important effects on the action of these drugs *(39)*.

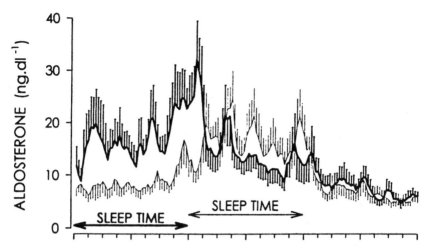

Fig. 3. Effect of an 8-h shift in sleep period cycle on 24-h profiles for plasma aldosterone in seven subjects. Blood was sampled at 10-min intervals. In the daytime sleep condition, the amplitude of the aldosterone pulses was significantly enhanced during the sleep period. Values are expressed as mean ± SEM. Adapted with permission *(41)*.

Plasma Aldosterone

Plasma aldosterone secretion follows a pattern such that mean hormone concentrations are highest during the night and early morning *(20–23,40)*. Plasma aldosterone values during a 24-h time period appear to be coupled to PRA, with renin secretion being either simultaneous with or preceding aldosterone secretion by 10–20 min, with this temporal coupling enhanced in a low-sodium state *(40)*. Under basal conditions, the relative contribution of sleep processes and circadian rhythm to plasma aldosterone levels remains poorly defined, particularly as relates to those systems that cojointly control aldosterone release (renin-angiotensin, adrenocorticotropic, and dopaminergic systems).

Heretofore, any timewise change in the 24-h profile of aldosterone was viewed simplistically as a circadian event. More recently, it has been recognized that the pattern of aldosterone release is influenced by sleep architecture *(41)*. Recent studies, employing an experimental design of abruptly shifting sleep by 8 h, show sleep processes to have a stimulatory effect on aldosterone release, as demonstrated by high mean levels together with high pulse amplitude and pulse frequency observed during the sleep period and reduced levels during sleep deprivation (Fig. 3). This pattern of secretion is similar to that observed with PRA *(26)*. The large increase in plasma aldosterone levels and pulse amplitude following awakening from nocturnal sleep is attributable to an increase in activity of the adrenocorticotropic axis, reflected by the surge in cortisol in the early morning. The issue of nocturnal aldosterone change is complex, with aldosterone pulses mainly related to PRA oscillations during the sleep periods, whereas aldosterone pulses are associated with cortisol pulses during the waking periods.

The influence of aldosterone circadian patterns on BP and, in particular, nocturnal BP is poorly defined. Little meaningful information exists that might permit an assessment of the role of aldosterone antagonism in modifying circadian BP patterns.

Sympathetic Nervous System

In both normotensive and hypertensive individuals, the BP fluctuates according to the level of both mental and physical activities. BP, HR, and SNS activity are typically highest when a hypertensive patient is awake and/or active. Conversely, these values reach a nadir between midnight and 3:00 AM *(42–44)*. Although the exact interplay of all physiologic and pathophysiologic mediators of the diurnal rhythm remains unclear, nocturnal BP and HR seems to track SNS activity best—but not entirely so. Experiments with autonomic blocking agents provide some insight into the importance of the SNS in diurnal BP rhythms. For example, the BP rhythm in high spinal cord transected patients (with complete tetraplegia) is nonexistent, despite HR variability being preserved (presumably because cardiac vagal innervation remains intact) *(45)*. Paraplegics and incomplete tetraplegics typically have a normal diurnal BP pattern. These findings are consistent with the thesis that central SNS outflow is an important determinant of the normal diurnal rhythm of BP.

Attempts to define the role of the SNS in determining nocturnal BP changes are complicated by methodologic constraints. This being said, SNS activity typically diminishes while asleep, with changes in the *sympathoadrenal* branch (epinephrine) being governed in a dual fashion by both posture and sleep and the *noradrenergic* branch (norepinephrine) being regulated more so by posture *(44)*. Diurnal changes in plasma catecholamine values, as markers of SNS activity, are subject to considerable sampling error and require careful interpretation as to the study conditions under which they were obtained. Plasma epinephrine concentrations and/or SNS activity decline during sleep (particularly during NREM sleep) and begin to increase in conjunction with morning awakening *(44,46,47)* and/or episodically during episodes of REM sleep (Fig. 4) *(48)*. Plasma norepinephrine concentrations trend downward when asleep and do not significantly increase until a postural stimulus to norepinephrine release, such as the upright position, is added to changes accompanying the arousal process *(44,46)*. Morning plasma norepinephrine concentrations, although typically higher than sleep values, are not necessarily the highest values attained during a 24-h time interval *(46,47)*. Finally, microneurography, a specific marker of muscle SNS activity, fails to show any increased neural activity in normal volunteers when performed between the hours of 6:30 AM and 8:30 AM, a time parenthetically when the rate of myocardial infarction is highest. This suggests that the early morning peak in

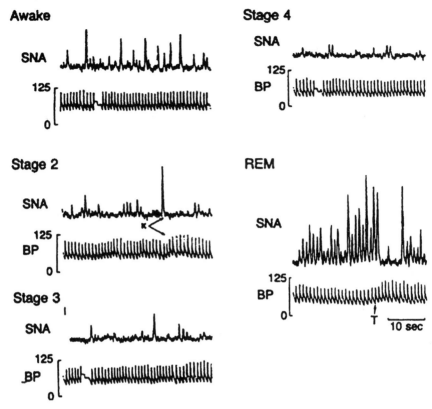

Fig. 4. Recordings of sympathetic nerve activity (SNA) and mean blood pressure (BP) in a single subject while awake and while in stages 2, 3, and 4 and REM sleep. As non-REM sleep deepens (stages 2–4), SNA gradually decreases and BP (mmHg) and variability in BP are gradually reduced. Arousal stimuli elicited K complexes on the electrocardiogram (not shown) were accompanied by increases in SNA and BP (indicated by the arrows, stage 2 sleep). In contrast to the changes during non-REM sleep, heart rate, BP, and BP variability increased during REM sleep, together with a profound increase in both the frequency and amplitude of SNA. There was a frequent association between REM twitches (momentary periods of restoration of muscle tone, denoted by T on the tracing) and abrupt inhibition of SNA and increases in BP. Adapted with permission *(48)*. Copyright 1993 Massachusetts Medical Society.

myocardial infarction and/or sudden cardiac death could, in part, reflect exaggerated end-organ responsiveness to norepinephrine following the relative sympathetic withdrawal that occurs during sleep *(49)*.

Nocturnal BP can assume a number of different and now well-characterized patterns: extreme dipping (an approximate 30% ↓ in BP while asleep), normal dipping (a 10–20% ↓ in nighttime BP), and nondipping (minimal drop in nocturnal BP or a rise in BP at night) *(7,50)*. Of these BP patterns, attention has recently centered on the significance of a nighttime nondipping BP pattern, because it is believed to be associated with more rapid progression of renal failure *(51)* and/ or a greater degree of left ventricular hypertrophy *(52)*. Aging, salt sensitivity, and African-American ethnicity are viewed as relevant demographic markers for this phenomenon *(7)*.

Little is known about the pathophysiology of nocturnal nondipping in either normotensive or essential hypertensives, although important clues to the origin of this phenomenon can be extracted from an analysis of sleep patterns. Sleep architecture and SNS activity are important determinants of nocturnal BP and HR. During NREM sleep, there is a tendency for HR to slow and BP to fall, a process characterized by a relative increase in parasympathetic or vagal activity *(53–55)*. It is now fairly well accepted that alterations in SNS activity may lead to relevant effects on the pathophysiology of sleep, as well as influence the diurnal BP profile. Derangements in autonomic nervous system activity, sleep-disordered breathing, and alterations in sleep architecture and duration are well-recognized causes of change in the circadian BP profile *(54)*. In addition, sleep disturbances are reported to influence the circadian BP profile. Schillaci et al. showed that the reported duration of sleep was significantly shorter for hypertensive "nondippers" than it was for "dippers" both in males and females *(56)*. Kario et al. found nondippers to have increased nocturnal physical activity, as determined by actigraphy *(57)*. Thus, the duration and quality of sleep should be considered in the interpretation of the diurnal BP profile.

Nutrition

The intake of Na^+ and/or K^+ is an important modulator of BP. The impact of such nutritional modification has most typically been assessed by evaluating change in casual BP determinations *(58,59)*, although more recently, ABP technology has been employed to delineate the 24-h pattern of change with such interventions *(60–64)*. Accordingly, it is only in the last decade that nocturnal BP patterns could serve as targets for dietary intervention *(60,64)*.

Prior research has identified demographic groups in whom the equilibrium point for Na^+ balance is set at a higher level of BP. For example, Weinberger et al. demonstrated that blacks and older individuals (>40 yr) poorly excrete a Na^+ load, and in order to achieve Na^+ balance, higher BP values are required for a longer period of time *(65)*. Falkner et al. have also reported that salt-sensitive adolescents with a positive family history of hypertension had greater increases in BP with salt loading than did adolescents who were either salt resistant or had a negative family history of hypertension *(66)*. Harshfield et al. have also demonstrated that Na^+ intake is an important determinant of ABP profiles in black children and adolescents *(67)*. Black subjects displayed a positive correlation between Na^+ excretion and asleep systolic BP, whereas Na^+ excretion was independent of asleep BP in white subjects.

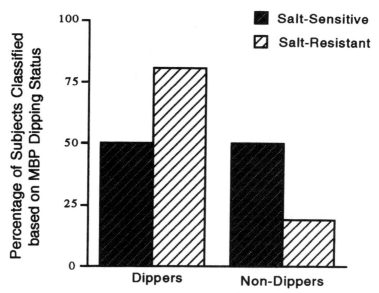

Fig. 5. Percentage of salt-sensitive versus salt-resistant normotensive adolescent blacks who were classified as dippers (>10% decline in nocturnal blood pressure) or nondippers (<10% decline in nocturnal blood pressure). Adapted with permission of Elsevier Science from ref. *(62)*. Copyright 1999 by American Journal of Hypertension Ltd.

Several investigators have probed the relationship between salt sensitivity and the nocturnal decline in ABP. Wilson et al. examined the relationship between salt sensitivity and ABP in healthy black adolescents *(62)*. They classified 30% of those studied as salt sensitive according to predetermined criteria for salt sensitivity, with the remaining subjects designated as salt resistant. Salt-sensitive subjects showed higher daytime diastolic and mean BP than did salt-resistant subjects. A significantly greater percentage of salt-sensitive subjects were classified as nondippers according to diastolic BP (<10% decrease in BP from awake to asleep) as compared to salt-resistant individuals (Fig. 5). These results were some of the first to indicate that salt sensitivity is associated with a nondipper nocturnal BP pattern in healthy black adolescents. These findings are consistent with prior observations by de la Sierra et al. *(63)*, which showed higher awake BP values in normotensive salt-sensitive adults as compared to salt-resistant adults, and a recent meta-analysis that found American blacks to experience a smaller dip in BP (higher levels of both systolic and diastolic BP) at night *(68)*.

The mechanism(s) by which Na⁺ sensitivity (or sodium loading) alters nocturnal BP (although incompletely elucidated) likely involves increased SNS activity *(65,69,70)*. Increased SNS activity, in turn, is known to modify Na⁺ handling, albeit in a mixed fashion. For example, Harshfield et al. have found that normotensive individuals differ in Na⁺ handling during SNS arousal *(71)*. In one group

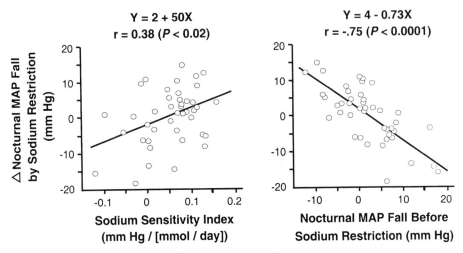

Fig. 6. Relationships of changes in nocturnal mean arterial pressure (MAP) fall induced by Na⁺ restriction with the sodium-sensitivity index as well as with nocturnal MAP fall before Na⁺ restriction. The sodium-sensitivity index, shown on the left, was calculated as the ratio of the change in MAP over the change in urine sodium excretion ($U_{Na}V$) produced by Na⁺ restriction (1–3 g NaCl/d). The nocturnal fall in MAP before Na⁺ restriction (on the right) was calculated as the difference between daytime and nighttime MAPs during high Na⁺ intake (12–15 g NaCl/d). The change in nocturnal MAP fall with Na⁺ restriction was calculated as the difference between low- and high-Na⁺ diets and had a positive relationship with the sodium-sensitivity index ($r = 0.38, p < 0.02$) and a negative relationship with the nocturnal MAP fall during the high-Na⁺ diet ($r = -0.75, p < 0.0001$) Adapted with permission *(60)*.

of adults, termed *excreters*, Na⁺ excretion increased during 1 h of behaviorally induced SNS arousal (competitive video games) with a return to baseline levels within 2 h of stimulation. In a second group of adults, termed *retainers*, Na⁺ excretion decreased in response to SNS arousal and remained below baseline values for at least 2 h following stimulation. The findings of Harshfield et al. *(71)*, as well as those of several other investigators, now suggest an important interactive role for SNS activation in Na⁺ retention and, by this process, a means by which nocturnal BP might be altered *(72,73)*.

The role of Na⁺ intake in the definition of nocturnal BP is evident from the studies of Uzu et al. *(60)* and Higashi et al. *(61)*. Uzu et al. found that a nondipper nocturnal BP pattern in salt-sensitive patients converted to a dipper pattern with Na⁺ restriction (Fig. 6) *(60)*. Higashi et al. *(61)* found that the nocturnal decline in mean BP was significantly smaller in salt-sensitive as compared to salt-resistant hypertensives during a Na⁺-loading protocol, sufficient to have elevated ABP levels (Fig. 7). In their studies, nondipping was also most commonly seen in those hypertensive patients who were salt sensitive and exposed to a high-Na⁺ diet. These findings suggest that a high-Na⁺ intake can now be considered as an

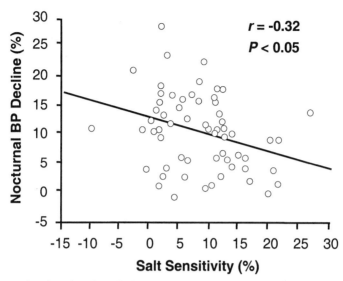

Fig. 7. Scatterplot showing the relationship between the nocturnal decline in blood pressure during a high-NaCl diet (340 mmol/d) (nocturnal BP decline) and the NaCl-induced increase in blood pressure (salt sensitivity). The NaCl-induced increase in BP was correlated with the nocturnal decline in BP during a high-NaCl diet but not during a low-NaCl diet. Adapted with permission *(61)*.

etiologic factor (among several others) for the failure of BP to decline at night in hypertensive patients, particularly in those who are salt sensitive.

Fewer investigations have examined the relationship between K⁺ intake and ABP responses *(7,64)*. A potential pathway by which K⁺ may influence ABP patterns involves K⁺-related natriuresis. For example, a number of studies have strongly suggested that a change in K⁺ intake alters Na⁺ balance, such that dietary K⁺ restriction results in Na⁺ retention and K⁺ supplementation produces a natriuretic response *(74,75)*. The effect of K⁺ on urinary Na⁺ excretion, plasma volume, and mean arterial pressure could also be evidence for a K⁺-mediated vasodilator effect on BP. For example, it is well established that the local intra-arterial infusion of K⁺ decreases forearm vascular resistance and increases forearm blood flow in a dose-dependent fashion *(76,77)*. It has also been demonstrated that K⁺ supplementation given in combination with a high-Na⁺ diet suppresses the increase in catecholamines, which typically occurs in response to Na⁺ loading *(70)*.

Theoretical premises such as these led Wilson et al. to examine the effects of a 3-wk increase in K⁺ on ABP responses in healthy black adolescents. Subjects were classified as dippers or nondippers according to whether they sustained a >10% decrease from awake to asleep BP, and were randomized to either a high-K⁺ diet or a usual diet control group. A significant proportion of nondippers switched from a nondipper to dipper status in response to the high-potassium diet

(7). Although this study did not show a change in nocturnal BP, a subsequent study, which specifically examined for this effect in salt-sensitive subjects, did show a reversal in nighttime BP as a consequence of a high-K^+ diet in salt-sensitive individuals *(64)*. These studies strongly suggest that K^+ intake may have a substantial influence on diurnal patterns of BP responses.

SUMMARY

How a nocturnal BP pattern presents is a consequence of both intrinsic circadian rhythms and the quantity and quality of sleep. Although a range of neuro-humoral factors can influence the circadian BP pattern, abnormal SNS activity is most commonly linked to a disappearance of the normal decline in nocturnal BP. Nutritional intake, such as either a high-Na^+ or a low-K^+ intake, can also erase the normal decline in nocturnal BP. The impact of nutrition on nocturnal BP change is most prominent in salt-sensitive individuals. Additional studies of an integrative nature will be necessary to more completely define the dynamic interplay between nutrition and various neuro-humoral axes in how nocturnal BP patterns are expressed.

REFERENCES

1. Bevan AT, Honor AJ, Stott FD. Direct arterial pressure reading in unrestricted man. Clin Sci 1969;36:329–344.
2. Pickering TG, Harshfield GA, Kleinert H, Blank S, Laragh JH. Blood pressure during normal daily activities, sleep, and exercise: comparison of values in normal and hypertensive subjects. JAMA 1982;47:992–996.
3. Pickering TG. Sleep, circadian rhythms and cardiovascular disease. Cardiovasc Rev Rep 1980;1:37–47.
4. Staessen JA, Fagard RH, Lijnen PJ, et al. Mean and range of ambulatory blood pressure in normotensive subjects from a meta-analysis of 23 studies. Am J Cardiol 1991;67:723–727.
5. Staessen JA, Bieniaszewski L, O'Brien E, et al. Nocturnal blood pressure fall on ambulatory monitoring in a large international base. Hypertension 1997;27:30–39.
6. Fogari R, Ambrosoli S, Corradi L, et al. 24-Hour blood pressure control by once-daily administration of irbesartan assessed by ambulatory blood pressure monitoring. J Hypertens 1997;15: 1511–1518.
7. Wilson DK, Sica DA, Devens M, et al. The influence of potassium intake on dipper and nondipper blood pressure status in an African-American adolescent population. Blood Pressure Monitor 1996;1:447–455.
8. Gill JR, Gullner HG, Lake CR, et al. Plasma and urinary catecholamines in salt-sensitive idiopathic hypertension. Hypertension 1988;11:312–319.
9. Staessen JA, Birkenhager W, Bulpitt CJ, et al. The relationship between blood pressure and sodium and potassium excretion during the day and night. J Hypertens 1003;11:443–447.
10. Solomon R, Weinberg MS, Dubey A. The diurnal rhythm of plasma potassium: relationship to diuretic therapy. J Cardiovasc Pharmacol 1991;17:854–859.
11. Struthers AD, Reid JL, Whitesmith R, et al. Effect of intravenous adrenaline on electrocardiogram, blood pressure and plasma potassium. Br Heart J 1983;49:90–93.
12. Bulpitt CJ, Shipley MJ, Semmence A. Blood pressure and plasma sodium and potassium. Clin Sci 1981;61:85s–87s.

13. Goto A, Yamada K, Nagoshi H, et al. Relation of 24-h ambulatory blood pressure with plasma potassium in essential hypertension. J Hypertens 1997;10:337–340.
14. Guasti L, Grimoldi P, Ceriani L, et al. Atrial natriuretic peptide and 24 h blood pressure. Blood Pressure Monitor 1997;2:89–92.
15. Kario K, Nishikimi T, Yoshihara F, et al. Plasma levels of natriuretic peptides and adreno-medullin in elderly hypertensive patients: relationship to 24-h blood pressure. J Hypertens 1998;16:1253–1259.
16. Chiang FT, Tseng CD, Hsu KL, et al. Circadian variation of atrial natriuretic peptide in normal people and its relationship to arterial blood pressure, plasma renin activity and aldosterone level. Int J Cardiol 1994;46:229–233.
17. Portaluppi F, Bagni B, degli Uberti E, et al. Circadian rhythms of atrial natriuretic peptide, renin, aldosterone, cortisol, blood pressure and heart rate in normal and hypertensive subjects. J Hypertens 1990;8:85–95.
18. Cugini P, Lucia P, Di Palma L, et al. Effect of aging on circadian rhythm of atrial natriuretic peptide, plasma renin activity, and plasma aldosterone. J Gerontol 1992;47:B214–B219.
19. Gordon RD, Wolfe LK, Island DP, et al. A diurnal rhythm in plasma renin activity in man. J Clin Invest 1966;45:1587–1592.
20. Katz FH, Romph P, Smith JA. Diurnal variation of plasma aldosterone, cortisol and renin activity in supine man. J Clin Endocrinol Metab 1975;40:125–134.
21. Kawasaki T, Cugini P, Uezono K, et al. Circadian variations of total renin, active renin, plasma renin activity and plasma aldosterone in clinically healthy young subjects. Horm Metab Res 1990;22:636–639.
22. Modlinger RS, Sharif-Zadeh K, Ertel NH, et al. The circadian rhythm of renin. J Clin Endocrinol Metab 1976;43:1276–1282.
23. Lightman SL, James VHT, Linsell C, et al. Studies of diurnal changes in plasma renin activity, and plasma noradrenaline, aldosterone and cortisol concentration in man. Clin Endocrinol (Oxf) 1981;14:213–223.
24. Mullen PE, James VHT, Lightman C, et al. A relationship between plasma renin activity and the rapid eye movement phase of sleep in man. J Clin Endocrinol Metab 1980;50:466–469.
25. Brandenberger G, Follenius M, Nuzet A, et al. Ultradian oscillations in plasma renin activity: their relationships to meals and sleep stages. J Clin Endocrinol Metab 1985;61:280–284.
26. Brandenberger G, Follenius M, Goichot B, et al. Twenty-four-hour profiles of plasma renin activity in relation to the sleep-wake cycle. J Hypertens 1994;12:277–283.
27. Brandenberger G, Follenius M, Simon C, et al. Nocturnal oscillations in plasma renin activity and REM–NREM sleep cycles in humans: a common regulatory mechanism. Sleep 1988; 11:242–250.
28. Brandenberger G, Krauth MO, Erhart J, et al. Modulation of episodic renin release during sleep in humans. Hypertension 1990;15:370–375.
29. Follenius M, Krieger J, Krauth MO, et al. Obstructive sleep apnea treatment: peripheral and central effects of plasma renin activity and aldosterone. Sleep 1991;14:211–217.
30. Kool MJ, Wijnen JA, Derkx FH, et al. Diurnal variation in prorenin in relation to other humoral factors and hemodynamics. Am J Hypertens 1994;7:723–730.
31. Watson RDS, Stallard TJ, Flinn RM, et al. Factors determining direct arterial pressure and its variability in hypertensive men. Hypertension 1980;2:333–341.
32. Chau NP, Chanudet X, Larroque P. Inverse relationship between upright plasma renin activity and 24-hour blood pressure variability in borderline hypertension. J Hypertens 1990;8: 913–918.
33. Harshfield GA, Pulliam DA, Alpert BS, et al. Renin–sodium profiles influence ambulatory blood pressure patterns in children and adolescents. Pediatrics 1990;87:94–100.
34. DeLeeuw PW, Van Leeuwen SJ, Birkenhager WH. Effect of sleep on blood pressure and its correlates. Clin Exp Hypertens A 1985;7:179–186.

35. Weisser K, Schloos J, Lehmann K, et al. Pharmacokinetics and converting enzyme inhibition after morning and evening administration of oral enalapril to healthy subjects. Eur J Clin Pharmacol 1991;40:95–99.

36. Palatini P, Racioppa A, Raule G, et al. Effect of timing of administration on the plasma ACE inhibitory activity and the antihypertensive effect of quinapril. Clin Pharmacol Ther 1992; 52:378–383.

37. Palatini P, Mos L, Motolese M, et al. Effect of evening versus morning benazepril on 24-hour blood pressure: a comparative study with continuous intraarterial monitoring. Int J Clin Pharmacol Toxicol 1993;31:295–300.

38. Witte K, Weisser K, Neubeck M, et al. Cardiovascular effects pharmacokinetics, and converting enzyme inhibition of enalapril after morning versus evening administration. Clin Pharmacol Ther 1993;54:177–186.

39. Morgan T, Anderson A, Jones E. The effect on 24 h blood pressure control of an angiotensin converting enzyme inhibitor (perindopril) administered in the morning or at night. J Hypertens 1997;15:205–211.

40. Vieweg WV, Veldhuis JD, Carey RM. Temporal pattern of renin and aldosterone secretion in men: effects of sodium balance. Am J Physiol 1992;31:F871–F877.

41. Charloux A, Gronfier C, Lonsdorfer-Wolf E, et al. Aldosterone release during the sleep-wake cycle in humans. Am J Physiol 1999;276:E43–E49.

42. Pickering TG, James GD. Determinants and consequences of the diurnal rhythm of blood pressure. Am J Hypertens 1993;6:166S–169S.

43. Millar-Craig MW, Bishop CN, Raftery EB. Circadian variation of blood pressure. Lancet 1978;1:795–797.

44. Dodt C, Breckling U, Derad I, et al. Plasma epinephrine and norepinephrine concentrations of healthy humans associated with nighttime sleep and morning arousal. Hypertension 1997; 30:71–76.

45. Nitsche B, Perschak H, Curt A, et al. Loss of circadian blood pressure variability in complete tetraplegia. J Hum Hypertens 1996;10:311–317.

46. Linsell CR, Lightman SL, Mullen PE, et al. Circadian rhythm of epinephrine and norepinephrine in man. J Clin Endocrinol Metab 1985;60:1210–1215.

47. Stene M, Panagiotis N, Tuck MI, et al. Plasma norepinephrine levels are influenced by sodium intake, glucocorticoid administration, and circadian changes in normal man. J Clin Endocrinol Metab 1980;51:1340–1345

48. Somers VK, Dyken ME, Mark AL, et al. Sympathetic nerve activity during sleep in normal subjects. N Engl J Med 1993;328:303–307.

49. Middlekauff HR, Sontz EM. Morning sympathetic nerve activity is not increased in humans. Implications for mechanisms underlying the circadian pattern of cardiac risk. Circulation 1995; 91:2549–2555.

50. Fernandez A, Sica DA, Wilson DK, Gehr TWB, White W. Extreme dipping—a definitional dilemma. Am J Hypertens 1999;12:150A.

51. Bianchi S, Bigazzi R, Campese VM. Altered circadian blood pressure profile and renal damage. Blood Pressure Monitor 1997;6:339–346.

52. Palatini P, Penzo M, Racioppa A. Clinical relevance of nighttime blood pressure and of daytime blood pressure variability. Arch Intern Med 1992;152:1855–1860.

53. Billman GE, Dujardin JP. Dynamic changes in cardiac vagal tone as measured by time-series analysis. Am J Physiol 1990;258:H896-H902.

54. Portaluppi F, Cortelli P, Provini F. Alterations of sleep and circadian blood pressure profile. Blood Pressure Monitor 1997;6:301–313.

55. Baumgart P. Circadian rhythm of blood pressure: internal and external time triggers. Chronobiol Int 1991;8:444–450.

56. Schillaci G, Verdecchia P, Borgioni C, et al. Predictors of diurnal blood pressure changes in 2042 subjects with essential hypertension. J Hypertens 1996;14:1167–1173.
57. Kario K, Pickering TG, Schwartz JE. Physical activity as a determinant of diurnal blood pressure variation. Am J Hypertens 1999;12:31A.
58. Moore TJ, Malarick C, Olmedo A, et al. Salt restriction lowers resting blood pressure but not 24-h ambulatory blood pressure. Am J Hypertens 1991;4:410–415.
59. Elliott P, Stamler J, Nichols R, et al. Intersalt revisited: further analyses of 24-hour sodium excretion and blood pressure within and across populations. Br Med J 1996;312:1249–1253.
60. Uzu T, Ishikawa K, Fujita T, et al. Sodium restriction shifts circadian rhythm of blood pressure from nondipper to dipper in essential hypertension. Circulation 1997;96:1859–1862.
61. Higashi Y, Oshima T, Ozono R, et al. Nocturnal decline in blood pressure is attenuated by NaCl loading in salt-sensitive patients with essential hypertension. Hypertension 1997;30(Part 1): 163–167.
62. Wilson DK, Sica DA, Miller SB. Ambulatory blood pressure non-dipping status in salt-sensitive and salt-resistant black adolescents. Am J Hypertens 1999;12:159–165.
63. de la Sierra A, del Mar Lluch M, Coca A, et al. Assessment of salt-sensitivity in essential hypertension by 24-h ambulatory blood pressure monitoring. Am J Hypertens 1995;8:970–977.
64. Wilson DK, Sica DA, Miller SB. Effects of potassium on blood pressure in salt-sensitive and salt-resistant adolescents. Hypertension 1999;34:181–186.
65. Weinberger MH, Miller JZ, Luft FC, et al. Definitions and characteristics of sodium sensitivity and blood pressure resistance. Hypertension 1986;8:II127–II134.
66. Falkner B, Kushner H, Khalsa DK, et al. Sodium sensitivity, growth and family history of hypertension in young blacks. J Hypertens 1986;4(Suppl 5): S381-S383.
67. Harshfield GA, Alpert BS, Pulliam DA, et al. Electrolyte excretion and racial differences in nocturnal blood pressure. Hypertension 1991;18:813–818.
68. Profant J, Dimsdale JE. Race and diurnal blood pressure patterns. Hypertension 1999;33: 1099–1104.
69. Yo Y, Nagano M, Moriguchi A, Nakamura F, Kobayashi R, Okuda N, et al. Predominance of nocturnal sympathetic nervous activity in salt-sensitive normotensive subjects. Am J Hypertens 1996;9:726–731.
70. Campese VM, Romoff MS, Levitan D, et al. Abnormal relationship between Na$^+$ intake and sympathetic nervous activity in salt-sensitive patients with essential hypertension. Kidney Int 1982;21:371–378.
71. Harshfield GA, Pulliam DA, Alpert BS. Patterns of sodium excretion during sympathetic nervous system arousal. Hypertension 1991;17:1156–1160.
72. Light KC, Koepke JP, Obrist PA, et al. Psychological stress induces sodium and fluid retention in men at high risk for hypertension. Science 1983;229:429–431.
73. Grignolo AJ, Koepke JP, Obrist PA. Renal function, heart rate, and blood pressure during exercise and avoidance in dogs. Am J Physiol 1982;2:R482–R490.
74. Krishna GG, Miller E, Kapoor S. Increased blood pressure during potassium depletion in normotensive man. N Engl J Med 1989;320:1177–1182.
75. Weinberger MH, Luft FC, Block R, Henry DP, Pratt JH, et al. The blood pressure-raising effects of high dietary sodium intake: racial differences in the role of potassium. J Am Coll Nutr 1982;1:139–148.
76. Linas SL. The role of potassium in the pathogenesis and treatment of hypertension. Kidney Int 1991;39:771–786.
77. Fujita T, Ito Y. Salt loads attenuate potassium-induced vasodilation of forearm vasculature in humans. Hypertension 1993;21:772–778.

9 Prognostic Value of Ambulatory Blood Pressure Monitoring

Paolo Verdecchia, MD
and Giuseppe Schillaci, MD

CONTENTS

INTRODUCTION

High blood pressure (BP) is a potent risk factor for cardiovascular disease in the general population. Unfortunately, however, the standard sphygmomanometric measurements of BP, taken as an index of the average BP load, have a quite weak predictive power in the single individual. One possible reason for that is the high variability of BP, with consequent need of several measurements in order to provide a more representative estimate of the average BP load to which a given person is exposed over a given time interval. On this assumption, clinically hypertensive subjects may benefit from ambulatory BP monitoring (ABPM),

From: *Contemporary Cardiology:*
Blood Pressure Monitoring in Cardiovascular Medicine and Therapeutics
Edited by: W. B. White © Humana Press Inc., Totowa, NJ

a procedure which gathers several BP measurements over time, when a main condition is fulfilled:

The difference in cardiovascular disease risk among different categories generated by ABPM should be greater than the difference among risk categories generated by the standard measurement of BP. As a result, statistical models including different measures of ABPM should lead, after adjustment for concomitant risk factors, to a lesser unexplained risk of cardiovascular disease than models including different measures of clinic BP.

In other words, ABPM should allow a clinically superior stratification of cardiovascular risk when compared with the standard sphygmomanometric measurements of BP. Once this point has been fulfilled on the basis of the results of one single session of the procedure, the next logical step would be the assessment of the prognostic value of serial changes of that procedure over time. An association between serial changes of the procedure and future occurrence of disease would make the procedure not only a predictor but also a surrogate measure of disease.

Once these aspects have been clarified, the procedure may be ready for intervention trials designed to see whether therapeutic interventions targeted on different risk categories generated by the new procedure are more effective in terms of disease reduction and/or cost-effectiveness than interventions on categories generated by the existing procedures.

There is evidence from clinical studies published over the last few years and discussed in this review that one single session of ABPM provides clinically useful information that improves cardiovascular risk stratification based on clinic BP and other traditional risk factors.

PROGNOSTIC VALUE OF AMBULATORY BLOOD PRESSURE

The available observational studies on the prognostic value of ambulatory BP have been conducted in tertiary care centers on subjects with essential hypertension either untreated (1–15) or treated (16) at the time of execution of ABPM or in the general population (17–20) (Table 1). In these studies, cardiovascular morbidity and mortality were the main outcome measures and one single session of ABPM allowed the definition of risk groups, which differed in their long-term outcome even after adjustment for several potential confounders.

Table 2 provides an overview of the results obtained by several independent research groups. Because some groups produced more that one report on partially overlapped populations, each group is represented in Table 2 with its largest contribution in terms of patient-years of observation.

We are involved in the PIUMA study (Progetto Ipertensione Umbria Monitoraggio Ambulatoriale) for 12 yr, an ongoing observational registry of morbidity and mortality in white adult subjects with essential hypertension. The study pro-

Table 1
Setting of Prognostic Studies
with Ambulatory Blood Pressure Monitoring

Referred untreated subjects with essential hypertension *(1–15)*
Referred treated subjects with resistant hypertension *(16)*
General population *(17–20)*

Table 2
Observational Prognostic Studies with Ambulatory Blood Pressure Monitoring:
Contributions by Different Centers

Author (ref.)	Country	Year	No. of subjects	Kind of population	Follow-up (yr)	Total events	Fatal events
Full papers							
Perloff et al. *(1)*	USA	1983	1076	RPH, U	5	153	75
Zweiker et al. *(13)*	Austria	1994	116	RPH, U	3	5	3
Ohkubo et al. *(17)*	Japan	1997	1542	GP, U, T	5.1	n.r.	93
Redon et al. *(16)*	Spain	1998	86	RPH, T	4	21	n.r.
Yamamoto et al. *(15)*	Japan	1998	105	RPS, T, U	3.2	15	n.r.
Khattar et al. *(12)*	UK	1998	479	RPH, U	9.1	98	38
Verdecchia et al. *(8)*	Italy	1998	2010	RPH, U	3.8	200	36
Staessen et al. *(26)*	Europe	1999	808	RPH, U	4.4	98	68
Abstracts							
Pickering and James *(11)*	USA	1994	573	RPH, U	5	18	n.r.
Suzuki et al. *(14)*	Japan	1996	132	RPH, U	4	25	n.r.
Total			6927		4.7	633	313

Note: RPH = Referred patients with hypertension; GP = general population; RPS = referred patients with stroke; U = untreated, T = treated, n.r. = not reported.

tocol has been reported in detail *(3–10)*. Follow-up is performed by family doctors in cooperation with our outpatient clinic, and subjects are treated with the goal of reducing clinic BP below 140/90 mmHg using standard lifestyle and pharmacological measures. There are periodical contacts with family doctors and telephone interviews with enrolled subjects in order to ascertain the vital status and the occurrence of major cardiovascular complications.

Contrary to the generally perceived opinion of paucity of observational prognostic studies on ABPM, Table 2 reveals an unsuspected high number of examined subjects (more than 6000) and subsequent outcome events (more than 500, at least 245 of which are fatal) across different studies.

Moreover, the survival analyses of other large databases, including the Cornell Study (Pickering, personal communication), the OvA study *(21)*, and the ELSA study *(22)*, are expected in a near future. For now, the existing database allows one to consider the prognostic value of ABPM according to eight different approaches to data analysis (Table 3).

Table 3
Prognostic Studies
with Ambulatory Blood Pressure Monitoring:
Different Analytical Approaches

Ambulatory BP as a continuous variable *(16.18.19)*
Observed versus predicted ambulatory BP *(1,2,23)*
"White coat" hypertension *(3,11,12,24)*
"White coat" effect *(6)*
Day–night BP changes *(3,4,10,13–15,19,25)*
Ultradian BP variability *(26)*
Ambulatory heart rate *(7)*
Ambulatory pulse pressure *(8)*

AMBULATORY BLOOD PRESSURE
AS A CONTINUOUS VARIABLE

An assessment of the prognostic value of ambulatory BP considered as a continuous variable has been carried out in the setting of the Ohasama study *(18–20)*, which is a general-population study in ambulant subjects aged 20 yr or more living in a Japanese rural area. Some of the subjects were untreated and some were being treated at the time of ABPM. During follow-up, which lasted an average of 5 yr, there were 93 fatal cardiovascular events. After adjustment for age, sex, smoking status, clinic BP, and use of antihypertensive medications, the risk of cardiovascular mortality was significantly increased in the highest quintile of the distribution of average 24-h systolic BP, whereas no independent relation was found between clinic BP and mortality. There was a U-shaped relationship between cardiovascular mortality and average 24-h systolic and diastolic BP, which may be interpreted as a possible expression of the link between low BP levels and various morbid conditions in the general population.

A limit of this study, which was the first to address the prognostic value of ABPM in the general population, is the lack of statistical adjustment for the potential confounding effect of diabetes, serum cholesterol, and a family history of premature coronary heart disease, three potent prognostic predictors.

Another relevant study is that by Redon et al. *(16)*. In this study, 86 patients with diastolic BP > 100 mmHg despite treatment with three or more drugs, including a diuretic, underwent 24-h ABPM. During an average follow-up period of 4 yr, 21 patients developed a first cardiovascular morbid event. After adjustment for age, sex, smoking, left ventricular hypertrophy, and clinic BP, the event rate was higher ($p < 0.02$) in the upper (13.6 events per 100 patient-years) than in the middle (9.5 events per 100 patient-years) and lowest (2.2 events per 100 patient-years) tertile of daytime diastolic BP. Despite some limitations, including the

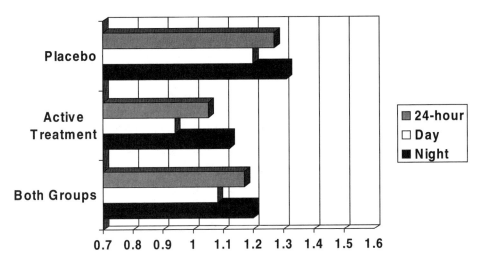

Fig. 1. Relative hazard rates for total cardiovascular events for every 10 mmHg increase in systolic blood pressure after adjustment for age, sex, smoking, office systolic blood pressure, previous cardiovascular events, and residence in western Europe.

small sample size and the lack of statistical adjustment for the potential confounding effect of factors like serum cholesterol and family history of premature coronary heart disease, this study is the first to support an independent predictive value of ABPM in patients with resistant hypertension.

Ambulatory BP has been examined as a continuous variable in the Systolic Hypertension in Europe (Syst-Eur) study *(26)*. In that study, ambulatory BP monitoring was carried out at randomization in 808 untreated patients. Of these, 98 developed a cardiovascular event over the follow-up period. After statistical adjustment for age, sex, office BP, active treatment, previous events, cigaret smoking, and residence in western Europe, nighttime systolic BP was an independent predictor of total, cardiac, and cerebrovascular events, whereas the average daytime BP did not achieve significance (Fig. 1). In the subjects randomized to placebo, for every 10% higher night/day ratio of systolic BP, the risk of events increased by 41% (95% confidence cardiovascular intervals: 3–94%; $p = 0.03$). These findings strongly support the prognostic value of ambulatory BP, in particular for BP levels recorded during the night.

OBSERVED VERSUS PREDICTED
AMBULATORY BLOOD PRESSURE

If we plot (Fig. 2) clinic BP vis-à-vis the average daytime ambulatory BP in a large population of subjects with essential hypertension, it is apparent that for any given value of clinic BP, the observed ABP is seldom that predicted by a linear regression equation, whereas it is often considerably higher or lower than

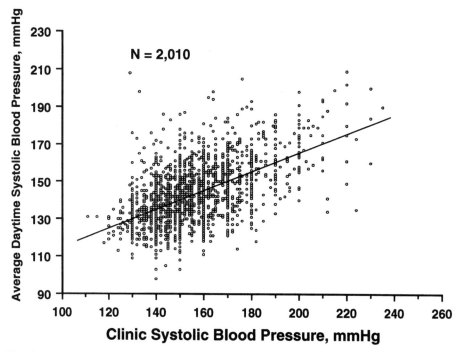

Fig. 2. The plot shows the association between clinic blood pressure and average daytime ambulatory blood pressure in 2010 untreated subjects with essential hypertension (PIUMA database).

predicted. For example, in patients with clinic systolic BP of 140–150 mmHg, the average daytime ABP may swing between less than 100 to about 190 mmHg.

Following this analytical approach, the ambulatory BP averages are not considered in absolute terms, but in relation to the values of clinic BP in that particular subject. Hence, a given ABP average may be that predicted by the regression equation if it coincides with the regression line, or it may be lower or higher than predicted. Dorothee Perloff, Maurice Sokolow, and colleagues, the pioneers of clinical use of ABPM, were the first to note that for any given value of clinic BP, the target organ damage in hypertension was more consistent in the patients with higher-than-predicted ABP than in those with lower-than-predicted ABP *(1,2)*. Subsequently, they followed for an average of 5 yr, 1076 patients with essential hypertension and detected 153 cardiovascular morbid events, 75 of which were fatal. The risk of events was significantly higher in the subset with higher-than-predicted ABP than in that with lower-than-predicted ABP, particularly in subjects with stage I hypertension. This study is limited by the lack of a normotensive control group, the lack of nocturnal blood pressure monitoring (resulting from the use of manually activated recorders), the lack of serum cholesterol, and cigaret smoking among the potential confounders in the multivariate analysis. Despite these limitations, this landmark study clearly showed for the first time the enormous potential clinical value of noninvasive ABPM and opened the way toward a larger use of this diagnostic technology in the clinical setting.

It is important to clarify that the subjects with lower-than-predicted ABP do not have a "normal" ABP. Hence, their cardiovascular risk should not be considered analogous to that of clinically normotensive subjects. In a word, the two concepts of "lower-than-predicted ABP" and "white coat" hypertension (discussed next) must be kept separate. On the other hand, the subjects with higher-than-predicted ABP are clearly characterized by office underestimation of the usual levels of BP. This high-risk group would remain undiagnosed with the sole use of clinic BP.

Some years ago, we have shown (27) that cigaret smoking is an important determinant of a higher-than-predicted ambulatory BP. In fact, clinic BP is less likely to be affected by smoking (usually, patients quit smoking shortly before the clinical visit), contrary to what happens to ambulatory BP, and the effect of smoking on ambulatory BP may lead to left ventricular (LV) hypertrophy (27). To clarify the prognostic impact of this phenomenon, we have recently analyzed the outcome of 841 subjects with essential hypertension JNC VI stage I who were followed for about 4 yr. During this period, the rate of cardiovascular morbid events was about 1 per 100 patient-years in the lowest quintile versus about 3 per 100 patient-years in the highest quintile of the difference between observed and predicted ABP (log-rank test: $p = 0.012$). However, such a difference did not remain significant in a multivariate survival analysis, which included cigaret smoking, age, 24-h pulse pressure, white coat hypertension, and a nondipping pattern as independent prognostic determinants (23).

Taken together, all these data suggest that a higher-than-predicted ABP should be considered a univariate prognostic predictor in subjects with stage I hypertension. Its adverse impact, however, is less strong than that of aging, cigaret smoking, and other more predictive components of ambulatory BP.

WHITE COAT HYPERTENSION

White coat hypertension, also referred to as office hypertension or isolated clinic hypertension, is generally defined by a persistently elevated office BP together with a normal pressure outside the office. Although the usual definition of elevated office BP is out of discussion ($\geq$140 mmHg systolic and/or 90 mmHg diastolic) (28,29), there is great deal of controversy about the definition of normal BP outside the office. As shown in Table 4, it is hard to find two studies using the same definition of white coat hypertension based on results of ABPM. Some studies use lower cutoff points, whereas others use higher cutoff points; the definition is based on systolic values in some studies and on diastolic values in other studies. Some studies use the average BP during daytime and other studies

Table 4
Different Definitions of White Coat Hypertension Based on ABPM

Pickering et al. *(30)*	< 134/90 mmHg (daytime ambulatory BP)
White et al. *(31)*	< 130/80 mmHg (daytime ambulatory BP)
Verdecchia et al. *(32)*	< 131/86 mmHg (W) or 136/87 mmHg (M) (daytime ambulatory BP)
Pierdomenico et al. *(33)*	< 135/85 mmHg (24-h ambulatory BP)
Kuwajima et al. *(34)*	< 140 mmHg (24-h ambulatory BP)
Cardillo et al. *(35)*	< 134/90 mmHg (daytime ambulatory BP)
Cerasola et al. *(36)*	< 134/90 mmHg (daytime ambulatory BP)
Glen et al. *(37)*	< 95 mmHg (daytime ambulatory BP)
Siegel et al. *(38)*	< 135/85 mmHg (daytime ambulatory BP)
Weber et al. *(39)*	< 85 mmHg (24-h ambulatory BP) and ≥ 5 mmHg < clinic BP
Hoegholm et al. *(40)*	< 90 mmHg (daytime ambulatory BP)
Marchesi et al. *(41)*	< 135/91 mmHg (daytime ambulatory BP)
Bidlingmeyer et al. *(42)*	< 140/90 mmHg (daytime ambulatory BP)
Rizzo et al. *(43)*	< 142/90 mmHg (daytime ambulatory BP)
Trenkwalder et al. *(44)*	< 146/87 mmHg (daytime ambulatory BP)
Staessen et al. *(45)*	< 133/82 mmHg (24-h ambulatory BP)
Amar et al. *(46)*	< 131/86 mmHg (W) or 136/87 mmHg (M) (daytime ambulatory BP)
Cuspidi et al. *(47)*	< 135/85 mmHg (24-h ambulatory BP)
Polonia et al. *(48)*	< 132/74 mmHg (daytime ambulatory BP)

W = women, M = men.

use the average 24-h BP. Still, some studies include a measure of the office–ambulatory BP difference in the definition.

At a first glance, the differences between the upper normal limits of ABP used to define white coat hypertension might seem small and of little clinical relevance. However, we have shown *(32)* that not only the prevalence of white coat hypertension but also LV mass at echocardiography and the prevalence of LV hypertrophy increased markedly when swinging from more restrictive (lower) to more liberal (higher) limits of ambulatory BP normalcy used for the definition of white coat hypertension (Fig. 3).

Inspection of Fig. 4, drawn from the PIUMA dataset *(49)*, indicates the importance of a restrictive definition of the upper normal limits of ambulatory BP in order to identify a population with characteristics of potentially low cardiovascular risk. The figure shows that the prevalence of LV hypertrophy, virtually absent below 120 mmHg and very modest below 130 mmHg (6%), increased to 10.5% when the limit was set to 140 mmHg. Thus, even modest swings over a relatively narrow range of presumably normal or nearly normal ambulatory BP result in considerable differences in the prevalence of subjects with increased LV mass and, because of its adverse prognostic value *(3,50,53)*, with potentially increased cardiovascular risk.

White et al. used a restrictive definition of white coat hypertension (i.e., average daytime ambulatory BP < 130/80 mmHg) and found normal values of LV

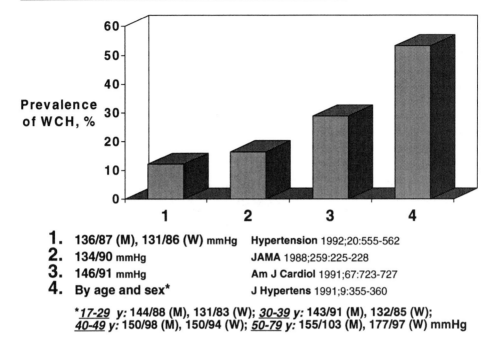

1. **136/87 (M), 131/86 (W)** mmHg   **Hypertension** 1992;20:555-562
2. **134/90** mmHg   **JAMA** 1988;259:225-228
3. **146/91** mmHg   **Am J Cardiol** 1991;67:723-727
4. **By age and sex***   **J Hypertens** 1991;9:355-360

   ***17-29** y:* **144/88 (M), 131/83 (W);** ***30-39** y:* **143/91 (M), 132/85 (W);**
   ***40-49** y:* **150/98 (M), 150/94 (W);** ***50-79** y:* **155/103 (M), 177/97 (W) mmHg**

Fig. 3. The bars show the prevalence of white coat hypertension according to the different criteria used to make diagnosis. Data from ref. *32*.

mass in these subjects *(31)*. Kuwajima et al. used a more liberal definition of white coat hypertension (i.e., average 24-h systolic BP < 140 mmHg, regardless of values of diastolic BP) and found an increased LV mass in 20 subjects with white coat hypertension compared with a normotensive control group *(34)*. Cardillo et al. *(35)* found a greater LV mass in a group of 20 subjects with white coat hypertension than in a control normotensive group, but the average daytime ambulatory BP was 12/13% higher in the group with white coat hypertension than in the normotensive group; hence, the different LV mass in the two groups might reflect the association between ambulatory BP and LV mass in the normotensive range *(54)*.

Overall, the normalcy of ambulatory BP and LV mass in the subjects with white coat hypertension suggests that their risk of future cardiovascular complications is potentially low.

In order to investigate the prognostic significance of white coat hypertension in the setting of the PIUMA study *(3)*, we followed for up to 7.5 yr 1187 adult subjects with essential hypertension and 205 healthy normotensive controls who had had baseline off-therapy 24-h noninvasive ABPM. The prevalence of white coat hypertension was 19.2%. Cardiovascular morbidity (number of combined fatal and nonfatal cardiovascular events per 100 patient-years), was 0.47 in the

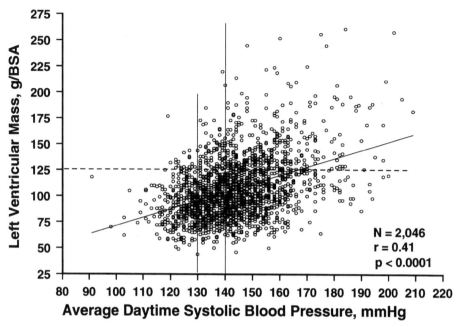

Fig. 4. The plot shows the association between average daytime ambulatory blood pressure and left ventricular mass at echocardiography in 2046 untreated subjects with essential hypertension (PIUMA database).

normotensive group, 0.49 in the group with white coat hypertension, 1.79 in dippers with ambulatory hypertension, and 4.99 in nondippers with ambulatory hypertension. After correcting for traditional risk factors, cardiovascular morbidity did not differ between the normotensive group and the group with white coat hypertension ($p = 0.83$). These data showed for the first time that cardiovascular morbidity is lower in white coat than in ambulatory hypertension and not dissimilar between white coat hypertension and clinical normotension.

Preliminary prospective data from the Cornell study seem to point in the same direction by showing a lesser cardiovascular morbidity in subjects with white coat hypertension than in those with ambulatory hypertension (11).

In a more recent analysis of the PIUMA database (24), including about 1500 hypertensive subjects followed for a mean of 4 yr and 157 major cardiovascular morbid events, the subgroup with white coat hypertension was divided up into 2 subsets with average daytime ABP < 130/80 mmHg or with intermediate values between 130/80 mmHg and 131/86 mmHg in women or 136/87 mmHg in men. Figure 5 shows that the rate of major cardiovascular morbid events, expressed per 100 persons per year, was 0.46 in a control group composed by healthy normotensive subjects, 0.67 in the white coat hypertension group defined more restrictively, 1.72 in the white coat hypertension group defined more liberally,

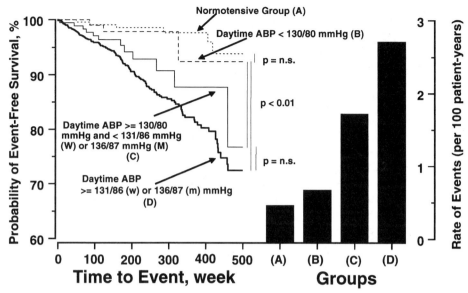

Fig. 5. The figure shows the rate of major cardiovascular morbid events in a normotensive group (A), two groups with white coat hypertension defined using a restrictive (B) or liberal (C) criterion, and a group with ambulatory hypertension (D). Reproduced with permission *(24)*.

and 2.71 in the group with ambulatory hypertension. These differences were not significant between the normotensive group and the group with white coat hypertension defined more restrictively, whereas they were significant between the normotensive group and the white coat hypertension group defined more liberally. These data support the use of a restrictive definition of white coat hypertension (i.e., average daytime ABP < 130/80 mmHg), in order to identify the minority of subjects not at increased risk of cardiovascular morbid events when compared with the normotensive subjects.

In this setting, a document issued by the American Society of Hypertension *(55)* suggests using restrictive upper limits to define normalcy of ambulatory BP (i.e., average daytime BP < 135 mmHg systolic and 85 mmHg diastolic). Also, the results of the PAMELA study, a cross-sectional study in a large general-population sample in northern Italy, suggest that the upper normal limits of daytime ABP should be set around 130 mmHg systolic and 80–85 mmHg diastolic *(56)*.

Khattar et al. *(12)* have recently completed a follow-up study of 479 patients examined with intra-arterial 24-h BP monitoring before the institution of therapy. It is widely established that intra-arterial blood pressure monitoring is the gold standard for BP measurement, although it is unsuitable for general clinical practice and most epidemiological studies. Khattar et al. defined white coat hypertension using an average 24-h ABP < 140/90 mmHg and found it in 26% of their patients. Over the subsequent follow-up period (9.1 yr on average), the rate of cardiovascular morbid events was 1.32 per 100 patient-years in the white coat hypertension group and 2.56 in the ambulatory hypertension group. These differences remained significant after adjustment for age, gender, race, and smoking, whereas clinic BP did not yield significance to enter the final multivariate model.

This important study merits two comments. First, the definition of white coat hypertension may not be comparable with that used in noninvasive ABPM studies because intra-arterial BP averages may be higher than those resulting from noninvasive monitoring possibly because the former are taken under fully ambulant conditions (57). Hence, it would be incorrect to extend such a definition to studies using the noninvasive ABPM. Second, despite the absence of a normotensive control group, the risk of cardiovascular complications was substantially lower in the subset with white coat hypertension than in that with ambulatory hypertension, thus confirming the results of studies with noninvasive ABPM.

For the time being, it is reasonable to consider the possibility that antihypertensive drug treatment may be useless in many subjects with white coat hypertension. Fagard et al. have shown that in subjects with high clinic BP and normal ambulatory BP, the antihypertensive drug treatment fails to reduce ambulatory BP (58) and this point is important since the reduction of target organ damage is more closely associated with the changes in ambulatory BP than with the changes in clinic BP (53,59–61).

We should not forget, however, that some of the subjects with white coat hypertension may have concomitant independent risk factors such as diabetes, cigaret smoking, elevated cholesterol levels, or a family history of premature coronary artery disease. Withholding drug treatment in these subjects on the basis of a low ambulatory BP in the setting of a high clinic BP may not be acceptable in the absence of convincing epidemiological evidence about the safety of such an intervention.

Therefore, although recognizing the importance of prospective intervention studies in white coat hypertension aimed at testing the equivalence of a no-drug regimen with a standard regimen based on clinic BP, we (49) proposed a temporary verdict of innocence for this categorization of low-risk subjects with essential hypertension, on condition of a correct definition, absence of important comorbid conditions, and adequate follow-up.

WHITE COAT EFFECT

The measurement of BP in the clinical environment may trigger an alerting reaction leading to a pressor rise in the patient (62,63). The rise in intra-arterial BP during the clinical visit is, on average, 27/14 mmHg; it is maximal during the first 4 min of the visit, disappears within about 10 min and persists over several visits *(64,65)*, even under treatment *(66)*. The transient rise in BP from before to during the visit is usually referred to as "white coat effect" or "white coat phenomenon," whereas the coexistence of persistently high clinic BP with normal ABP is often referred to as white coat hypertension.

Contrary to a commonly perceived feeling, white coat effect and white coat hypertension are different entities that markedly differ in their definition, pathophysiologic mechanisms, and clinical significance. The former is a measure of BP change from before to during the visit *(64,65)*, whereas the latter is an attempt to define a low-risk stratum of clinically hypertensive subjects with normal BP levels out of the medical setting *(49,67)*.

A reliable estimate of the white coat effect is possible through intra-arterial or noninvasive techniques that allow a beat-by-beat measurement of the BP rise from immediately before to during the visit. The white coat effect has also been estimated by the difference between clinic BP and average daytime ambulatory BP, based on the unproved assumption that average daytime ambulatory BP reflects the BP immediately before the visit. Parati et al. demonstrated that there is no association between the BP rise from before to during the visit, determined beat-to-beat using the Finapres method, and the difference between clinic and daytime ambulatory BP *(68)*.

In a recent analysis of the PIUMA database *(6)*, we addressed the prognostic significance of the clinic–ambulatory BP difference in a large cohort of subjects with essential hypertension. During a follow-up period of up to 9 yr, there were 157 major cardiovascular morbid events, 32 of which were fatal. The rate of total cardiovascular morbid events (Fig. 6) did not differ (log-rank test) among the four quartiles of the distribution of the clinic–ambulatory BP difference. Also, the rate of fatal cardiovascular events did not differ among the four quartiles of the distribution of the clinic–ambulatory BP difference. These data indicate that the clinic–ambulatory BP difference, taken as a measure of the white coat effect, is not a predictor of cardiovascular morbidity and mortality in subjects with essential hypertension.

The prognostic significance of the true white coat effect, defined as the rise in BP from before to during the visit as detected with intra-arterial or noninvasive beat-to-beat BP monitoring, has not yet been established.

DAY–NIGHT BLOOD PRESSURE CHANGES

The blood pressure shows cyclical fluctuations in humans, with different and superimposed periods and amplitudes. The fluctuations may last seconds to minutes or may last longer (diurnal variability, seasonal variability). The investigation of short-term variability, which has been made possible by using the invasive beat-to-beat monitoring, disclosed three major frequency components: high frequency (0.14–0.40 Hz, linked to respiratory rate), mid-frequency (0.07–0.14 Hz,

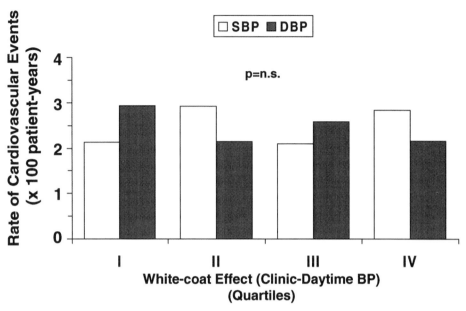

Fig. 6. The bars show the rate of cardiovascular morbid events in the four quartiles of the distribution of the white coat effect, expressed as the difference between office blood pressure and average daytime ambulatory blood pressure. Data from ref. *(6)*.

corresponding to the classic Mayer waves, and related to sympathetic activity), and low-frequency (0.02–0.07 Hz, linked to a variety of cardio-respiratory mechanisms) *(69)*. BP fluctuations occurring with frequencies less than 0.02 Hz (very low frequency) are largely unexplained *(70)*.

As far as the day–night BP variability is concerned, we know from the classic invasive studies by the Oxford and Milan groups that the BP falls by approximately 20–25% from day to night *(71–73)*.

In the last few years, 24-h noninvasive ambulatory BP monitoring has been increasingly used to investigate the diurnal BP changes associated with the sleep–wake cycle. Usually, the 24-h interval is divided into two periods of day and night (or wakefulness and sleep), and daytime and nighttime BP averages are then calculated. Day and night may be defined using the waking and sleeping periods as resulting from the patient's diary, or through arbitrarily defined fixed time intervals, both wide (0600–2200 h and 2200–0060 h) and narrow (1000–2000 h and midnight to 0600 h). The use of narrow fixed intervals excludes the morning and evening transitional periods, during which a variable proportion of subjects actually is awake or asleep, and may be preferable to wide fixed time intervals because it gives more accurate estimates of the actual BP values during sleep and wakefulness, at least in subjects going to bed and arising in reasonably well-defined time intervals *(74–76)*.

A potential objection to the use of noninvasive ambulatory BP monitoring is that frequent cuff inflations could disturb sleep *(77)*, with consequent possible overestimation of nighttime BP. Independent laboratories, however, have shown *(78,79)* that the intra-arterial BP profile is similar in the absence and in the presence of concomitant noninvasive BP monitoring.

The dippers–nondippers classification is based on the hypothesis that for any given value of daytime BP, target organ damage and prognosis may be worse when the BP load is persistent throughout the 24 h than when it is limited to the daytime hours. This terminology was first introduced by O'Brien et al. *(80)*, who noted a more frequent history of stroke in nondippers than in dippers.

Generally, nondippers are defined by a reduction in systolic and diastolic BP (or in mean arterial pressure) by less that x from day to night, whereas dippers are defined by a reduction in systolic or diastolic BP by more than x. The suggested value of x may range from 10% *(81)*, or 10/5 mmHg *(80)*, up to 0% (i.e., no reduction at all in BP from day to night, or higher BP during the night than during the day). Of course, the prevalence of nondippers varied among different studies, depending on the definitions of day and night and of the division line between dippers and nondippers *(82)*.

Like all categorizations of continuous variables, the dipper–nondipper classification is open to criticism because it implies a dicotomization of a continuous value and also because the definitions of day and night and that of the partition line between dippers and nondippers are arbitrary. However, such a classification seems to be surviving critiques because a large body of evidence is showing that not only LV hypertrophy *(81,83–86)* but also silent cerebrovascular disease *(87,88)*, stroke *(80)*, microalbuminuria *(89,90)*, and progression of renal damage *(91)* are greater in subjects with blunted reduction in BP from day to night than in those with normal nocturnal BP reduction. Some years ago, we found that for every given value of ambulatory BP, LV mass was greater in nondippers than in dippers in women, but not in men *(92)*, and these findings have been confirmed by Schmieder et al. *(86)*. However, as correctly pointed out by Fagard et al. *(93)*, only a small part of the variance of LV mass is directly accounted for by its relationship with the day–night BP change.

In our experience, a greater LV mass in nondippers than in dippers was found only in hypertensive patients with increased ambulatory BP values, but not in normotensive subjects or in subjects with white coat hypertension *(94)*. In another study by our group *(95)*, the number and complexity of ventricular arrhythmias in never-treated hypertensive patients were greater in nondippers than in dippers also, after adjustment for the differences in LV mass, which was greater in nondippers than in dippers.

Rizzoni et al. *(83)* showed that not only LV mass but also peripheral vascular changes are greater in nondippers than in dippers, and these data have been confirmed in another laboratory *(96)*. A Japanese group found that the cerebral lacunae

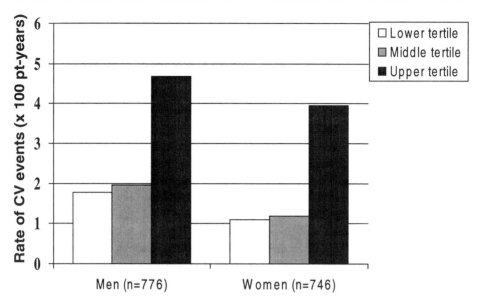

Fig. 7. The bars show the rate of major cardiovascular morbid events in the three tertiles of the distribution of the night–day ratio of systolic blood pressure. Data from ref. *(4)*.

detected with magnetic resonance, a possible expression of silent ischemia, are increased in nondippers than in dippers *(87,88)*. The number of lacunae had a J-shaped appearance, with an increase of lacunae in extreme dippers as compared with dippers *(88)*, probably as a result of nocturnal hypotension with consequent cerebral ischemia as a result of defective autoregulation of cerebral blood flow.

When dippers and nondippers are compared, proper covariance should be arranged for imbalances between the groups in the average 24-h ambulatory BP. If the two groups are matched by daytime BP only, the average 24-h values will be higher in nondippers than in dippers. We found that women who are non-dippers have a greater LV mass than their dippers counterparts also, after adjustment for 24-h BP, whereas no significant difference was detected in men after correcting for daytime or 24-h BP values *(97)*.

In the PIUMA study *(3)*, among subjects with ambulatory hypertension, women who were nondippers at the baseline evaluation had a higher cardiovascular morbidity during follow-up than dippers, and this difference held after adjustment for the other independent covariates in a Cox proportional hazard model. A not significant (possibly reflecting a type II error) trend in the same direction was found in men *(3)*. In order to further examine this point, we recently reanalyzed our database *(4)* in order to assess the relation between cardiovascular morbidity and the night–day BP ratio, a continuous way of expressing the nocturnal BP reduction. The rate of cardiovascular events increased markedly from the second to the third tertile of the night–day ratio of systolic and diastolic BP (Fig. 7).

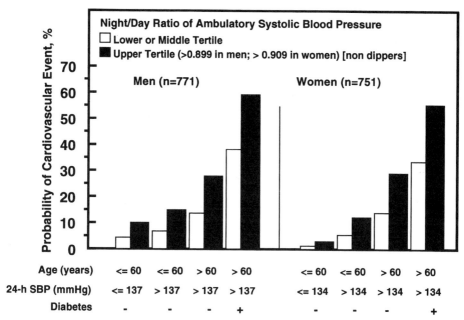

Fig. 8. The bars show the probability of a major cardiovascular morbid event in dippers and nondippers (nondippers defined by a night–day ratio of systolic blood pressure in the upper tertile) at different levels of concomitant risk markers. Data from ref. *(4)*.

The adverse predictive value of a blunted nocturnal reduction in BP (night–day ratio of systolic BP >0.90 in men and >0.91 in women) remained significant after adjustment for other independent covariates, including age, diabetes, and 24-h systolic BP (Fig. 8). These results confirm that the worse outcome in non-dippers is independent of the average 24-h levels of ambulatory BP.

Other studies support the adverse prognostic significance of a blunted day–night rhythm of BP. In the Ohasama study, Ohkubo et al. *(20)* found an increased cardiovascular mortality in nondippers (relative risk 2.56, $p = 0.02$) and inverted dippers (relative risk 3.69, $p = 0.04$) in comparison with dippers.

In a small study carried out in 116 hypertensive subjects followed for an average of 31 mo, Zweiker et al. *(13)* noted a significantly higher rate of cardiovascular complications in nondippers than in dippers.

Similar findings have been obtained by Suzuki et al. in a Japanese elderly population *(14)*. These authors found that age >75 yr, the male sex and a nondipping pattern (relative risk vs dippers: 2.9) were independent predictors of 25 total cardiovascular events in 132 elderly subjects followed for an average of 4 yr *(14)*.

In another study from Japan *(15)*, 105 patients with a symptomatic lacunar infarct were studied with 24-h ABPM and followed for a mean of 3.2 yr. The magnitude of the reduction in BP from day to night at the baseline assessment was significantly smaller in the group with future cerebrovascular events than in that with no future events and no development of silent lacunae.

Taken together, all these findings indicate that the assessment of day–night BP variability through the use of 24-h noninvasive ABPM is important from a clinical standpoint in subjects with hypertension because it allows an improvement in cardiovascular risk stratification provided by clinic BP and other traditional risk markers.

Because 24-h ABPM is the only practical way to assess the circadian rhythm of BP, the results of these prognostic studies should have considerable bearing on future guidelines regarding indications for ABPM in the clinical practice.

ULTRADIAN BLOOD PRESSURE VARIABILITY

Several years ago, Parati et al. found that for every given value of ambulatory BP, the frequency and severity of target organ damage were greater in association with a high BP variability than with a low BP variability (98). These findings were confirmed by Palatini et al. (85) in a study with noninvasive ABPM.

We have recently investigated (99) the association between ultradian BP variability (standard deviation of ambulatory BP averages, one reading every 15 min during the day and night) and LV mass in 1822 untreated hypertensive subjects from the PIUMA database. Subjects were divided into quartiles of the distribution of average 24-h SBP. Within each quartile, the subjects with a standard deviation of daytime and nighttime SBP below or above the median were classified at low or high BP variability. Within each quartile, LV mass did not differ between the groups at low SBP variability versus those at high SBP variability (all p = n.s.). Overall, age-adjusted LV mass was 115 and 115 g/m^2 in men at low and high daytime SBP variability (p = n.s.), and 116 and 114 g/m^2 in men at low and high nighttime SBP variability (p = n.s.). Corresponding values in women were 98 and 99 g/m^2 (p = 0.53) and 98 and 99 g/m^2 (p =n.s.). These findings suggest that when the effects of age and average 24-h BP are taken into account, short-term BP variability assessed with noninvasive BP monitoring is unrelated to LV mass in subjects with essential hypertension.

We have also used the PIUMA database to assess the prognostic significance of ultradian BP variability (49). The rate of major cardiovascular morbid events was higher in the subjects with a high variability of daytime and nighttime systolic BP (defined as the standard deviation of daytime, or nighttime, systolic BP above the group mean) than in those with low variability. However, this difference did not remain significant in a Cox multivariate analysis after correction for age, diabetes, previous cardiovascular events, and ambulatory BP (5).

On the basis of these findings it is not possible to speculate whether an increased BP variability is a cause or simply an index of target organ damage. Vascular structural changes may reduce baroceptor sensitivity in subjects with hypertension (100) and the inverse relation between BP variability and baroceptor sensitivity *(101,102)* seems to be independent of the reduction in baroceptor sensitivity associated with BP and age *(101)*. A unifying explanation could be that the overall impact of factors associated with vascular damage and reduced baroceptor sensitivity such as aging, severity of hypertension and diabetes could be reflected by a rise in BP variability detectable with noninvasive BP monitoring.

Anyway, the univariate association between BP variability and cardiovascular morbid events was largely spurious and resulting from the overwhelming predictive effect of age, BP, diabetes mellitus, and previous cardiovascular morbid events, all potential markers of increased vascular damage and reduced baroceptor sensitivity. The possible prognostic advantage of beat-to-beat techniques for assessment of the BP variability remains to be determined.

AMBULATORY HEART RATE

There is strong evidence of an association between resting heart rate and subsequent incidence of cardiovascular and noncardiovascular complications *(103)*. According to these findings, tachycardia should not be considered simply a benign marker of short-lived anxiety triggered by the clinical visit, but a clinically relevant risk marker *(103)*.

In subjects with essential hypertension, a 36-yr follow-up analysis from the Framingham Study showed that resting heart rate is an independent risk marker for all-cause mortality and, to a lesser extent, cardiovascular mortality *(104)*. However, clinic heart rate is highly variable becauase the alerting reaction to the visit evokes not only a BP rise but also a tachycardic effect, which may vary considerably from patient to patient *(64,65)*.

Consequently, we have analyzed the PIUMA database *(7)* in order to investigate the association between clinic and ambulatory heart rate with cardiovascular and noncardiovascular complications. For an average of 3.6 yr, we followed 1942 initially untreated and uncomplicated subjects with essential hypertension and all subjects underwent simultaneous assessment of ambulatory BP and heart rate, one reading every 15 min for 24 h. During follow-up, there were 74 deaths from all causes (1.06 per 100 person-years) and 182 total (fatal + nonfatal) cardiovascular morbid events (2.66 per 100 person-years). There was no association between clinic, average 24-h, daytime, and nighttime heart rate and total mortality. However, the subjects who subsequently died showed a blunted reduction of heart rate from day to night at the baseline examination. After adjustment for age, diabetes, and average 24-h systolic BP, for each 10% reduction in the heart rate from day to night, the risk of mortality increased by 30% (95% CI: 2–65; $p = 0.04$). Death rates were 0.38, 0.71, 0.94, and 2.00 per 100 person-years in the four quartiles of the distribution of the percent reduction in heart rate from day to night. For every given level of clinic heart rate or average 24-h heart rate, the all-cause mortality increased with the progressive flattening of the 24-h heart-rate profile (Fig. 9).

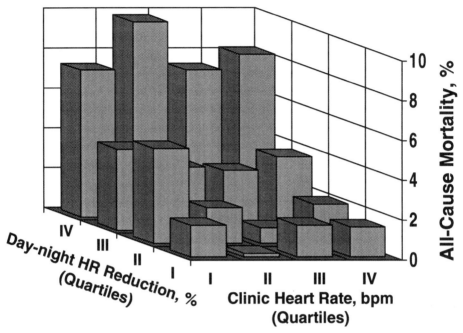

Fig. 9. The bars show the rate of fatal events in the four quartiles of the distribution of office heart rate and of the reduction in heart rate from day to night. Reproduced with permission *(7)*.

How can we explain the lack of association between clinic or ambulatory heart rate and prognosis? First, the relatively short duration of follow-up (3.6 yr on average) could have precluded the disclosure of such an association. An increase in the heart rate might require a long time to produce major clinical complications. Furthermore, clinic and ambulatory BP and heart rate values at entry were significantly higher in the subjects who were subsequently given β-blockers during follow-up, as compared with those who were not. It is known that β-blockers might retard progression of atherosclerosis *(105,106)* and exert a primary prevention of cardiovascular complications *(107)*. In our study, the preferential administration of β-blockers to the more tachycardic subjects may have interfered with the possible relation between tachycardia and adverse prognosis. In this setting, it is interesting to note that most of the studies that showed an association between heart rate and prognosis had been carried out when β-blockers were not available for clinical use. Finally, we excluded subjects with concomitant heart disease by using echocardiography in the majority of subjects and other diagnostic tools, including radionuclide techniques and coronary angiography when clinically indicated. Hence, more subjects with subclinical heart disease, possibly reflected by tachycardia, could have been excluded from our study but included in the previous studies showing an association between tachycardia and adverse cardiovascular events.

From a pathophysiological standpoint, a blunted circadian rhythm of heart rate may reflect a lesser ability of heart rate to accelerate in response to sympathetic stimulation and/or a lesser ability of the heart rate to decelerate in response to vagal stimulation. Of course, we could not establish whether alterations of the sympatho-vagal balance were prognostic determinants in our study.

A blunted tachycardic response to an exercise test, which might be considered an analog to a blunted heart rate increase from night to day, identified a subset of apparently healthy subjects at increased risk of mortality (108). In a study in elderly individuals, subjects with higher ratings for subcortical gray matter hyperintensities showed a smaller fall in heart rate from day to night (109).

In conclusion, we suggest that a flattened diurnal rhythm of heart rate can be considered a novel adverse risk marker, which merits further epidemiological assessment.

AMBULATORY PULSE PRESSURE

An important basic mechanism of the rise in pulse pressure with age is believed to be the progressive stiffening of large elastic arteries (110–112). A significant association has been noted in several studies between pulse pressure and subsequent rate of cardiovascular morbid events and such an association was independent of systolic and diastolic BP (113–117). In a previous study from our laboratory, such an association was also independent of LV mass at echocardiography and white coat hypertension (3).

However, pulse pressure may be affected by the alerting reaction evoked by the clinical visit. Mancia et al. (64,65) showed that the rise in intra-arterial systolic and diastolic BP during the physician's visit is 4–75 mmHg (mean, 27) and 1–36 mmHg (mean, 15), respectively. The larger rise in systolic than diastolic BP implies an increase in pulse pressure of about 12 mmHg from before to during the visit. Hence, the clinic pulse pressure may overestimate the usual levels of pulse pressure. In this setting, some cross-sectional studies suggest that ambulatory pulse pressure correlates with organ damage more closely than clinic pulse pressure does (22,118,119). In order to investigate the prognostic value of ambulatory pulse pressure, we followed for an average of 3.8 yr, 2010 initially untreated and uncomplicated subjects with essential hypertension from the PIUMA database (8). The rate of total cardiovascular events (per 100 persons per year) in the 3 tertiles of the distribution of office pulse pressure was 1.38, 2.12, and 4.34, respectively, and that of fatal events was 0.12, 0.30, and 1.07 (log-rank test: both $p < 0.01$). In the three tertiles of the distribution of average 24-h pulse pressure, the rate of total cardiovascular events was 1.19, 1.81, and 4.92, and that of fatal events was 0.11, 0.17, and 1.23 (log-rank test: both $p < 0.01$). After controlling for the effect of concomitant risk factors, survival data were better fitted by the model containing ambulatory pulse pressure than by that containing clinic pulse pressure. In each of the three tertiles of clinic pulse pressure, cardiovascular

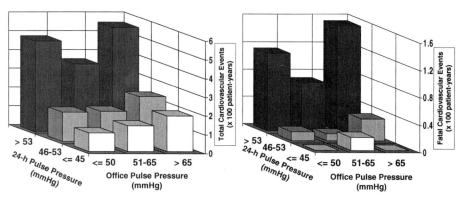

Fig. 10. The bars show the rate of total (left) and fatal (right) cardiovascular morbid events in the three tertiles of the distribution of office and average 24-h pulse pressure. Reproduced with permission *(8)*.

morbidity and mortality (Fig. 10) increased from the first to the third tertile of average 24-h ambulatory pulse pressure (log-rank test: all *p* < 0.01).

These data indicate that the alerting reaction to office BP measurement weakens the relation between pulse pressure and total cardiovascular risk, and that ambulatory pulse pressure provides a more precise estimate of risk.

This and other *(3,113–117)* demonstrations of the prognostic value of pulse pressure provide a strong rationale to investigate in prospective outcome trials whether pulse pressure is equivalent or superior to systolic and diastolic BP as a guide for antihypertensive strategy.

CONCLUSIONS

Inspection of Table 2 shows the dramatic rise of prognostic studies with ABPM published over the last few years. Other important prognostic studies *(21,22)* are about to be completed. Thus, we may anticipate that a consensus will be probably reached over the next few years on how to interpret the results of ABPM in order to get the best prognostic information from this procedure.

With ABPM, we now stand at a step similar to that we get reached several years ago with clinic BP, when the results of observational studies on the prognostic value of clinic BP justified the execution of the first intervention studies in patients with severe hypertension. Now, the stage is set for intervention studies with ABPM. We should urgently begin studies aimed to determine if the following hold:

- A standard management, based solely on clinic BP, is equivalent (in terms of progression of organ damage and, hopefully, prognosis) to a no-drug management in low-risk subjects with white coat hypertension.
- A standard management, based solely on clinic BP and without any execution of ABPM, is superior (in terms of progression of organ damage and, hopefully, prognosis) to a management targeted on results of ABPM.

ACKNOWLEDGMENTS

We gratefully thank Mr. Paolo De Luca and Mr. Mariano Cecchetti for their nurse and technical assistance.

REFERENCES

1. Perloff D, Sokolow M, Cowan R. The prognostic value of ambulatory blood pressure. JAMA 1983;249:2792–2798.
2. Perloff D, Sokolow M, Cowan RM, Juster RP. Prognostic value of ambulatory blood pressure measurements: further analyses. J Hypertens 1989;7(Suppl 3):S3–S10.
3. Verdecchia P, Porcellati C, Schillaci G, Borgioni C, Ciucci A, Battistelli M, et al. Ambulatory blood pressure: an independent predictor of prognosis in essential hypertension. Hypertension 1994;24:793–801.
4. Verdecchia P, Schillaci G, Borgioni C, Ciucci A, Gattobigio R, Porcellati C. Nocturnal pressure is the true pressure. Blood Pressure Monit 1996;1(Suppl 2):S81–S85.
5. Verdecchia P, Borgioni C, Ciucci A, Gattobigio R, P, Schillaci G, Sacchi N, et al. Prognostic significance of blood pressure variability in essential hypertension. Blood Pressure Monit 1996;1:3–11.
6. Verdecchia P, Schillaci G, Borgioni C, Ciucci A, Porcellati C. Prognostic significance of the white-coat effect. Hypertension 1997;29:1218–1224.
7. Verdecchia P, Schillaci G, Borgioni C, Ciucci A, Telera MP, Pede S, et al. Adverse prognostic value of a blunted circadian rhythm of heart rate in essential hypertension. J Hypertens 1998;16:1335–1343.
8. Verdecchia P, Schillaci G, Borgioni C, Ciucci A, Pede S, Porcellati C. Ambulatory pulse pressure. A potent predictor of total cardiovascular risk in hypertension. Hypertension 1998; 32:983–988.
9. Verdecchia P. Clinical significance of day-night blood pressure changes in essential hypertension. Ther Res 1996;17:4600–4611.
10. Verdecchia P, Schillaci G, Gatteschi C, Zampi I, Battistelli M, Bartoccini C, et al. Blunted nocturnal fall in blood pressure in hypertensive women with future cardiovascular morbid events. Circulation 1993;88:986–992.
11. Pickering TG, James GD. Ambulatory blood pressure and prognosis. J Hypertens 1994; 12(Suppl 8):S29–S33.
12. Khattar RS, Senior R, Lahiri A. Cardiovascular outcome in white-coat versus sustained mild hypertension: a 10 year follow-up study. Circulation 1998;98:1892–1897.
13. Zweiker R, Eber B, Schumacher M, Toplak H, Klein W. "Non dipping" related to cardiovascular events in essential hypertensive patients. Acta Med Austriaca 1994;21:86–89.
14. Suzuki Y, Kuwajima I, Aono T, Toyoshima T, Ozawa T. Prognostic value of ambulatory blood pressure in elderly hypertensive patients: dipper vs nondipper. Abstract 16th Scientific Meeting of the International Society of Hypertension, June 1996, p. S381 (abstract).
15. Yamamoto Y, Akiguchi I, Oiwa K, Hayashi M, Kimura J. Adverse effect of nighttime blood pressure on the outcome of lacunar infarct patients. Stroke 1998;29:570–576.
16. Redon J, Campos C, Narciso ML, Rodicio JL, Pascual JM, Ruilope LM. Prognostic value of ambulatory blood pressure monitoring in refractory hypertension. A prospective study. Hypertension 1998;31:712–718.
17. Ohkubo T, Imai Y, Tsuji I, Nagai K, Kato J, Kikuchi N, et al. Home blood pressure measurement has a stronger predictive power for mortality than does screening blood pressure: a population-based observation in Ohasama, Japan. J Hypertens 1998;16:971–975.
18. Imai Y, Ohkubo T, Tsuji I, Nagai K, Satoh H, Hisamichi S, et al. Prognostic value of ambulatory and home blood pressure measurements in comparison to screening blood pressure measurements: a pilot study in Ohasama. Blood Pressure Monit 1996;1(Suppl 2):S51–S58.

19. Ohkubo T, Imai Y, Tsuji I, Nagai K, Watanabe N, Minami N, et al. Prediction of mortality by ambulatory blood pressure monitoring versus screening blood pressure measurements: a pilot study in Ohasama. J Hypertens 1997;15:357–364.

20. Ohkubo T, Imai Y, Tsuji I, Nagai K, Watanabe N, Minami N, et al. Relation between nocturnal decline in blood pressure and mortality. The Ohasama study. Am J Hypertens 1997;10: 1201–1207.

21. Clement DL, De Buyzere M, on behalf of the OvA investigators. Office versus Ambulatory (OvA) recording of blood pressure, a European multicenter study: inclusion and early follow-up characteristics. Blood Pressure Monit 1998;3:167–172.

22. Zanchetti A, Bond G, Henning M, Neiss A, Mancia G, Dal Palù C, et al., on behalf of the ELSA investigators. Risk factors associated with alterations in carotid intima-media thickness in hypertension: baseline data from the European Lacidipine Study on Atherosclerosis. J Hypertens 1988;16:949–961.

23. Porcellati C, Verdecchia P, Schillaci G, Borgioni C, Ciucci A, Zampi I, et al. Prognostic impact of office underestimation of usual blood pressure in essential hypertension, submitted.

24. Verdecchia P, Schillaci G, Borgioni C, Ciucci A, Porcellati C. White-coat hypertension. Lancet 1996;348:1444–1445.

25. Khattar RS, Parsons A, Kinsey C, Senior R, Lahiri A. Ambulatory systolic blood pressure is superior to clinic measurement for the prediction of future cardiovascular events in essential hypertension: a 10-year follow-up study. Circulation 1998;96:I–337 (abstract).

26. Staessen JA, Thijs L, Fagard R, O'Brien ET, Clement D, de Leeuw PW, et al., for the Systolic Hypertension in Europe (Syst-Eur) Trial Investigators. Predicting cardiovascular risk using conventional vs ambulatory blood pressure in older patients with systolic hypertension. JAMA 1999;282:539–546

27. Verdecchia P, Schillaci G, Borgioni C, Ciucci A, Zampi I, Battistelli M, et al. Cigarette smoking, ambulatory blood pressure and cardiac hypertrophy in essential hypertension. J Hypertens 1995;13:1209–1215.

28. Guidelines Sub-Committee. 1993 guidelines for the management of mild hypertension: memorandum from a World Health Organization/International Society of Hypertension meeting. J Hypertens 1993;11:905–918.

29. Joint National Committee on Detection, Evaluation and Treatment of High Blood Pressure. The Sixth Report of the Joint National Committee on Detection, Evaluation and Treatment of High Blood Pressure (JNC VI). National Institute of Health, Washington, DC, 1997.

30. Pickering TG, James GD, Boddie C, Harshfield GA, Blank S, Laragh JH. How common is white-coat hypertension? JAMA 1988;259:225–228.

31. White WB, Schulman P, McCabe EJ, Dey HM. Average daily blood pressure, not office pressure, determines cardiac function in patients with hypertension. JAMA 1989;261: 873–877.

32. Verdecchia P, Schillaci G, Boldrini F, Zampi I, Porcellati C. Variability between current definitions of 'normal' ambulatory blood pressure. Implications in the assessment of white-coat hypertension. Hypertension 1992;20:555–562.

33. Pierdomenico SD, Lapenna D, Guglielmi MD, Antidormi T, Schiavone C, Cuccurullo F, et al. Target organ status and serum lipids in patients with white-coat hypertension. Hypertension 1995;26:801–807.

34. Kuwajima I, Miyao M, Uno A, Suzuki Y, Matsushita S, Kuramoto K. Diagnostic value of electrocardiography and echocardiography for white-coat hypertension in the elderly. Am J Cardiol 1994;73:1232–1234.

35. Cardillo C, De Felice F, Campia U, Folli G. Psychophysiological reactivity and cardiac end-organ changes in white-coat hypertension. Hypertension 1993;21:836–844.

36. Cerasola G, Cottone S, Nardi E, D'Ignoto G, Volpe V, Mulè G, et al. White-coat hypertension and cardiovascular risk. J Cardiovasc Risk 1995;2:545–549.

37. Glen SK, Elliot HL, Curzio JL, Lees KR, Reid JL. White-coat hypertension as a cause of cardiovascular dysfunction. Lancet 1996;348:654–657.
38. Siegel WC, Blumenthal JA, Divine GW. Physiological, psycological and behavioural factors and white-coat hypertension. Hypertension 1990;16:140–146.
39. Weber MA, Neutel JM, Smith DHG, Graettinger WF. Diagnosis of mild hypertension by ambulatory blood pressure monitoring. Circulation 1994;90:2291–2298.
40. Hoegholm A, Kristensen KS, Bang LE, Nielsen JW, Nielsen WB, Madsen NH. Left ventricular mass and geometry in patients with established hypertension and white-coat hypertension. Am J Hypertens 1993;6:282–286.
41. Marchesi E, Perani G, Falaschi F, Negro C, Catalano O, Ravetta V, et al. Metabolic risk factors in white-coat hypertensives. J Hum Hyertens 1994;8:475–479.
42. Bidlingmeyer I, Burier M, Bidlingmeyer M, Waeber B, Brunner HR. Isolated office hypertension: a prehypertensive state? J Hypertens 1996;14:327–332.
43. Rizzo V, Cicconetti P, Bianchi A, Lorido A, Morelli S, Vetta F, et al. White-coat hypertension and cardiac organ damage in elderly subjects. J Hum Hypertens 1996;10:293–298.
44. Trenkwalder P, Plaschke M, Steffes-Tremer I, Lydtin H. "White-coat" hypertension and alerting reaction in elderly and very elderly hypertensive patients. Blood Pressure 1993;2: 262–271.
45. Staessen J, O'Brien E, Atkins N, Amery A. Short report: ambulatory blood pressure in normotensive compared with hypertensive subjects. J Hypertens 1993;11:1289–1297.
46. Amar J, Bieler L, Salvador M, Chamontin B. Intima-media thickness of carotid artery in white-coat and ambulatory hypertension. Arch Mal Coeur Vaiss 1997;90:1075–1078.
47. Cuspidi C, Marabini M, Lonati L, Sampieri L, Comerio G, Pelizzoli S, et al. Cardiac and carotid structure in patients with established hypertension and white-coat hypertension. J Hypertens 1995;13:1707–1711.
48. Polonia JJ, Santos AR, Gama GM, Basto F, Bettencourt PM, Martins LR. Follow-up clinic and ambulatory blood pressure in untreated white-coat hypertensive patients (evaluation after 2–5 years). Blood Pressure Monit 1997;2:289–295.
49. Verdecchia P, Schillaci G, Borgioni C, Ciucci A, Porcellati C. White-coat hypertension: not guilty when correctly defined. Blood Pressure Monit 1998;3:147–152.
50. Casale PN, Devereux RB, Milner M, Zullo G, Harshfield GA, Pickering TG, et al. Value of echocardiographic measurement of left ventricular mass in predicting cardiovascular morbid events in hypertensive men. Ann Intern Med 1986;105:173–178.
51. Koren MJ, Devereux RB, Casale PN, Savage DD, Laragh JH. Relation of left ventricular mass and geometry to morbidity and mortality in uncomplicated essential hypertension. Ann Intern Med 1991;114:345–352.
52. Levy D, Garrison RJ, Savage DD, Kannel WB, Castelli WP. Prognostic implications of echocardiographically determined left ventricular mass in the Framingham heart study. N Engl J Med 1990;322:1561–1566.
53. Verdecchia P, Schillaci G, Borgioni C, Ciucci A, Gattobigio R, Zampi I, et al. Prognostic significance of serial changes in left ventricular mass in essential hypertension. Circulation 1998;97:48–54.
54. Porcellati C, Schillaci G, Verdecchia P, Battistelli M, Bartoccini C, Zampi I, et al. Diurnal blood pressure changes and left ven-tricular mass: Influence of daytime blood pressure. High Blood Pressure 1993;2:249–258.
55. Pickering T, for an American Society of Hypertension Ad Hoc Panel. Recommendations for the use of home (self) and ambulatory blood pressure monitoring. Am J Hypertens 1996;9: 1–11.
56. Mancia G, Sega R, Bravi C, De Vito G, Valagussa F, Cesana G, et al. Ambulatory blood pressure normality: results from the PAMELA study. J Hypertens 1995;13:1377–1390.
57. Hunyor SN, Flynn JM, Cochineas C. Comparison of performance of various sphygmomanometers with intra-arterial blood pressuse recordings. Br Med J 1978;2:159–162.

58. Fagard RH, Bielen E, Staessen JA, Thijs L, Amery A. Response of ambulatory blood pressure to antihypertensive therapy guided by clinic pressure. Am J Hypertens 1993;6:648–653.
59. Porcellati C, Verdecchia P, Schillaci G, Boldrini F, Motolese M. Long-term effects of benazepril on ambulatory blood pressure, left ventricular mass, diastolic filling and aotic flow in essential hypertension. Int J Clin Pharmacol Ther Toxicol 1991;29:187–197.
60. Mancia G, Zanchetti A, Agabiti Rosei E, Benemio G, De Cesaris R, Fogari R, et al., for the SAMPLE Study Group. Ambulatory blood pressure is superior to clinic blood pressure in predicting treatment-induced regression of left ventricular hypertrophy. Circulation 1997;95: 1464–1470.
61. Fagard RH, Staessen J, Thijs L. Relationship between changes in left ventricular mass and in clinic and ambulatory blood pressure in response to antihypertensive therapy. J Hypertens 1997;15:1493–1502.
62. Riva Rocci S. La tecnica della sfigmomanometria. Gazz Med Torino 1897;10:181–191.
63. Ayman D, Goldshine AD. Blood pressure determinations by patients with essential hypertension: the difference between clinic and home readings before treatment. Am J Med Sci 1940; 200:465–474.
64. Mancia G, Bertineri G, Grassi G, Parati G, Pomidossi G, Ferrari A, et al. Effects of blood pressure measured by the doctor on patient's blood pressure and heart rate. Lancet 1983;2: 695–698.
65. Mancia G. Parati G, Pomidossi G, Grassi G, Casadei R, Zanchetti A. Alerting reaction and rise in blood pressure during measurement by physician and nurse. Hypertension 1987;9: 209–215.
66. Omboni S, Parati G, Santucciu C, Mutti E, Groppelli A, Trazzi S, et al. "White-coat" effect and patient's response to antihypertensive treatment. J Hypertens 1994;12(Suppl 3):S10 (abstract).
67. Pickering TG. White-coat hypertension in a changing era of medical care. Blood Pressure Monit 1996;1(Suppl 2):S27–S32.
68. Parati G, Ulian L, Santucciu C, Omboni S, Mancia G. The difference between clinic and daytime blood pressure is not a measure of the "white-coat effect." Hypertension 1998;31: 1185–1189.
69. Parati G, Saul JP, Di Rienzo M, Mancia G. Spectral analysis of blood pressure and heart rate variability in evaluating cardiovascular regulation: a critical reappraisal. Hypertension 1995; 25:1276–1286.
70. Malliani A, Pagani M, Lombardi F, Cerutti S. Cardiovascular neural regulation explored in the frequency domain. Circulation 1991;84(2):482–492.
71. Richardson DW, Honour AJ, Goodman AC. Changes in arterial pressure during sleep in man. Hypertension 1968;16:62–78.
72. Littler WA, West MJ, Honour AJ, Sleight P. The variability of arterial pressure. Am Heart J 1978;95:180–186.
73. Mancia G, Ferrari A, Gregorini L, et al. Blood pressure and heart rate variabilities in normotensive and hypertensive human beings. Circ Res 1983;53:96–104.
74. van Ittersum FJ, Ijzerman RG, Stehouwer CDA, Donker AJM. Analysis of twenty-four-hour ambulatory blood pressure monitoring: what time period to assess blood pressures during waking and sleeping? J Hypertens 1995;13:1053–1058.
75. Fagard R, Brguljan J, Thijs L, Staessen J. Prediction of the actual awake and asleep blood pressures by various methods of 24h pressure analysis. J Hypertens 1996;14:557–563.
76. Pickering TG. How should the diurnal changes of blood pressure be expressed? Am J Hypertens 1995;8:681–682.
77. Degaute J-P, van de Borne P, Kerkhofs M, Dramaix M, Linkowski P. Does non-invasive blood pressure monitoring disturb sleep? J Hypertens 1992;10:879–885.
78. Parati G, Pomidossi G, Casadei R, et al. Ambulatory blood pressure does not interfere with the haemodynamic effects of sleep. J Hypertens 1985;3(Suppl 2):S107–S109.

79. Brigden G, Broadhurst P, Cashman P, Raftery E. Effects of non-invasive ambulatory blood pressure devices on blood pressure. Am J Cardiol 1991;66:1396–1398.

80. O'Brien E, Sheridan J, O'Malley K. Dippers and non-dippers. Lancet 1988;2:397.

81. Verdecchia P, Schillaci G, Guerrieri M, et al. Circadian blood pressure changes and left ventricular hypertrophy in essential hypertension. Circulation 1990;81:528–536.

82. Verdecchia P, Porcellati C. Day–night changes of ambulatory blood pressure: another risk marker in essential hypertension? G Ital Cardiol 1992;22:879–886 (in Italian).

83. Rizzoni D, Muiesan ML, Montani G, Zulli R, Calebich S, Agabiti-Rosei E. Relationship between initial cardiovascular structural changes and daytime and nighttime blood pressure monitoring. Am J Hypertens 1992;5:180–186.

84. Kuwajima I, Suzuki Y, Shimosawa T, Kanemaru A, Hoshino S, Kuramoto K. Diminished nocturnal decline in blood pressure in elderly hypertensive patients with left ventricular hypertrophy. Am Heart J 1992;67:1307–1311.

85. Palatini P, Penzo M, Racioppa A, et al. Clinical relevance of nighttime blood pressure and of daytime blood pressure variability. Arch Intern Med 1992;152:1855–1860.

86. Schmieder RE, Rockstroh JK, Äpfelbacher F, Schulze B, Messerli FH. Gender-specific cardiovascular adaptation due to circadian blood pressure variations in essential hypertension. Am J Hypertens 1995;8:1160–1166.

87. Shimada K, Kawamoto A, Matsubayashi K, Nishinaga M, Kimura S, Ozawa T. Diurnal blood pressure variations and silent cerebrovascular damage in elderly patients with hypertension. J Hypertens 1992;10:875–878.

88. Kario K, Matsuo T, Kobayashi H, Imiya M, Matsuo M, Shimada K. Nocturnal fall of blood pressure and silent cerebrovascular damage in elderly hypertensive subjects: advanced silent cerebrovascular damage in extreme dippers. Hypertension 1996;27:130–135.

89. Redon J, Liao Y, Lozano JV, Miralles A, Pascual JM, Cooper RS. Ambulatory blood pressure and microalbuminuria in essential hypertension: role of circadian variability. J Hypertens 1994;12:947–953.

90. Bianchi S, Bigazzi R, Baldari G, Sgherri G, Campese VM. Diurnal variations of blood pressure and microalbuminuria in essential hypertension. Am J Hypertens 1994;7:23–29.

91. Timio M, Venanzi S, Lolli S, et al. Night-time blood pressure and progression of renal insufficiency. High Blood Pressure Cardiovasc Prev 1994;3:39–44.

92. Verdecchia P, Schillaci G, Boldrini F, Guerrieri M, Porcellati C. Sex, cardiac hypertrophy and diurnal blood pressure variations in essential hypertension. J Hypertens 1992;10:683–692.

93. Fagard RH, Staessen JA, Thijs L. The relationships between left ventricular mass and daytime and night-time blood pressures: a meta-analysis of comparative studies. J Hypertens 1995;13:823–829.

94. Porcellati C, Schillaci G, Verdecchia P, et al. Diurnal blood pressure changes and left ventricular mass: influence of daytime blood pressure. High Blood Pressure Cardiovasc Prev 1993;2:249–258.

95. Schillaci G, Verdecchia P, Borgioni C, et al. Association between persistent pressure overload and ventricular arrhythmias in essential hypertension. Hypertension 1996;28:284–289.

96. Pierdomenico SD, Guglielmi MD, Lapenna D, et al. Arterial disease in dippers and non-dippers. Am J Hypertens 1996;9:61A (abstract).

97. Verdecchia P, Schillaci G, Borgioni C, et al. Gender, day–night blood pressure changes and left ventricular mass in essential hypertension: dippers and peakers. Am J Hypertens 1995;8:193–196.

98. Parati G, Pomidossi G, Albini F, Malaspina D, Mancia G. Relationship of 24-h blood pressure mean and variability to severity of target organ damage in hypertension. J Hypertens 1987;5:93–98.

99. Schillaci G, Verdecchia P, Borgioni C, Ciucci A, Porcellati C. Lack of association between blood pressure variability and left ventricular mass in essential hypertension. Am J Hypertens 1998;11:515–522.

100. Angell-James JE. Characteristics of single aortic and right subclavian fiber activity in rabbits with chronic renal hypertension. Circ Res 1973;32:149–155.

101. Watson RDS, Stallard TJ, Flinn RM, Littler WA. Factors determining arterial pressure and its variability in hypertensive man. Hypertension 1980;2:333–341.

102. Floras JS, Hassan MO, Vann Jones J, Osikowska BA, Sever PS, Sleight P. Factors influencing blood pressure and heart rate variability in hypertensive humans. Hypertension 1988;11: 273–281.

103. Palatini P, Julius S. Heart rate and cardiovascular risk. J Hypertens 1997;15:3–17.

104. Gillam MW, Kannel WB, Belanger A, D'Agostino RB. Influence of heart rate on mortality among persons with hypertension: the Framingham study. Am Heart J 1993;125:1148–1154.

105. Beere PA, Glagov S, Zarins CK. Retarding effect of lowered heart rate on coronary atherosclerosis. Science 1984;226:180–182.

106. Kaplan JR, Manuck SB, Adams MR, Weingand KW, Clarkson TB. Inhibition of coronary atherosclerosis by propranolol in behaviorally predisposed monkeys fed an atherogenic diet. Circulation 1987;76:1364–1372.

107. Wikstrand J, Warnold I, Olsson G, Tuomilehto J, Elmfeldt D, Berglund G, on behalf of the Advisory Committee. Primary prevention with metoprolol in patients with hypertension. Mortality results from the MAPHY study. JAMA 1988;259:1976–1982.

108. Erikssen J, Rasmussen K, Forfang K, Storstein O. Exercise ECG and case history in the diagnosis of latent coronary heart disease among presumably healthy middle-aged men. Eur J Cardiol 1977;5:463–476.

109. Goldstein IB, Bartzokis G, Hance DB, Shapiro D. Relationship between blood pressure and subcortical lesions in healthy elderly people. Stroke 1998;29:765–772.

110. Sleight P. Blood pressures, hearts, and U-shaped curves. Lancet 1988;i:235.

111. Safar ME. Pulse pressure in essential hypertension: clinical and therapeutic implications. J Hypertens 1989;7:769–776.

112. Franklin SS, Sutton-Tyrrel K, Belle S, Weber M, Kuller LH. The importance of pulsatile components of hypertension in predicting carotid stenosis in older adults. J Hypertens 1997; 15:1143–1150.

113. Dyer AR, Stamler J, Shekelle RB, Schoenberger JA, Stamler R, Shekelle S, et al. Pulse pressure—III. Prognostic significance in four Chicago epidemiological studies. J Chronic Dis 1982;35:283–294.

114. Darné B, Girerd X, Safar ME, Cambien F, Guize L. Pulsatile versus steady component of blood pressure: a cross-sectional and prospective analysis of cardiovascular mortality. Hypertension 1989;13:392–400.

115. Madhavan S, Ooi WL, Cohen H, Alderman MH. Relation of pulse pressure and blood pressure reduction to the incidence of myocardial infarction. Hypertension 1994;23:395–401.

116. Benetos A, Safar M, Rudnichi A, Smulyan H, Richard J-L, Ducimetière P, et al. Pulse pressure. A predictor of long-term cardiovascular mortality in a French male population. Hypertension 1997;30:1410–1415.

117. Mitchell GF, Moyé LA, Braunwald E, Rouleau J-L, Bernstein V, Geltman EM, et al., for the SAFE Investigators. Sphygmomanometrically determined pulse pressure is a powerful independent predictor of recurrent events after myocardial infarction in patients with impaired left ventricular function. Circulation 1997;96:4254–4260.

118. James MA, Watt PAC, Potter JF, Thurston H, Swales JD. Pulse pressure and resistance artery structure in the elderly. Hypertension 1995;26:301–306.

119. Khattar RS, Acharya DU, Kinsey C, Senior R, Lahiri A. Longitudinal association of ambulatory pulse pressure with left ventricular mass and vascular hypertrophy in essential hypertension. J Hypertens 1997;15:737–743.

10 Circadian Rhythm of Myocardial Infarction and Sudden Cardiac Death

Craig A. Chasen, MD
and James E. Muller, MD

CONTENTS

INTRODUCTION

In the early 1900s, Russian authors Obraztsov and Strazhesko *(1)* reported that climbing stairs and emotional distress might trigger a myocardial infarction (MI). However, the prevailing belief throughout most of this century was that activities are of little importance in causing cardiac disease onset. This chapter will review the recent clinical data that support the role of triggering by proving that in many cases, acute myocardial infarction and sudden cardiac death occur in a nonrandom fashion with circadian (daily), circaseptan (weekly), and circannual (seasonal) variations.

From: *Contemporary Cardiology:*
Blood Pressure Monitoring in Cardiovascular Medicine and Therapeutics
Edited by: W. B. White © Humana Press Inc., Totowa, NJ

MYOCARDIAL INFARCTION

Circadian Variation of Myocardial Infarction

In many instances, myocardial infarction is not a random clinical event. The onset of myocardial infarction has a distinct daily pattern with a peak incidence in the hours after awakening and arising *(2)*. Using the serum creatine phosphokinase (CPK) measurements obtained from 703 subjects in the Multicenter Investigation of Limitation of Infarct Size study *(3)*, our group was able to objectively derive the time of onset of MI. A marked circadian variation in the incidence of MI was noted with a threefold increase at 9 AM (45 MIs) as compared to 11 PM (15 MIs). In the Intravenous Streptokinase in Acute Myocardial Infarction Study (ISAM) *(4)*, Willich et al. used clinical criteria and serial CPK measurements to identify the time of onset of MI in all 1741 patients enrolled. A morning peak in the onset of MI was reported with a 3.8-fold increase in frequency noted between 8 AM and 9 AM as compared to midnight and 1 AM. The authors also stated that the morning was a risk period for patients with mild as well as severe coronary artery disease. Goldberg et al. *(5)* examined the times of onset of acute MI (AMI) in relation to awakening in 137 patients with confirmed AMI. Approximately 23% of patients reported onset of initial symptoms of MI within 1 h after awakening. Willich et al. *(6)*, using the community-based Triggers and Mechanisms of Myocardial Infarction pilot data, supported this finding with the observation that the increased incidence of MI occurred within the first 3 h after awakening. Of the 3339 patients entered into the Thrombolysis in Myocardial Infarction II Trial (TIMI II) *(7)*, 34.4% of the heart attacks occurred between 6 AM and noon versus 15.4% between midnight and 6 AM. Genes et al. *(8)* reviewed the data on 2563 patients entered into the USIK trial and noted that 30.6% of the acute cardiac events occurred between 6 AM and noon and only 20.1% occurred between midnight and 6 AM. The morning peak was blunted in smokers and in patients with previous infarction.

Cannon and associates *(9)* examined the time of onset of myocardial ischemic pain in 7731 patients who were prospectively identified in the Thrombolysis in Myocardial Ischemia (TIMI) III Registry. The authors documented a statistically significant ($p < 0.001$) circadian variation in the incidence of onset of unstable angina and evolving non-Q-wave myocardial infarction with a peak occurrence rate between 6 AM and noon.

In the ISAM *(4)* and TIMI II *(7)* trials, the subgroup of patients receiving β-adrenergic receptor blocking therapy prior to the event did not show a morning excess in the incidence of myocardial infarction. Hjalmarson et al. *(10)*, after reviewing 4796 cases of acute myocardial infarction, confirmed the above findings and noted that the subgroups of congestive heart failure and prior infarction also had no morning increase in the occurrence of MI. Ridker et al. *(11)* noted that physicians randomized to aspirin therapy experienced a selective 59% reduction in MI during the morning hours compared with a 34.1% reduction for the remaining hours of the day.

Thompson et al. *(12)* and others *(10,13–17)* have suggested that in the evening hours (between 6 PM and midnight), a secondary peak of onset of myocardial infarction is present. This may relate to the evening meal or other triggers concentrated in those hours.

Weekly Variations of Acute MI

Numerous authors have reported a circaseptan (weekly) variation of MI with a peak incidence on Monday *(18–25)*. Willich et al. *(22)* noted this increase to be primarily in the working population with a 33% increase in relative risk of MI on this day of the week. In contrast, Spielberg et al. *(18)* observed a Monday increase in both the working and retired subgroups of patients that were studied.

Some researchers noted an increased incidence of MI on the weekend *(20,25, 26)*, whereas others identified a weekend nadir *(22–24,27)*. Sayer et al. *(28)* and Genes et al. *(8)* reported no significant circaseptan variation in the incidence of MI onset.

Seasonal Variations of Acute MI
and Coronary Artery Disease Deaths

Several investigators have reported a circannual (seasonal) variation in the incidence of onset of acute myocardial infarction with a peak in winter *(18,28–31)*. Of the 83,541 subjects entered into the National Registry of Myocardial Infarction (NRMI) database between 1990 and 1993, 10% more acute cardiac events occurred in winter or spring than in summer ($p < 0.05$) *(30)*. Spencer et al. *(29)* reviewed the data on 259,891 patients reported to the second National Registry of Myocardial Infarction (NRMI-2) during the 25-mo period beginning July 1, 1994. The authors noted that over 50% more cases of MI were reported in the winter (peak in January) than during the summer (nadir in July).

Sayer et al. *(28)* prospectively obtained data on 1225 consecutive patients with acute myocardial infarction admitted to a general hospital. Overall, a winter peak in the incidence of onset of MI was noted. However, the subgroups of patients who were diabetic, South Asian, or taking β-blockers or aspirin on admission did not demonstrate a seasonal variation. Marchant et al. *(31)* noted a winter peak in the 633 consecutive patients with AMI admitted to the CCU during a 4-yr period. Interestingly, the authors noted an excess of infarctions on colder days in both winter and summer, suggesting an effect of environmental temperature on the onset of this disease. Colder weather has been shown to alter hemodynamic (blood pressure [BP], sympathetic tone) and hematologic (platelet count, fibrinogen) factors favoring arterial thrombosis *(32–35)*.

Ku et al. *(27)* and Ahlbom *(36)* did not identify a significant seasonal variation in the incidence of MI. Ku et al. *(27)* speculated that the warm, stable climate of a subtropical region, as opposed to the temperature swings of a temperate climate, may have played a role his findings.

A circannual (seasonal) variation in cardiac mortality with an increased incidence during the winter months has been noted by several investigators *(31,37–39)*.

Acute Myocardial Infarction and Sleep

In the United States, annually, more than 250,000 acute myocardial infarctions and >38,000 sudden cardiac deaths (SCD) occur at night during sleep. This rate is less than observed during the daytime hours and the distribution of onset of cardiac events at night during sleep is nonuniform. Lavery et al. *(40)* performed an extensive literature review on the incidence of acute cardiac episodes between the hours of midnight and 5:59 AM and compiled 19 published studies on acute myocardial infarction, 7 published studies on automatic implantable cardioverter–defibrillator (AICD) discharges, and 12 published studies on sudden cardiac death. The peak incidence of myocardial infarction and AICD discharge occurred between midnight and 0:59 AM, and the peak incidence of SCD took place between 1:00 and 1:59 AM. The lowest incidence of MI and AICD discharge occurred between 3:00 and 3:59 AM, and the trough for SCD was between 4:00 and 4:59 AM.

Normal sleep is a dynamic process involving complex regulation of autonomic nervous system activity punctuated by episodes of rapid-eye-movement (REM) sleep and catecholamine secretion that rivals the awakened state *(41)*. Further research on sleep-state-dependent fluctuations in autonomic nervous system activity may make it possible to reduce acute cardiac events during this time period.

MECHANISMS OF ACTION

Individually or in combination, a variety of factors may create the milieu at the level of the coronary plaque that leads to an increased incidence of onset of myocardial infarction in the morning hours. These factors include, but are not limited to, peripheral arterial blood pressure surge *(42)*, increase in coronary vasomotor tone *(43)*, and shear stress *(44)*, and alterations in blood coagulation components that favor thrombosis.

A growing body of evidence supports a role for hemostatic factors in triggering cardiovascular events. Higher levels of fibrinogen *(45–47)*, factor VII *(48)*, factor VIII *(45,49)*, plasminogen activator inhibitor (PAI) *(47,50–55)*, tissue plasminogen activator (TPA) *(55,56)*, and von Willebrand factor *(45–47,49,52,56)* have been documented in patients with atherosclerotic cardiovascular disease. Thompson et al. *(57)* conducted a prospective multicenter trial enrolling 3043 patients with angina pectoris who underwent coronary arteriography and were followed for 2 yr. An increased risk of myocardial infarction and sudden cardiac death was associated with higher baseline concentrations of fibrinogen, von

Willebrand factor antigen, and tissue plasminogen activator antigen. Interestingly, despite the arteriographic evidence of CAD and symptomatic angina pectoris, low serum fibrinogen concentrations correlated with a low risk of cardiac events. The authors suggested that impaired fibrinolysis, as well as endothelial cell injury, and inflammatory activity play a pathogenetic role in the progression of CAD.

Enhanced platelet activity has been implicated in the pathogenesis of acute coronary syndromes. Platelet aggregability (58) and in vitro platelet responsiveness to adenosine diphosphate and epinephrine (59) increase only after the patient awakens and assumes the upright posture. During this same time period, plasma levels of catecholamines rise, which stimulate the release of platelets from the spleen and amplify platelet activity.

Blood viscosity (60), factor VII activity and PAI levels (61), heparin potency (62), and thrombolytic drug efficacy (63) follow a circadian variation that favors morning hypercoagulability and hypofibrinolysis.

CARDIOVASCULAR TRIGGERS

The circadian, circaseptan, and circannual variations in the incidence of onset of MI strongly support the concept that the patient can trigger the onset of an acute myocardial infarction at any time. The Myocardial Infarction Onset Study (MIOS) investigators have identified four triggers of onset of MI: start of activity in the morning, anger, heavy physical exertion, and sexual activity (64–66). These four triggers alone account for over 15% of infarctions, totaling more than 250,000 events in the United States each year.

Anger

The Determinants of Myocardial Infarction Onset Study investigators interviewed 1623 subjects approximately 4 d after an acute myocardial infarction to assess the intensity and timing of anger (and other triggers) during the 26 h before the acute event (66). Anger was objectively assessed by the onset anger scale (a single-item, seven-level, self-report scale) and the state anger subscale of the State-Trait Personality Inventory. The onset anger scale identified 39 patients (2.4%) who experienced anger within the 2 h prior to onset of MI. This corresponded to a relative risk of MI of 2.3, using the case-crossover study design developed by Maclure (67). The state anger subscale corroborated these findings with a relative risk of 1.9.

The risk of anger triggering myocardial infarction can be modulated. Regular users of aspirin had a relative risk of 1.4, which was significantly lower than nonusers (66). Increasing levels of educational attainment are associated with a reduced risk of anger-induced MI. The relative risk was twice as high among patients with less than high school education (3.3) compared with those with some college education (1.6) (68).

Verrier and Mittleman *(69)* attribute the lethal effects of anger to its activation of high-gain central neurocircuitry and the sympathetic nervous system, leading to acute sinus tachycardia, hypertension, impaired myocardial perfusion, and a high degree of cardiac electrical instability. Reich et al. *(70)* noted that anger was the probable trigger for 15% of the life-threatening arrhythmias identified in 117 patients. Fear, anxiety and bereavement have also been implicated in increased vulnerability to cardiac events *(71)*

Heavy Exertion

In the MILIS *(72)*, TIMI-2 *(7)*, and MIOS *(64)* trials, heavy physical exertion was identified as a trigger of acute myocardial infarction. In the Multicenter Investigation of Limitation of Infarct Size (MILIS) trial *(72)*, 14% of patients engaged in moderate physical activity and 9% engaged in heavy physical activity prior to sustaining a myocardial infarction.

In the TIMI-2 trial *(7)*, moderate or marked physical activity was reported to occur at onset of MI in 18.7% of patients. Compared with patients whose infarction occurred at rest or during mild activity, those with exertion-related infarction had fewer coronary vessels with $\geq$60% stenosis ($p = 0.002$) and were more likely to have an occluded infarct-related vessel after thrombolytic therapy ($p = 0.01$). The profile of the patient with exertion-related infarction was a non-smoking, caucasian male with pre-existing exertional angina, who did not use nitrates or calcium blockers in the 24 h prior to infarction.

Fifty-four (4.4%) of 1228 patients enrolled in the MIOS trial *(64)* reported heavy exertion (six or more metabolic equivalent units [METS]) within 1 h of the onset of myocardial infarction. The cardiac symptoms often began during the activity. The estimated relative risk of MI in the hour after heavy physical activity, as compared with less strenuous or no physical exertion, was 5.9. Among people who usually exercised less than one, one to two, three to four, or five or more times per week, the respective relative risks were 107, 19.4, 8.6, and 2.4. Therefore, habitually sedentary individuals were at greatest risk of MI after heavy exertion and increasing levels of regular physical exercise were associated with progressively lower coronary risk. This same relationship appears to hold true for heavy physical exertion and sudden cardiac death *(73,74)*.

Sexual Activity

The MIOS trial also identified 3% of patients who experienced the onset of myocardial infarction within 2 h after sexual activity. Case-crossover analysis calculated a relative risk of 2.5 for onset of MI during this time period *(65)*. Nine percent of the patients engaged in sexual relations within 24 h of symptom onset. The relative risk of MI during sexual activity is no different for patients with known cardiac disease than for people without heart disease—a finding that may reassure patients during cardiac rehabilitation. In addition, the absolute, as opposed to relative, risk increase is very low.

Potential Trigger Mechanisms

Triggers may induce the onset of infarction by multiple concomitant pathways. Significant physical activity or emotional stress may lead to (1) hemodynamic stress of hypertension and tachycardia from sympathetic stimulation, (2) endothelial dysfunction-induced coronary vasoconstriction with increased shear forces, and (3) a prothrombotic state *(75)* characterized by platelet activation and a reduced fibrinolytic response and reduced prostacyclin release. It is not known if physical exertion leads directly to plaque rupture, or whether the exertion merely adds a thrombotic or vasoconstrictive element to the causal pathway.

Physical Activity: More Friend Than Foe

Physical activity has a favorable effect on the lipid profile by lowering total serum cholesterol and triglycerides and raising high-density lipoprotein (HDL) cholesterol. In addition, physical activity is associated with reduced blood pressure, improved glucose tolerance, increased insulin sensitivity, and reduced blood coagulability *(76)*.

Although anger, heavy physical exertion, and sexual activity have been identified as triggers of the onset of MI, the absolute risk of infarction with each trigger is low, because baseline risk is low. For example, the risk of MI may double in the 2 h after sexual activity, but because the baseline risk of MI for a healthy 50-yr-old male in any given hour is 1 in 1 million, the absolute risk increases only to 2 in 1 million. Similarly, the risk of sudden cardiac death (SCD) in people engaging in vigorous exercise is 10 times higher in cardiac patients than in apparently healthy people. As the baseline risk is very low in the healthy individual (1:565,000 person-hours), the absolute risk of SCD in the cardiac patient is also low (1:60,000 person-hours) *(77)*.

The higher rate of infarction in the morning hours has raised concerns about the desirability of physical activity during this time period. Murray and colleagues *(78)* found no difference in risk of cardiac events between individuals who attended cardiac rehabilitation programs in the morning and those who attended in the afternoon.

Mental Stress

People who possess a high potential for hostility in response to a mental stress and an inability to express that anger outwardly appear to be at significant risk for the development of coronary artery disease *(79)*. Acute mental stress may be a trigger of transient myocardial ischemia *(80,81)*, myocardial infarction *(82)*, and sudden cardiac death *(83–86)*.

Bairey et al. *(80)* noted that 75% of 29 patients with CAD and exercise-induced myocardial ischemia also demonstrated mental-stress-induced wall motion abnormalities by radionuclide ventriculography. Barry et al. *(81)* performed ambulatory electrocardiographic monitoring with diary in 28 subjects with CAD and identified 372 episodes of ST-segment depression over a span of 5–6 wk. At least 22% of the ischemic episodes occurred at high levels of mental stress but low physical activity. In addition, transient ischemia was more likely to occur as the intensity level of mental activity increased.

Behar et al. *(82)* studied 1818 consecutive patients with acute MI. Exceptional heavy physical work, a violent quarrel at work or at home, and unusual mental stress were the three most frequent possible triggers of MI that occurred within 24 h of symptom onset. Within the first week of missile attacks on Israel during the 1991 Iraqi war, 20 people developed an acute myocardial infarction at one hospital compared to eight MIs during a control period *(87)*. Leor and Kloner *(88)* identified a 35% increase in the number of hospital admissions for acute myocardial infarction in Southern California in the week following the 1994 Northridge earthquake. Most of these events were associated with mental rather than physical stress.

Numerous authors have noted an increase in sudden cardiac death triggered by mental stress [(i.e., psychological *(89)*, occupational *(90)*, natural disasters *(91,92)*] probably the result of neural/neuro-hormonal activation and sympathetic stimulation *(84–86)* precipitating malignant arrhythmias *(93.94)* in the presence of structural heart disease.

An increase in coagulation factors VII and VIII, fibrinogen, von Willebrand factor, and platelet activity has also been observed in patients subjected to mental stress and may play a role in precipitating acute cardiac events *(94,95)*.

GENERAL THEORY OF THROMBOSIS

Our group has proposed the addition of the concept of triggering activities *(96)* to the role of thrombosis in acute coronary syndromes advanced by Falk *(97)* and others *(98–100)*. This creates a new general theory of onset of coronary thrombosis. The concepts of *vulnerable plaques*, *triggers,* and *acute risk factors* are essential to this hypothesis. The type of coronary plaque most vulnerable to rupture is lipid rich and has a thin fibrous cap that is weakest at its junction with the intima *(101)*, probably the result of increased macrophage activity with elaboration of metalloproteinases *(102,103)*. The triggers, either physical or mental, provoke disruption of the vulnerable plaque. The acute risk factor is defined as the pathophysiological change (vasoconstrictive, hemodynamic, or hemostatic) potentially leading to occlusive coronary thrombosis.

An acute coronary syndrome might be triggered by a stress that produces a hemodynamic response sufficient to cause a major plaque disruption, exposing collagen and atheromatous core contents to coronary blood, that results in thrombus formation at the site of the plaque. If the thrombus is large, yet does not totally obstruct coronary blood flow, unstable angina or non-Q-wave MI may result clinically. If the thrombus is large and totally occludes the coronary vessel, acute myocardial infarction often occurs. A synergistic combination of triggering activities may account for thrombosis in a setting in which each activity alone may not exceed the threshold for causation of infarction. For example, heavy physical exertion producing a minor plaque disruption in a sedentary cigaret smoker [associated with an increase in coronary artery vasoconstriction and a hypercoagulable state (104)] may be needed to cause occlusive thrombosis and disease onset. However, in a patient with an extremely vulnerable plaque, even the nonstrenuous activities of daily living may be sufficient to trigger the cascade leading to the cardiovascular event.

Given the compelling data on the circadian variation of myocardial event onset, it is prudent to provide pharmacological protection during the morning hours for patients already receiving anti-ischemic and antihypertensive therapy. As tolerated, therapies should include antiplatelets (aspirin, ticlopidine, clopidogrel), β-blockers, and regular aerobic exercise. HMG-CoA reductase inhibitors have had early favorable effects in reducing cardiac events, presumably through plaque stabilization (105).

SUDDEN CARDIAC DEATH

Introduction

Sudden cardiac death (SCD) accounts for approximately 25% of deaths from ischemic heart disease (106), totaling over 300,000 fatalities per year in the United States alone (107). This often lethal event can result from the interplay between structural abnormalities of the heart, transient functional disturbances, and the specific electrophysiologic events responsible for fatal arrhythmias (108).

Clinical Variables Associated with SCD

Medical information obtained by history and physical examination may identify a patient at increased risk for sudden cardiac death. Sexton et al. (109) identified diabetes mellitus, current cigaret smoking, and family history of ischemic heart disease as independent risk factors for sudden unexpected cardiac death. Wannamethee et al. (110) reported that elevated heart rate, heavy drinking, and arrhythmia emerged as factors that appear to be particular to SCD. Gillum (111) reported a marked racial and gender disparity in people succumbing to sudden cardiac death in the United States. Age-adjusted rates per 100,000 were highest in African-American males and lowest in Hispanic women (black men, 209; white men, 166; Hispanic men, 75; black women, 108; white women, 74; Hispanic women, 35).

The 12-lead electrocardiogram (ECG) may contain abnormalities that identify patients at risk for sudden cardiac death, such as the long QT-syndrome
(112). Brugada et al. *(113)* also noted a high rate of sudden death in patients with
right bundle branch block and ST-segment elevation in leads V1–V3. Recently,
Yi et al. *(114)* noted that patients after MI appear to be at increased risk of SCD
if the QT-interval is prolonged or the QT-interval displays blunted or abolished
circadian variation.

In patients with heart disease, the risk of SCD may be identified by investigat-
ing the following: coronary anatomy, global and regional left ventricular function, the presence of ischemia during rest and/or exercise, the presence of late
potentials by signal-averaged ECG, the presence of spontaneous ventricular tachycardia, and the results of electrophysiologic testing *(115,116)*.

Exposure to physical or mental stress may trigger the onset of SCD. Hayashi
et al. *(117)* found the incidence of SCD was low while sleeping, resting or doing
light work and was high while using the toilet, engaged in sports, or performing
heavy work. Maron et al. *(118)* noted the incidence of SCD in highly trained
athletes, such as marathon runners, was exceedingly small (approximately 1 in
50,000). Young athletes in the United States who do suffer SCD during strenuous
physical exertion usually have underlying occult structural heart disease such
as hypertrophic cardiomyopathy, coronary artery anomalies, or myocarditis *(119–
122)*. The major earthquake that occurred in Northridge, California in 1994
caused extreme mental stress in the city's inhabitants and precipitated 24 SCDs
in 24 h, a sharp increase from the average of 4.6 SCDs per day usually seen
(92). Sudden cardiac death may be triggered by the inhalation of fuel gases and
exposure to dry-cleaning fluid, possibly by sensitizing the heart to circulating
catecholamines *(123)*.

CIRCADIAN VARIATION
OF OUT-OF-HOSPITAL SUDDEN CARDIAC DEATH

Evidence in the United States

Many studies of the timing of the onset of sudden cardiac death have revealed
nonrandom circadian (daily), circaseptan (weekly), and circannual (seasonal)
distributions with a peak incidence in the morning hours, Saturday to Monday,
and winter, respectively.

Data from the Framingham Heart Study *(124)* revealed a significant circadian
variation in the occurrence of sudden cardiac death, with a peak incidence from
7 AM to 9 AM ($p < .01$) and a nadir from 9 AM to 1 PM. The risk of sudden cardiac
death was at least 70% higher during the peak period than was the average risk
during the other times of the day. Our group *(125)* reviewed the death certificates
of 2203 individuals dying out of the hospital in Massachusetts in 1983 and noted a

prominent circadian variation of sudden cardiac death with a low incidence during the night and an increased incidence from 7 to 11 AM. Levine and co-workers *(126)* identified a morning peak of sudden cardiac death in out-of-hospital cardiac arrests in the City of Houston Emergency Medical Services. Willich et al. *(127)* prospectively reviewed 94 cases of SCD in 4 cities and towns in Massachusetts. A circadian variation in the incidence of SCD was demonstrated with a peak from 9 AM to noon. The authors noted that the incidence of SCD during the first 3 h after awakening carried a relative risk of 2.6 compared with the rest of the day. Thakur et al. *(128)* retrospectively reviewed 2250 consecutive patients with witnessed cardiac arrest during a 5-yr period. A circadian variation in the occurrence of sudden cardiac death was demonstrated with a 2.4-fold increase between the hours of 6 AM to noon. This circadian rhythm persisted despite gender, age (above or below 70 yr), and initial cardiac arrest rhythms and was not evident in the rate of successful resuscitation or the rate of survival.

Sudden cardiac death may occur in as many as 40% of all patients who suffer from heart failure *(129)*. The multicenter trial Veterans Affairs Congestive Heart Failure–Survival Trial of Antiarrhythmic Therapy (CHF-STAT) documented a morning increase of sudden cardiac death in patients with CHF *(130)*. The Cardiac Arrhythmia Suppression Trial (CAST) revealed that patients randomized to flecainide, encainide, and moricizine experienced a significant increase in the morning peak of sudden cardiac death, as compared to placebo *(131)*. Cohen et al. *(132)* performed a meta-analysis on the circadian variation of acute cardiovascular events and noted that 1 out of every 15 SCDs are attributable to the morning excess incidence.

Very recently, Peckova et al. *(133)* explored the temporal variation of SCD in 6603 out-of-hospital cardiac arrests attended by the Seattle Fire Department. A circadian variation in the occurrence of SCD was noted with two nearly equal peaks at 8 AM to 11 AM and at 4 PM to 7 PM. The evening peak was attributed primarily to ventricular fibrillation.

The incidence of sudden cardiac death from noncoronary causes may also show circadian variation. Maron et al. *(134)* studied 94 patients with hypertrophic cardiomyopathy who died suddenly and whose time of death could be ascertained accurately to the nearest hour. A circadian variation in the incidence of SCD was seen with 46% of the fatalities occurring between 7 AM and 1 PM. A second but smaller peak was noted between 8 PM and 10 PM. Thirty-nine percent of the sudden cardiac deaths occurred during periods of severe exertion.

Beard et al. *(39)* studied the records of 1054 cases of SCD in Rochester, Minnesota during the years 1950–1975. A circaseptan variation was noted with a peak incidence on Saturday. In contrast, Rabkin et al. *(135)* noted an excess proportion of SCDs on Monday in subjects without clinical evidence of CAD. Patients with ischemic heart disease had a more uniform incidence of SCD through-out the week.

Evidence Outside the United States

Mifune and Takeda *(136)* reviewed 90 consecutive patients with prehospital sudden cardiac arrest and noted a circadian pattern, with many cases occurring during the day and few at night. Goudevenos et al. *(137)* prospectively studied 223 sudden cardiac deaths that occurred in a closed population in northwest Greece over a 3.5-yr period. Family physicians and/or relatives of the deceased were interviewed within 12 d of SCD. A circadian variation in the incidence of SCD was noted with the apex occurring between 9 AM and noon. Assanelli et al. *(138)* observed a circadian variation in the incidence of SCD in subjects less than 45 yr of age, with a peak incidence in the morning hours. Pasqualetti et al. *(139)* reviewed 269 cases of sudden cardiac death over a 17-yr period (1970–1987) in Italy. The authors noted circadian, circaseptan, and circannual variations in the incidence of SCD with an increased incidence in the morning hours, Saturday to Monday, and October to January, respectively.

Numerous investigators have identified a bimodal distribution of sudden cardiac deaths during the day. Ishida et al. *(140)* reviewed 531 cases of sudden cardiac death in Kanagawa Prefecture spanning 10 yr. In ischemic heart disease, deaths most frequently occurred between 12 AM and 1 AM and between 5 PM and 6 PM. Deaths resulting from acute cardiac failure occurred during sleep. Goto et al. *(141)* investigated 303 patients who suffered SCD in Yamagata city from 1984 to 1987. There was a tendency for sudden death to occur in the early morning, evening, and winter season. Arntz et al. *(142)* studied 703 consecutive patients who suffered SCD during 1988–1990 in Berlin, Germany. The determination of time of day of the event was based on the arrival time of the rescue squad. A striking circadian rhythm was identified with a peak incidence between 6 AM and noon and a secondary peak between 3 PM and 7 PM ($p < 0.0001$). Martens et al. *(143)* studied the time of the day of calls received for out-of-hospital cardiac arrests prospectively registered by seven major Belgian emergency medical services. An intraday variation in the incidence of calls for cardiac arrests was observed with a peak incidence between 6 AM and noon, a smaller crest in the early afternoon, and a nadir at night. Hayashi et al. *(144)* noted a bimodal distribution in the daily incidence of SCD with peaks between 6 AM and 8 AM and between 6 PM and 8 PM.

Even nocturnal deaths appear to have a nonrandom distribution. Tatsanavivat et al. *(145)* conducted a survey by mail of sudden and unexplained death in sleep that occurred in 60 adults in northeast Thailand during 1988–1989. These deaths were found to have a circannual variation, with 38% occurring between March and May and 10% between September and October.

Prevention of SCD

Out-of-hospital sudden cardiac death in the Beta-blocker Heart Attack Trial also demonstrated a marked morning increase in the placebo group with 38% of the SCDs occurring between 5 AM and 11 AM. However, patients randomized to propranolol therapy received a major protective effect during that same time period *(146)*. A recent analysis of the Danish Verapamil Infarction Trials (DAVIT I and II) suggests that verapamil is associated with a preferential reduction in morning sudden cardiac deaths *(147)*. The recently reported Cardiac Insufficiency Bisoprolol II (CIBIS II) trial *(148)* showed that patients with NYHA Class III & IV congestive heart failure randomized to active treatment (bisoprolol) received a 45% reduction in sudden cardiac death (3.6% vs 6.4%). The study of the patterns of sudden cardiac death may yield important clues to the pathophysiology of the disease process *(149)*.

CIRCADIAN VARIATION OF ARRHYTHMIAS

Malignant tachyarrhythmias are the most common cause of sudden cardiac death. Olshausen et al. *(150)* analyzed the Holter Monitor tapes of 61 patients who experienced sudden cardiac death while being monitored. Monomorphic ventricular tachycardia was seen in 43%. Other rhythm disturbances noted were polymorphic ventricular tachycardia (including torsades de pointes), primary ventricular fibrillation, and 1:1 conducting atrial tachycardia. Cellular hypertrophy compensating for cell loss due to ischemia, intraventricular hypertension, cardiomyopathy, and myocarditis might play a role in arrhythmogenesis, as evidenced by the fact that experimental induction and regression of hypertrophy are paralleled by changes in the inducibility of ventricular tachyarrhythmias *(151)*.

Canada et al. *(152)* noted that ventricular ectopy reveals a prominent peak during the daytime hours and a trough at night. Twidale et al. *(153)* observed that the peak incidence of sustained symptomatic ventricular tachycardia in 68 patients occurred between 10 AM and noon. Valkama et al. *(154)* reviewed 24-h long-term electrocardiographic recordings in 34 patients with known coronary artery disease. A circadian rhythm was identified for spontaneous ventricular tachycardia (VT) (four or more beats of VT) with a peak incidence at 6 AM. Rebuzzi et al. *(155)* studied 406 patients with 24-hr ambulatory electrocardiographic monitoring to assess the time of incidence of VT. A nonrandom daily distribution of this arrhythmia was described with a peak incidence between 11 AM and noon.

Lampert et al. *(156)* studied 32 subjects with an implantable cardioverter–defibrillator (ICD) in whom 2558 episodes of VT were recorded. D'Avila et al. *(157)* noted that in 22 patients with an ICD, 42% of the total appropriate defibrillator shocks occurred during the morning hours. Behrens et al. *(158)* also noted a circadian variation ($p < 0.001$) of ventricular tachyarrhythmias with a primary morning peak between 7 AM and 11 AM and a secondary, much smaller peak between 4 PM and 8 PM. Mallavarapu et al. *(159)* analyzed the stored electrograms from 390 ICD recipients who sustained a total of 2692 episodes of VT or ventricular fibrillation (VF). The peak incidence of the arrhythmia occurred between 10 AM and 11 AM, with a nadir between 2 AM and 3 AM. This circadian pattern persisted despite age, gender, ejection fraction, or VT cycle length. Fries et al. *(160)* studied 119 consecutive patients after ICD implantation. Over a mean of 3 yr, 1849 ventricular arrhythmic events (VAE) were detected in 57 patients. The majority of both single episodes of VAE and short-term recurrent tachyarrhythmias were registered between 8 AM and noon and in the evening. Tofler et al. *(161)* studied 483 patients who had an ICD implanted in the early 1990s and noted that almost 22% of the ventricular tachyarrhythmias occurred between the hours of 9 AM and noon. Venditti et al. *(162)* analyzed defibrillation thresholds (DFTs) at different times of day in 134 patients with an ICD. The morning DFT (8 AM to noon) was 15 J versus 13 J in the mid-afternoon (noon to 4 PM) and late (4 PM to 8 PM) afternoon, ($p < 0.02$). In a separate group of 930 patients implanted with an ICD system with date and time stamps for each therapy, Venditti and colleagues reviewed 1238 episodes of ventricular tachyarrhythmias treated with shock therapy. There was a significant peak in failed first shocks in the morning compared with other time intervals, supporting the concept that greater amounts of energy are required for termination of morning tachyarrhythmias. Fries et al. *(163)* noted that in 138 recipients of ICDs, the worst antitachycardia pacing success rates occurred during the time period with the highest episode frequency (the morning hours). McClelland et al. *(164)* studied 162 subjects with CAD and found that the time of day during which ventricular stimulation protocols were performed did not affect test results. The absence of a morning increase could be explained by the supine posture in which all tests are conducted.

Nanthakumar et al. *(165)* reviewed 54 patients with an ICD that experienced 1012 episodes of ventricular tachycardia (VT) with and 102 episodes of VT without antiandrenergic medications. As anticipated, the episodes of VT without β-blockade followed a circadian variation with a peak incidence of onset at 9 AM, followed by a secondary peak at 4 PM. In contrast to Behrens et al. *(166)*, the presence of a β-blocker did not affect this circadian rhythm.

Not all studies revealed a morning peak in the incidence of malignant ventricular arrhythmias. Wood et al. *(167)* followed 43 patients with an ICD for a mean of 226 d. The daily distribution of the 830 ventricular tachyarrhythmia episodes recorded was nonrandom with a peak incidence between 2 PM and 3 PM. Interestingly, this pattern was not observed in subjects receiving antiarrhythmic drug therapy. Lucente et al. *(168)* utilized Holter electrocardiographic recordings to document the time of onset of ventricular tachycardia in 94 subjects with CAD. A circadian variation in the incidence of VT was noted with a peak occurrence rate between 2 PM and 3 PM in patients with a recent MI and between noon and 1 PM in patients with an old MI.

The underlying structural heart disease may influence the type and temporal distribution of clinically significant arrhythmias. Wolpert et al. *(169)* studied 28 patients with CAD and 11 subjects with nonischemic dilated cardiomyopathy who had implantable cardioverter–defibrillators over a mean period of 2 yr. Patients with CAD manifested a circadian variation in the frequency of malignant ventricular arrhythmias (MVA) with a peak incidence between 9 AM and 10 AM. A circaseptan variation was also noted with a peak incidence on Saturday. In contrast, the peak incidence of arrhythmias in the subjects with cardiomyopathy occurred in the late afternoon and early evening. In addition, the peak incidence of arrhythmias during the week occurred on Mondays and Wednesdays.

With further epidemiological, clinical, and basic science research, we may achieve a better understanding of the mechanisms that provoke the onset of acute cardiovascular disease. This knowledge would help investigators design effective preventive therapies for these disorders.

REFERENCES

1. Obraztsov VP, Strazhesko ND. The symptomatology and diagnosis of coronary thrombosis. In: Vorobeva VA, Konchalovski MP, eds. Works of the First Congress of Russian Therapists. Comradeship Typography of A.E. Mamontov, 1910, pp. 26–43.
2. Muller JE, Tofler GH. Circadian variation and cardiovascular disease [editorial;comment]. N Engl J Med 1991;325:1038–1039.
3. Muller JE, Stone PH, Turi ZG, Rutherford JD, Czeisler CA, Parker C, et al. Circadian variation in the frequency of onset of acute myocardial infarction. N Engl J Med 1985;313: 1315–1322.
4. Willich SN, Linderer T, Wegscheider K, Leizorovicz A, Alamercery I, Schroder R. Increased morning incidence of myocardial infarction in the ISAM Study: absence with prior beta-adrenergic blockade. ISAM Study Group. Circulation 1989;80:853–858.
5. Goldberg RJ, Brady P, Muller JE, Chen ZY, de Groot M, Zonneveld P, et al. Time of onset of symptoms of acute myocardial infarction. Am J Cardiol 1990;66:140–144.
6. Willich SN, Lowel H, Lewis M, Arntz R, Baur R, Winther K, et al. Association of wake time and the onset of myocardial infarction. Triggers and mechanisms of myocardial infarction (TRIMM) pilot study. TRIMM Study Group. Circulation 1991;84:VI62–VI67.
7. Tofler GH, Muller JE, Stone PH, Forman S, Solomon RE, Knatterud GL, et al. Modifiers of timing and possible triggers of acute myocardial infarction in the Thrombolysis in Myocardial Infarction Phase II (TIMI II) Study Group. J Am Coll Cardiol 1992;20:1049–1055.
8. Genes N, Vaur L, Renault M, Cambou JP, Danchin N. Circadian rhythm in myocardial infarct in France. Results of the USIK study. Presse Med 1997;26:603–608.
9. Cannon CP, McCabe CH, Stone PH, Schactman M, Thompson B, Theroux P, et al. Circadian variation in the onset of unstable angina and non-Q-wave acute myocardial infarction (the TIMI III Registry and TIMI IIIB). Am J Cardiol 1997;79:253–258.
10. Hjalmarson A, Gilpin EA, Nicod P, Dittrich H, Henning H, Engler R, et al. Differing circadian patterns of symptom onset in subgroups of patients with acute myocardial infarction. Circulation 1989;80:267–275.
11. Ridker PM, Manson JE, Buring JE, Muller JE, Hennekens CH. Circadian variation of acute myocardial infarction and the effect of low-dose aspirin in a randomized trial of physicians. Circulation 1990;82:897–902.
12. Thompson DR, Blandford RL, Sutton TW, Marchant PR. Time of onset of chest pain in acute myocardial infarction. Int J Cardiol 1985;7:139–148.
13. Peters RW, Zoble RG, Liebson PR, Pawitan Y, Brooks MM, Proschan M. Identification of a secondary peak in myocardial infarction onset 11 to 12 hours after awakening: the Cardiac Arrhythmia Suppression Trial (CAST) experience. J Am Coll Cardiol 1993;22:998–1003.

14. Fernandes E, Candeias O. Circadian rhythm at the onset of symptoms in clinical cases of myocardial infarction. Our first five hundred cases. Acta Med Port 1995;8:667–669.
15. Hansen O, Johansson BW, Gullberg B. Circadian distribution of onset of acute myocardial infarction in subgroups from analysis of 10,791 patients treated in a single center. Am J Cardiol 1992;69:1003–1008.
16. Kono T, Morita H, Nishina T, Fujita M, Hirota Y, Kawamura K, et al. Circadian variations of onset of acute myocardial infarction and efficacy of thrombolytic therapy. J Am Coll Cardiol 1996;27:774–778.
17. Thompson DR, Sutton TW, Jowett NI, Pohl JE. Circadian variation in the frequency of onset of chest pain in acute myocardial infarction [see comments]. Br Heart J 1991;65:177–178.
18. Spielberg C, Falkenhahn D, Willich SN, Wegscheider K, Voller H. Circadian, day-of-week, and seasonal variability in myocardial infarction: comparison between working and retired patients. Am Heart J 1996;132:579–585.
19. Gnecchi-Ruscone T, Piccaluga E, Guzzetti S, Contini M, Montano N, Nicolis E. Morning and Monday: critical periods for the onset of acute myocardial infarction. The GISSI 2 Study experience. Eur Heart J 1994;15:882–887.
20. Massing W, Angermeyer MC. Myocardial infarction on various days of the week. Psychol Med 1985;15:851–857.
21. Thompson DR, Pohl JE, Sutton TW. Acute myocardial infarction and day of the week. Am J Cardiol 1992;69:266–267.
22. Willich SN, Lowel H, Lewis M, Hormann A, Arntz HR, Keil U. Weekly variation of acute myocardial infarction. Increased Monday risk in the working population. Circulation 1994; 90:87–93.
23. Ohlson CG, Bodin L, Bryngelsson IL, Helsing M, Malmberg L. Winter weather conditions and myocardial infarctions. Scand J Soc Med 1991;19:20–25.
24. Peters RW, Brooks MM, Zoble RG, Liebson PR, Seals AA. Chronobiology of acute myocardial infarction: cardiac arrhythmia suppression trial (CAST) experience. Am J Cardiol 1996;78:1198–1201.
25. van der Palen J, Doggen CJ, Beaglehole R. Variation in the time and day of onset of myocardial infarction and sudden death. NZ Med J 1995;108:332–334.
26. Zhou RH, Xi B, Gao HQ, Liu XQ, Li YS, Cao KJ, et al. Circadian and septadian variation in the occurrence of acute myocardial infarction in a Chinese population. Jpn Circ J 1998;62: 190–192.
27. Ku CS, Yang CY, Lee WJ, Chiang HT, Liu CP, Lin SL. Absence of a seasonal variation in myocardial infarction onset in a region without temperature extremes. Cardiology 1998;89: 277–282.
28. Sayer JW, Wilkinson P, Ranjadayalan K, Ray S, Marchant B, Timmis AD. Attenuation or absence of circadian and seasonal rhythms of acute myocardial infarction. Heart 1997;77: 325–329.
29. Spencer FA, Goldberg RJ, Becker RC, Gore JM. Seasonal distribution of acute myocardial infarction in the second National Registry of Myocardial Infarction. J Am Coll Cardiol 1998; 31:1226–1233.
30. Ornato JP, Peberdy MA, Chandra NC, Bush DE. Seasonal pattern of acute myocardial infarction in the National Registry of Myocardial Infarction. J Am Coll Cardiol 1996;28: 1684–1688.
31. Marchant B, Ranjadayalan K, Stevenson R, Wilkinson P, Timmis AD. Circadian and seasonal factors in the pathogenesis of acute myocardial infarction: the influence of environmental temperature. Br Heart J 1993;69:385–387.
32. Kawahara J, Sano H, Fukuzaki H, Saito K, Hirouchi H. Acute effects of exposure to cold on blood pressure, platelet function and sympathetic nervous activity in humans. Am J Hypertens 1989;2:724–726.

33. Keatinge WR, Coleshaw SR, Cotter F, Mattock M, Murphy M, Chelliah R. Increases in platelet and red cell counts, blood viscosity, and arterial pressure during mild surface cooling: factors in mortality from coronary and cerebral thrombosis in winter. Br Med J 1984;289: 1405–1408.

34. Woodhouse PR, Khaw KT, Plummer M, Foley A, Meade TW. Seasonal variations of plasma fibrinogen and factor VII activity in the elderly: winter infections and death from cardiovascular disease [see comments]. Lancet 1994;343:435–439.

35. Bull G, Brozovic M, Chakrabarti R, Mead T, Morton J, North W, et al. Relationship of air temperature to various chemical, haematological, and haemostatic variables. J Clin Pathol 1979;32:16–20.

36. Ahlbom A. Seasonal variations in the incidence of acute myocardial infarction in Stockholm. Scand J Soc Med 1979;7:127–130.

37. Baker-Blocker A. Winter weather and cardiovascular mortality in Minneapolis–St. Paul. Am J Public Health 1982;72:261–265.

38. Rogers WJ, Bowlby LJ, Chandra NC, French WJ, Gore JM, Lambrew CT, et al. Treatment of myocardial infarction in the United States (1990 to 1993). Observations from the National Registry of Myocardial Infarction. Circulation 1994;90:2103–2114.

39. Beard CM, Fuster V, Elveback LR. Daily and seasonal variation in sudden cardiac death, Rochester, Minnesota, 1950–1975. Mayo Clin Proc 1982;57:704–706.

40. Lavery CE, Mittleman MA, Cohen MC, Muller JE, Verrier RL. Nonuniform nighttime distribution of acute cardiac events: a possible effect of sleep states. Circulation 1997;96: 3321–3327.

41. Verrier RL, Muller JE, Hobson JA. Sleep, dreams, and sudden death: the case for sleep as an autonomic stress test for the heart. Cardiovasc Res 1996;31:181–211.

42. Millar-Craig MW, Bishop CN, Raftery EB. Circadian variation of blood-pressure. Lancet 1978;1:795–797.

43. Panza JA, Epstein SE, Quyyumi AA. Circadian variation in vascular tone and its relation to alpha-sympathetic vasoconstrictor activity [see comments]. N Engl J Med 1991;325:986–990.

44. Vita JA, Treasure CB, Ganz P, Cox DA, Fish RD, Selwyn AP. Control of shear stress in the epicardial coronary arteries of humans: impairment by atherosclerosis [see comments]. J Am Coll Cardiol 1989;14:1193–1199.

45. Hamsten A, Blomback M, Wiman B, Svensson J, Szamosi A, de Faire U, et al. Haemostatic function in myocardial infarction. Br Heart J 1986;55:58–66.

46. Agewall S, Wikstrand J, Wendelhag I, Tengborn L, Fagerberg B. Femoral artery wall morphology, hemostatic factors and intermittent claudication: ultrasound study in men at high and low risk for atherosclerotic disease. Haemostasis 1996;26:45–57.

47. Woodburn KR, Lowe GD, Rumley A, Love J, Pollock JG. Relation of haemostatic, fibrinolytic, and rheological variables to the angiographic extent of peripheral arterial occlusive disease. Int Angiol 1995;14:346–352.

48. Broadhurst P, Kelleher C, Hughes L, Imeson JD, Raftery EB. Fibrinogen, factor VII clotting activity and coronary artery disease severity. Atherosclerosis 1990;85:169–173.

49. Meade TW, Cooper JA, Stirling Y, Howarth DJ, Ruddock V, Miller GJ. Factor VIII, ABO blood group and the incidence of ischaemic heart disease. Br J Haematol 1994;88:601–607.

50. Hamsten A, Wiman B, de Faire U, Blomback M. Increased plasma levels of a rapid inhibitor of tissue plasminogen activator in young survivors of myocardial infarction. N Engl J Med 1985;313:1557–1563.

51. Estelles A, Tormo G, Aznar J, Espana F, Tormo V. Reduced fibrinolytic activity in coronary heart disease in basal conditions and after exercise. Thromb Res 1985;40:373–383.

52. Andreotti F, Roncaglioni MC, Hackett DR, Khan MI, Regan T, Haider AW, et al. Early coronary reperfusion blunts the procoagulant response of plasminogen activator inhibitor-1 and von Willebrand factor in acute myocardial infarction. J Am Coll Cardiol 1990;16:1553–1560.

53. Gray RP, Yudkin JS, Patterson DL. Plasminogen activator inhibitor: a risk factor for myocardial infarction in diabetic patients. Br Heart J 1993;69:228–232.
54. Munkvad S, Jespersen J, Gram J, Kluft C. Interrelationship between coagulant activity and tissue-type plasminogen activator (t-PA) system in acute ischaemic heart disease. Possible role of the endothelium. J Intern Med 1990;228:361–366.
55. Chandler WL, Stratton JR. Laboratory evaluation of fibrinolysis in patients with a history of myocardial infarction. Am J Clin Pathol 1994;102:248–252.
56. Blann AD, Dobrotova M, Kubisz P, McCollum CN. von Willebrand factor, soluble P-selectin, tissue plasminogen activator and plasminogen activator inhibitor in atherosclerosis. Thromb Haemost 1995;74:626–630.
57. Thompson SG, Kienast J, Pyke SD, Haverkate F, van de Loo JC. Hemostatic factors and the risk of myocardial infarction or sudden death in patients with angina pectoris. European Concerted Action on Thrombosis and Disabilities Angina Pectoris Study Group [see comments]. N Engl J Med 1995;332:635–641.
58. Tofler GH, Brezinski D, Schafer AI, Czeisler CA, Rutherford JD, Willich SN, et al. Concurrent morning increase in platelet aggregability and the risk of myocardial infarction and sudden cardiac death. N Engl J Med 1987;316:1514–1518.
59. Brezinski DA, Tofler GH, Muller JE, Pohjola-Sintonen S, Willich SN, Schafer AI, et al. Morning increase in platelet aggregability. Association with assumption of the upright posture. Circulation 1988;78:35–40.
60. Ehrly AM, Jung G. Circadian rhythm of human blood viscosity. Biorheology 1973;10:577–583.
61. Kapiotis S, Jilma B, Quehenberger P, Ruzicka K, Handler S, Speiser W. Morning hypercoagulability and hypofibrinolysis. Diurnal variations in circulating activated factor VII, prothrombin fragment F1+2, and plasmin–plasmin inhibitor complex. Circulation 1997;96:19–21.
62. Decousus H, Boissier C, Perpoint B, Page Y, Mismetti P, Laporte S, et al. Circadian dynamics of coagulation and chronopathology of cardiovascular and cerebrovascular events. Future therapeutic implications for the treatment of these disorders? Ann NY Acad Sci 1991;618:159–165.
63. Kurnik PB. Circadian variation in the efficacy of tissue-type plasminogen activator [see comments]. Circulation 1995;91:1341–1346.
64. Mittleman MA, Maclure M, Tofler GH, Sherwood JB, Goldberg RJ, Muller JE. Triggering of acute myocardial infarction by heavy physical exertion. Protection against triggering by regular exertion. Determinants of Myocardial Infarction Onset Study Investigators [see comments]. N Engl J Med 1993;329:1677–1683.
65. Muller JE, Mittleman A, Maclure M, Sherwood JB, Tofler GH. Triggering myocardial infarction by sexual activity. Low absolute risk and prevention by regular physical exertion. Determinants of Myocardial Infarction Onset Study Investigators [see comments]. JAMA 1996;275:1405–1409.
66. Mittleman MA, Maclure M, Sherwood JB, Mulry RP, Tofler GH, Jacobs SC, et al. Triggering of acute myocardial infarction onset by episodes of anger. Determinants of Myocardial Infarction Onset Study Investigators [see comments]. Circulation 1995;92:1720–1725.
67. Maclure M. The case-crossover design: a method for studying transient effects on the risk of acute events. Am J Epidemiol 1991;133:144–153.
68. Mittleman MA, Maclure M, Nachnani M, Sherwood JB, Muller JE. Educational attainment, anger, and the risk of triggering myocardial infarction onset. The Determinants of Myocardial Infarction Onset Study Investigators. Arch Intern Med 1997;157:769–775.
69. Verrier RL, Mittleman MA. Life-threatening cardiovascular consequences of anger in patients with coronary heart disease. Cardiol Clin 1996;14:289–307.
70. Reich P, DeSilva RA, Lown B, Murawski BJ. Acute psychological disturbances preceding life-threatening ventricular arrhythmias. JAMA 1981;246:233–235.

71. Verrier RL, Mittelman MA. Cardiovascular consequences of anger and other stress states. Baillieres Clin Neurol 1997;6:245–259.
72. Tofler GH, Stone PH, Maclure M, Edelman E, Davis VG, Robertson T, et al. Analysis of possible triggers of acute myocardial infarction (the MILIS study). Am J Cardiol 1990;66: 22–27.
73. Siscovick DS, Weiss NS, Fletcher RH, Lasky T. The incidence of primary cardiac arrest during vigorous exercise. N Engl J Med 1984;311:874–877.
74. Vuori I. The cardiovascular risks of physical activity. Acta Med Scand 1986;711(Suppl): 205–214.
75. Khanna PK, Seth HN, Balasubramanian V, Hoon RS. Effect of submaximal exercise on fibrinolytic activity in ischaemic heart disease. Br Heart J 1975;37:1273–1276.
76. Rauramaa R, Salonen JT, Kukkonen-Harjula K, Seppanen K, Seppala E, Vapaatalo H, et al. Effects of mild physical exercise on serum lipoproteins and metabolites of arachidonic acid: a controlled randomised trial in middle aged men. Br Med J 1984;288:603–606.
77. AHA. Cardiac rehabilitation programs. A statement for healthcare professionals from the American Heart Association. Circulation 1994;90:1602–1610.
78. Murray PM, Herrington DM, Pettus CW, Miller HS, Cantwell JD, Little WC. Should patients with heart disease exercise in the morning or afternoon? [see comments]. Arch Intern Med 1993;153:833–836.
79. Manuck SB, Kaplan JR, Matthews KA. Behavioral antecedents of coronary heart disease and atherosclerosis. Arteriosclerosis 1986;6:2–14.
80. Bairey CN, Krantz DS, Rozanski A. Mental stress as an acute trigger of ischemic left ventricular dysfunction and blood pressure elevation in coronary artery disease. Am J Cardiol 1990; 66:28G–31G.
81. Barry J, Selwyn AP, Nabel EG, Rocco MB, Mead K, Campbell S, et al. Frequency of ST-segment depression produced by mental stress in stable angina pectoris from coronary artery disease. Am J Cardiol 1988;61:989–993.
82. Behar S, Halabi M, Reicher-Reiss H, Zion M, Kaplinsky E, Mandelzweig L, et al. Circadian variation and possible external triggers of onset of myocardial infarction. SPRINT Study Group. Am J Med 1993;94:395–400.
83. Toyoshima H, Hayashi S, Tanabe N, Miyanishi K, Satoh T, Aizawa Y, et al. Sudden death of adults in Japan. Nagoya J Med Sci 1996;59:81–95.
84. Willich SN, Maclure M, Mittleman M, Arntz HR, Muller JE. Sudden cardiac death. Support for a role of triggering in causation. Circulation 1993;87:1442–1450.
85. Davis AM, Natelson BH. Brain–heart interactions. The neurocardiology of arrhythmia and sudden cardiac death. Tex Heart Inst J 1993;20:158–169.
86. Lown B, Verrier RL, Rabinowitz SH. Neural and psychologic mechanisms and the problem of sudden cardiac death. Am J Cardiol 1977;39:890–902.
87. Meisel SR, Kutz I, Dayan KI, Pauzner H, Chetboun I, Arbel Y, et al D. Effect of Iraqi missile war on incidence of acute myocardial infarction and sudden death in Israeli civilians [see comments]. Lancet 1991;338:660–661.
88. Leor J, Kloner RA. The Northridge earthquake as a trigger for acute myocardial infarction. Am J Cardiol 1996;77:1230–1232.
89. Frasure-Smith N, Lesperance F, Talajic M. Depression following myocardial infarction. Impact on 6-month survival [see comments]. JAMA 1993;270:1819–1825. Erratum: JAMA 1994;271(14)1082.
90. Eliot RS, Clayton FC, Pieper GM, Todd GL. Influence of environmental stress on pathogenesis of sudden cardiac death. Fed Proc 1977;36:1719–1724.
91. Trichopoulos D, Katsouyanni K, Zavitsanos X, Tzonou A, Dalla-Vorgia P. Psychological stress and fatal heart attack: the Athens (1981) earthquake natural experiment. Lancet 1983; 1:441–444.

92. Leor J, Poole WK, Kloner RA. Sudden cardiac death triggered by an earthquake [see comments]. N Engl J Med 1996;334:413–419.
93. Schwartz PJ, Zaza A, Locati E, Moss AJ. Stress and sudden death. The case of the long QT syndrome. Circulation 1991;83:II71–II80.
94. Frimerman A, Miller HI, Laniado S, Keren G. Changes in hemostatic function at times of cyclic variation in occupational stress. Am J Cardiol 1997;79:72–75.
95. Jern C, Eriksson E, Tengborn L, Risberg B, Wadenvik H, Jern S. Changes of plasma coagulation and fibrinolysis in response to mental stress. Thromb Haemost 1989;62:767–771.
96. Muller JE, Abela GS, Nesto RW, Tofler GH. Triggers, acute risk factors and vulnerable plaques: the lexicon of a new frontier. J Am Coll Cardiol 1994;23:809–813.
97. Falk E. Plaque rupture with severe pre-existing stenosis precipitating coronary thrombosis. Characteristics of coronary atherosclerotic plaques underlying fatal occlusive thrombi. Br Heart J 1983;50:127–134.
98. Davies MJ, Thomas A. Thrombosis and acute coronary-artery lesions in sudden cardiac ischemic death. N Engl J Med 1984;310:1137–1140.
99. Fuster V, Badimon L, Badimon JJ, Chesebro JH. The pathogenesis of coronary artery disease and the acute coronary syndromes (2). N Engl J Med 1992;326:310–318.
100. Willerson JT, Campbell WB, Winniford MD, Schmitz J, Apprill P, Firth BG, et al. Conversion from chronic to acute coronary artery disease: speculation regarding mechanisms. Am J Cardiol 1984;54:1349–1354.
101. Richardson PD, Davies MJ, Born GV. Influence of plaque configuration and stress distribution on fissuring of coronary atherosclerotic plaques [see comments]. Lancet 1989;2:941–944.
102. Davies MJ. The contribution of thrombosis to the clinical expression of coronary atherosclerosis. Thromb Res 1996;82:1–32.
103. Libby P. Molecular bases of the acute coronary syndromes. Circulation 1995;91:2844–2850.
104. Belch JJ, McArdle BM, Burns P, Lowe GD, Forbes CD. The effects of acute smoking on platelet behaviour, fibrinolysis and haemorheology in habitual smokers. Thromb Haemost 1984;51:6–8.
105. Brown BG, Zhao XQ, Sacco DE, Albers JJ. Lipid lowering and plaque regression. New insights into prevention of plaque disruption and clinical events in coronary disease. Circulation 1993;87:1781–1791.
106. Sexton PT, Jamrozik K, Walsh J. Sudden unexpected cardiac death among Tasmanian men. Med J Aust 1993;159:467–470.
107. Myerburg RJ, Kessler KM, Castellanos A. Sudden cardiac death. Structure, function, and time-dependence of risk. Circulation 1992;85:I2–I10.
108. Jimenez RA, Myerburg RJ. Sudden cardiac death. Magnitude of the problem, substrate/trigger interaction, and populations at high risk. Cardiol Clin 1993;11:1–9.
109. Sexton PT, Walsh J, Jamrozik K, Parsons R. Risk factors for sudden unexpected cardiac death in Tasmanian men. Aust NZ J Med 1997;27:45–50.
110. Wannamethee G, Shaper AG, Macfarlane PW, Walker M. Risk factors for sudden cardiac death in middle-aged British men. Circulation 1995;91:1749–1756.
111. Gillum RF. Sudden cardiac death in Hispanic Americans and African Americans. Am J Public Health 1997;87:1461–1466.
112. Brugada P, Geelen P. Some electrocardiographic patterns predicting sudden cardiac death that every doctor should recognize. Acta Cardiol 1997;52:473–484.
113. Brugada J, Brugada P. Further characterization of the syndrome of right bundle branch block, ST segment elevation, and sudden cardiac death. J Cardiovasc Electrophysiol 1997;8:325–331.
114. Yi G, Guo XH, Reardon M, Gallagher MM, Hnatkova K, Camm AJ, et al. Circadian variation of the QT interval in patients with sudden cardiac death after myocardial infarction. Am J Cardiol 1998;81:950–956.

115. Meinertz T, Hofmann T, Zehender M. Can we predict sudden cardiac death? Drugs 1991;2: 9–15.
116. Shen WK, Hammill SC. Survivors of acute myocardial infarction: who is at risk for sudden cardiac death? Mayo Clin Proc 1991;66:950–962.
117. Hayashi S, Toyoshima H, Tanabe N, Satoh T, Miyanishi K, Seki N, et al. Activity immediately before the onset of non-fatal myocardial infarction and sudden cardiac death. Jpn Circ J 1996;60:947–953.
118. Maron BJ, Poliac LC, Roberts WO. Risk for sudden cardiac death associated with marathon running. J Am Coll Cardiol 1996;28:428–431.
119. Maron BJ. Triggers for sudden cardiac death in the athlete. Cardiol Clin 1996;14:195–210.
120. Burke AP, Farb A, Virmani R, Goodin J, Smialek JE. Sports-related and non-sports-related sudden cardiac death in young adults. Am Heart J 1991;121:568–575.
121. Taylor AJ, Rogan KM, Virmani R. Sudden cardiac death associated with isolated congenital coronary artery anomalies. J Am Coll Cardiol 1992;20:640–647.
122. Phillips M, Robinowitz M, Higgins JR, Boran KJ, Reed T, Virmani R. Sudden cardiac death in Air Force recruits. A 20-year review. JAMA 1986;256:2696–2699.
123. Adgey AA, Johnston PW, McMechan S. Sudden cardiac death and substance abuse. Resuscitation 1995;29:219–221.
124. Willich SN, Levy D, Rocco MB, Tofler GH, Stone PH, Muller JE. Circadian variation in the incidence of sudden cardiac death in the Framingham Heart Study population. Am J Cardiol 1987;60:801–806.
125. Muller JE, Ludmer PL, Willich SN, Tofler GH, Aylmer G, Klangos I, et al. Circadian variation in the frequency of sudden cardiac death [see comments]. Circulation 1987;75: 131–138.
126. Levine RL, Pepe PE, Fromm RE Jr, Curka PA, Clark PA. Prospective evidence of a circadian rhythm for out-of-hospital cardiac arrests. JAMA 1992;267:2935–2937.
127. Willich SN, Goldberg RJ, Maclure M, Perriello L, Muller JE. Increased onset of sudden cardiac death in the first three hours after awakening. Am J Cardiol 1992;70:65–68.
128. Thakur RK, Hoffmann RG, Olson DW, Joshi R, Tresch DD, Aufderheide TP, et al. Circadian variation in sudden cardiac death: effects of age, sex, and initial cardiac rhythm. Ann Emerg Med 1996;27:29–34.
129. Uretsky BF, Sheahan RG. Primary prevention of sudden cardiac death in heart failure: will the solution be shocking? J Am Coll Cardiol 1997;30:1589–1597.
130. Behrens S, Ney G, Fisher SG, Fletcher RD, Franz MR, Singh SN. Effects of amiodarone on the circadian pattern of sudden cardiac death (Department of Veterans Affairs Congestive Heart Failure-Survival Trial of Antiarrhythmic Therapy). Am J Cardiol 1997;80:45–48.
131. Peters RW, Mitchell LB, Brooks MM, Echt DS, Barker AH, Capone R, et al. Circadian pattern of arrhythmic death in patients receiving encainide, flecainide or moricizine in the Cardiac Arrhythmia Suppression Trial (CAST). J Am Coll Cardiol 1994;23:283–289.
132. Cohen MC, Rohtla KM, Lavery CE, Muller JE, Mittleman MA. Meta-analysis of the morning excess of acute myocardial infarction and sudden cardiac death. Am J Cardiol 1997;79: 1512–1516.
133. Peckova M, Fahrenbruch CE, Cobb LA, Hallstrom AP. Circadian variations in the occurrence of cardiac arrests: initial and repeat episodes. Circulation 1998;98:31–39.
134. Maron BJ, Kogan J, Proschan MA, Hecht GM, Roberts WC. Circadian variability in the occurrence of sudden cardiac death in. J Am Coll Cardiol 1994;23:1405–1409.
135. Rabkin SW, Mathewson FA, Tate RB. Chronobiology of cardiac sudden death in men. JAMA 1980;244:1357–1358.
136. Mifune J, Takeda Y. Sudden cardiac arrest: clinical characteristics and predictors of survival. Jpn Circ J 1989;53:1536–1540.

137. Goudevenos JA, Papadimitriou ED, Papathanasiou A, Makis AC, Pappas K, Sideris DA. Incidence and other epidemiological characteristics of sudden cardiac death in northwest Greece. Int J Cardiol 1995;49:67–75.

138. Assanelli D, Bersatti F, Turla C, Restori M, Amariti ML, Romano A, et al. Circadian variation of sudden cardiac death in young people with and without coronary disease. Cardiologia 1997;42:729–735.

139. Pasqualetti P, Colantonio D, Casale R, Acitelli P, Natali G. The chronobiology of sudden cardiac death. The evidence for a circadian, circaseptimanal and circannual periodicity in its incidence. Minerva Med 1990;81:391–398.

140. Ishida K, Takagi T, Ohkura K, Yabuki S, Machii K, Ito M. Out-of-hospital sudden cardiac death: a comparative study spanning 10 years. J Cardiol 1989;19:765–773.

141. Goto T, Yokoyama K, Okada T, Araki T, Miura T, Saitoh H, et al. Sudden cardiac death in the emergency hospital. Kokyu To Junkan 1990;38:665–670.

142. Arntz HR, Willich SN, Oeff M, Bruggemann T, Stern R, Heinzmann A, et al. Circadian variation of sudden cardiac death reflects age-related variability in ventricular fibrillation. Circulation 1993;88:2284–2289.

143. Martens PR, Calle P, Van den Poel B, Lewi P. Further prospective evidence of a circadian variation in the frequency of call for sudden cardiac death. Belgian Cardiopulmonary Cerebral Resuscitation Study Group. Intensive Care Med 1995;21:45–49.

144. Hayashi S, Toyoshima H, Tanabe N, Miyanishi K. Daily peaks in the incidence of sudden cardiac death and fatal stroke. Jpn Circ J 1996;60:193–200.

145. Tatsanavivat P, Chiravatkul A, Klungboonkrong V, Chaisiri S, Jarerntanyaruk L, Munger RG, et al. Sudden and unexplained deaths in sleep (Laitai) of young men in rural northeastern Thailand. Int J Epidemiol 1992;21:904–910.

146. Peters RW, Muller JE, Goldstein S, Byington R, Friedman LM. Propranolol and the morning increase in the frequency of sudden cardiac death (BHAT Study). Am J Cardiol 1989;63: 1518–1520.

147. Andersen L, Sigurd B, Hansen J. Verapamil and circadian variation of sudden cardiac death. Am Heart J 1996;131:409–410.

148. Albert CM, Hennekens CH, O'Donnell CJ, Ajani UA, Carey VJ, Willett WC, et al. Fish consumption and risk of sudden cardiac death [see comments]. JAMA 1998;279:23–28.

149. Peters RW. Circadian patterns and triggers of sudden cardiac death. Cardiol Clin 1996;14: 185–194.

150. Olshausen KV, Witt T, Pop T, Treese N, Bethge KP, Meyer J. Sudden cardiac death while wearing a Holter monitor. Am J Cardiol 1991;67:381–386.

151. Henry PD, Pacifico A. Sudden cardiac death: still more questions than answers [editorial]. G Ital Cardiol 1997;27:1319–1324.

152. Canada WB, Woodward W, Lee G, DeMaria A, Low R, Mason DT, et al. Circadian rhythm of hourly ventricular arrhythmia frequency in man. Angiology 1983;34:274–282.

153. Twidale N, Taylor S, Heddle WF, Ayres BF, Tonkin AM. Morning increase in the time of onset of sustained ventricular tachycardia. Am J Cardiol 1989;64:1204–1206.

154. Valkama JO, Huikuri HV, Linnaluoto MK, Takkunen JT. Circadian variation of ventricular tachycardia in patients with coronary arterial disease. Int J Cardiol 1992;34:173–178.

155. Rebuzzi AG, Lucente M, Lanza GA, Coppola E, Manzoli U. Circadian rhythm of ventricular tachycardia. Prog Clin Biol Res 1987;277B:153–158.

156. Lampert R, Rosenfeld L, Batsford W, Lee F, McPherson C. Circadian variation of sustained ventricular tachycardia in patients with coronary artery disease and implantable cardioverter-defibrillators [see comments]. Circulation 1994;90:241–247.

157. d'Avila A, Wellens F, Andries E, Brugada P. At what time are implantable defibrillator shocks delivered? Evidence for individual circadian variance in sudden cardiac death [see comments]. Eur Heart J 1995;16:1231–1233.

158. Behrens S, Galecka M, Bruggemann T, Ehlers C, Willich SN, Ziss W, et al. Circadian variation of sustained ventricular tachyarrhythmias terminated by appropriate shocks in patients with an implantable cardioverter defibrillator. Am Heart J 1995;130:79–84.

159. Mallavarapu C, Pancholy S, Schwartzman D, Callans DJ, Heo J, Gottlieb CD, et al. Circadian variation of ventricular arrhythmia recurrences after cardioverter-defibrillator implantation in patients with healed myocardial infarcts. Am J Cardiol 1995;75:1140–1144.

160. Fries R, Heisel A, Huwer H, Nikoloudakis N, Jung J, Schafers HJ, et al. Incidence and clinical significance of short-term recurrent ventricular tachyarrhythmias in patients with implantable cardioverter–defibrillator. Int J Cardiol 1997;59:281–284.

161. Tofler GH, Gebara OC, Mittleman MA, Taylor P, Siegel W, Venditti FJ Jr, et al. Morning peak in ventricular tachyarrhythmias detected by time of implantable cardioverter/defibrillator therapy. The CPI Investigators. Circulation 1995;92:1203–1208.

162. Venditti FJ Jr, John RM, Hull M, Tofler GH, Shahian DM, Martin DT. Circadian variation in defibrillation energy requirements. Circulation 1996;94:1607–1612.

163. Fries R, Heisel A, Nikoloudakis N, Jung J, Schafers HJ, Schieffer H. Antitachycardia pacing in patients with implantable cardioverter–defibrillators: inverse circadian variation of therapy success and acceleration. Am J Cardiol 1997;80:1487–1489.

164. McClelland J, Halperin B, Cutler J, Kudenchuk P, Kron J, McAnulty J. Circadian variation in ventricular electrical instability associated with coronary artery disease. Am J Cardiol 1990;65:1351–1357.

165. Nanthakumar K, Newman D, Paquette M, Greene M, Rakovich G, Dorian P. Circadian variation of sustained ventricular tachycardia in patients subject to standard adrenergic blockade. Am Heart J 1997;134:752–757.

166. Behrens S, Ehlers C, Bruggemann T, Ziss W, Dissmann R, Galecka M, et al . Modification of the circadian pattern of ventricular tachyarrhythmias by beta-blocker therapy. Clin Cardiol 1997;20:253–257.

167. Wood MA, Simpson PM, London WB, Stambler BS, Herre JM, Bernstein RC, et al. Circadian pattern of ventricular tachyarrhythmias in patients with implantable cardioverter–defibrillators. J Am Coll Cardiol 1995;25:901–907.

168. Lucente M, Rebuzzi AG, Lanza GA, Tamburi S, Cortellessa MC, Coppola E, et al. Circadian variation of ventricular tachycardia in acute myocardial infarction. Am J Cardiol 1988;62:670–674.

169. Wolpert C, Jung W, Spehl S, Schumacher B, Omran H, Schimpf R, et al . Circadian and weekly distribution of malignant ventricular arrhythmias in patients with coronary heart disease or dilatative cardiomyopathy who have an implanted cardioverter–defibrillator. Dtsch Med Wochenschr 1998;123:140–145.

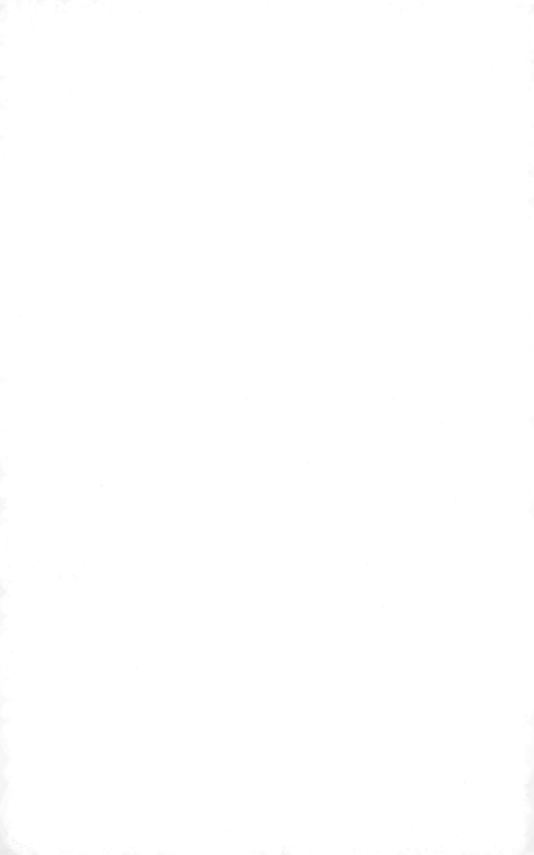

11 Seasonal, Weekly, and Circadian Variability of Ischemic and Hemorrhagic Stroke

Tudor D. Vagaonescu, MD, PHD,
Robert A. Phillips, MD, PHD,
and Stanley Tuhrim, MD

CONTENTS

INTRODUCTION

Circadian rhythms have been recognized in many biological phenomena, including secretion of hormones, activities of the autonomic nervous system, and various cardiovascular pathologies. Transient myocardial ischemia *(1,2)*, acute myocardial infarction *(3)*, embolism *(4)*, sudden cardiac death *(5)*, and death resulting from hypertension, ischemic heart disease, and cerebrovascular disease *(6)* have been shown to follow a certain circadian pattern; the same has been observed in the onset of stroke.

Stroke onset has been categorized into three general patterns according to their temporal distribution: circadian (rhythm length of approximately 24 h), circaseptan (rhythm length of about 1 wk), seasonal or circannual (rhythm with

From: *Contemporary Cardiology:*
Blood Pressure Monitoring in Cardiovascular Medicine and Therapeutics
Edited by: W. B. White © Humana Press Inc., Totowa, NJ

a period of about 1 yr). Newer methods of analyzing temporal variation include the single cosinor method, which adjusts, by least squares, a rhythmic function with a presumed period to data series, providing point and interval estimates of mesor (average values of rhythmic function fitted to the data), amplitude (half the total predictable change defined by the rhythmic function fitted to the data), and acrophase (lag from a given reference time of the rhythm's crest time, defined by the rhythmic function fitted to the data) (7). A summary of the most important studies in this area is provided in Table 1.

SEASONAL VARIABILITY

Seasonal variation in the occurrence of cerebrovascular diseases has been noted since ancient times. The Old Testament suggested that apoplexy ("struck violently") occured more often during hot weather (8). Over the past two centuries, several authors have addressed the topic of seasonal periodicity in the onset of stroke (7,9–31).

In the subtropical zone, patients of age 70 and above have been noted to have more cerebral infarcts on warmer days (26). This might be the result of increases in thromboembolic mechanisms secondary to physiological changes in response to heat: dehydration, increased blood viscosity and hemoconcentration, decrease in blood pressure, and increased concentration of platelets (27).

In both the Northern and Southern Hemispheres, stroke seems to be associated frequently with cold weather. The cold climate may contribute to a higher incidence of strokes by hemodynamic and nonhemodynamic mechanisms. Blood pressure (as the major hemodynamic factor) is higher during cold weather (32). In addition to increased vasoconstriction in the cold, poor control of hypertension in winter months may result because of delays in outpatient therapy during adverse weather conditions (18). Hypertension by itself is not the only responsible factor for the increased stroke rate in winter time, as normotensives have been noticed to have also a higher incidence of cerebral hemorrhage during winter (26). Other (nonhemodynamic) factors that might explain this finding are increased platelet and erythrocyte counts, blood viscosity, and catecholamine secretion, all increasing with the decrease in temperature (33). The possible relation of the seasonal variation of serum cholesterol (higher in winter months and lower in the summer) (34–37) with the seasonality of cerebrovascular disease has not been explained. Controversies exist about the seasonal variation observed within the different stroke categories and within different age groups. A seasonal variability for cerebral hemorrhage has been noted by some groups (16,18,22,23, 28,29) but not by others (19,20); thromboembolic stroke was shown to present with a seasonal pattern in most of the studies (7,13,14,19,20,22,23,26,31). The seasonal association with certain types of strokes seems to be dependent, at least partly, with the age of the patients in certain climates: in Japan, younger patients (less than 64 yr old) showed a higher seasonality than elderly patients *(23)*, whereas in Ireland, elderly patients presented a negative correlation between the occurrence of cerebrovascular accidents and the temperature during winter months *(24)*. The rupture of intracranial aneurysms has been reported to occur most often in late fall in men, and in late spring in women *(25)*. The differences may be explained by the very heterogeneous populations studied.

CIRCASEPTAN VARIABILITY

Few studies have concentrated on the circaseptan variability in cerebrovascular disease *(22,31,37,38)*. Weekly variability could be related to the change in behaviors that occur during certain periods of the week. The circaseptan variability has been identified as an increase in strokes on Saturday evenings (a result of the short-term lifestyle changes during the weekend) *(22)*, on Mondays (in working patients, associated with male sex, alcohol use, cigaret smoking, and hypertension) *(31)*, or on Wednesdays (in hospital-onset strokes when compared with community-onset strokes) *(32)* or Tuesdays (for large-vessel infarction) *(38)*.

CIRCADIAN VARIABILITY

Although earlier studies suggested that the onset of stroke was fairly evenly distributed among the 24 h of the day *(11)*, more recent studies suggest a circadian variability for all strokes as well as for certain stroke subtypes. However, contradictory data exists regarding the precise onset of stroke. This has been observed to occur more frequently

- In the early morning hours (midnight to 6 AM) *(39–41)*;
- During the late morning hours (6 AM to noon) *(7,14,28,31,42–51)*;
- Between 6 AM and 6 PM *(52–54)*.

The contradictory data presented are explained by the difficulties encountered in determining the exact time of stroke onset (self-report or report by family members, tendency to underreport strokes occurring during a certain time of the day, recalling stroke onset according to its severity) as well as the possible link between the stroke onset and the triggering event, which may be several hours away from the onset of stroke symptoms *(55,56)*.

Stroke categories seem to respect also a certain circadian pattern:

- Atherothrombotic stroke has been described more often between midnight and 6 AM *(41)* or between 6 AM and noon *(14,28,42)*;
- Intracerebral hemorrhage occurs more often between 6 AM and noon *(14,28,41–44)*; and
- Embolic stroke seems to occur more frequently between noon and 6 PM *(14,41)*.

Similar results were obtained in a large cohort of 1148 patients admitted to the Mount Sinai Medical Center in New York City over 6 yr, where the onset of stroke

Table 1

Summary of the Studies Assessing the Temporal Distribution of Stroke Onset

Author/year	Type of study	Location	No. of patients	Age	Temporal variability (peak month, day or hours)	Notes
Perkins (1933)	Hospital	Brooklyn, NY	801	N/A	Seasonal (September–January)	
Aring (1935)	Hospital	Boston, MA	245	N/A	Seasonal (November–March)	
Bokonjic (1968)	Hospital	Sarajevo, Yugoslavia	463	N/A	Seasonal (December–January)	
Mc Dowell (1970)	Hospital	New York, NY	1000	N/A	Seasonal (winter months)	
Alter (1970)	Hospital	Fargo, ND and Moorhead, MN	408	N/A	Seasonal (April and November)	
Hossmann (1971)	Hospital	Koln, Germany	127	N/A	Circadian (1 AM to 5 AM)	Embolic stroke (noon to midnight; March–May)
Olivares (1973)	Hospital	Mexico City, Mexico	206	65	Circadian (6 AM to noon) Seasonal (August–September)	
Agnoli (1975)	Hospital	Rome, Italy	256	N/A	Circadian (6 AM to 2 PM)	Infarct (midnight to 6 AM)
Marshall (1977)	Hospital	London, UK	707	N/A	Circadian (midnight to 6 AM)	Hemorrhage (noon to midnight)
Ramirez-Lassepas (1980)	Hospital	St Paul, MN	128	63	Seasonal (January–March)	
Brackenridge (1981)	Hospital and community	Melbourne, Australia	1630	68.8	Circaseptan (Wednesday) Seasonal (mid–July)	
Christie (1981)	Community	Melbourne, Australia		N/A	Seasonal (July)	
Haberman (1981)	Hospital and community	England and Wales, UK	864	N/A	Seasonal (January–March)	
Kaps (1983)	Hospital	Giessen, Germany	563	64	Circadian (7 AM to 7 PM)	
Jovicic (1983)	Hospital	Belgrad, Yugoslawia	85	N/A	Circadian (8 AM to 11 AM) Seasonal (September–November)	
Tsementzis (1985)	Hospital	West Midlands and Birmingham, UK	567	<70	Circadian (10 AM to noon)	SAH (10 AM to noon; 6 PM to 8 PM)
Suzuki (1987)	Hospital	Akita, Japan	2168	<67.1	Seasonal (December–February)	TIA (June–August)
Sobel (1987)	Hospital and community	Lehig Valley, PA	1944		Seasonal (none for all strokes)	Infarct (February–April)
Van der Windt (1988)	Hospital	Utrecht, Netherlands	66	N/A	Circadian (6 AM to 6 PM)	
Gill (1988)	Hospital	West Midlands, UK	30,679	N/A	Seasonal (January)	
Biller (1988)	Hospital	Iowa City, IA	2960	N/A	Seasonal (none for all strokes)	Cerebral Infarction (June–August) ICH (December–February)
Marler (1989)	Hospital	MD, MA, CA, IL	1167	68	Circadian (10 AM to noon)	
Marsh (1990)	Hospital	Iowa City, IA	151	63	Circadian (6 AM to noon)	

246

Study	Setting	Location	No.	Mean age	Temporal pattern	Stroke subtype pattern
Arboix (1990)	Hospital	Barcelona, Spain	206	N/A	Circadian (none for all strokes)	Thrombotic stroke (midnight to 6 AM); Intraparenchymal hemorrhage (6 AM to noon); Cardioembolic stroke (6 AM to 6 PM)
Argentino (1990)	Hospital	Rome, Italy	426	66	Circadian (6 AM to noon)	
Pasqualetti (1990)	Hospital	L'Aquila, Italy	732	N/A	Circadian (2 AM to 8AM); Circaseptan (Saturday–Tuesday); Seasonal (September–March)	
Shinkawa (1990)	Hospital and community	Hisayama, Japan	308	72	Seasonal (February)	Hemorrhage (January); Infarction (March)
Johansson (1990)	Hospital	Lund, Sweden	497	73	Circadian (9 AM to 1PM); Circaseptan (Tuesday); Seasonal (none for all strokes)	Infarction (July and December); Embolic Stroke (March and April)
Woo (1991)	Hospital	Shatin, Hong Kong	683	N/A	Seasonal (none)	
Ince (1992)	Hospital	Istanbul, Turkey	120	N/A	Circadian (6 AM to 6 PM)	
Wroe (1992)	Hospital and community	Oxfordshire, UK	675	N/A	Circadian (6 AM to noon)	Infarct (6 AM to noon; 2 PM to 4 PM); SAH (8 AM to 10 AM; 6 PM to 8 PM); ICH (10 AM to noon; 6 PM to 8PM); SAH (10 AM to noon; 2 PM to 4 PM)
Sloan (1992)	Hospital	MA, MD, NY, IL	480	61	Circadian (none for all strokes)	
Ricci (1992)	Community	Umbria, Italy	368	N/A	Circadian (6 AM to noon)	ICH (September–December)
Capon (1992)	Hospital	Brussels, Belgium	236	N/A	Seasonal (December–March)	
Pardiwalla (1993)	Hospital	Bombay, India	182	N/A	Seasonal (November–December)	
Chyatte (1993)	Hospital	Chicago, IL	1487	N/A	Circadian (6 AM to 2 PM); Seasonal (late spring women; late fall men)	Intracranial aneurysm
Gallerani (1993)	Hospital	Ferrara, Italy	977	NA	Circadian (7 AM to noon); Seasonal (October)	
Vinall (1994)	Hospital	14 countries	685	50	Seasonal (January–March)	SAH secondary to aneurysm rupture
Butchart (1994)	Hospital	Cardiff, UK	96	N/A	Seasonal (December–March); Circadian (6 AM to noon)	
Kelly–Hayes (1995)	Community and hospital	Framingham, MA	635	N/A	Circadian (8 AM to noon); Circaseptan (Monday); Seasonal (January and August)	
Lago (1998)	Hospital	Valencia and Castellon, Spain	1223	72	Circadian (1 AM to 6AM)	
Tuhrim (1998)	Hospital	New York, NY	1148	71	Seasonal (November–January); Circadian (6 AM to noon)	

Abbreviations: ICH = intracerebral hemorrhage; SAH = subarachnoidal hemorrhage; TIA = transient ischemic attack.

(caused by cerebral infarction as well as cerebral hemorrhage) has been observed to occur most frequently between 6 AM and noon (and between November and January) (Tuhrim et al., unpublished results).

Nevertheless, most data suggest that infarcts occur in the morning hours. By analyzing the data by the single cosinor method, the acrophase for all strokes has been described between 2 AM and 8 AM (22), between 7 AM and noon (7), and at 11 AM (38). For the different stroke categories, the acrophase has been described between 11 AM and noon for cerebral infarction (7,38), at 10:24 AM for cardioembolic stroke (38), at 12:41 PM for transient ischemic attacks (7), and at 5:16 PM for subarachnoid hemorrhage (38). No difference in circadian rhythm has been observed between first time and recurrent stroke (50). The circadian variability of stroke onset has been described also in patients with mitral valve replacement, who present a peak of cerebrovascular events (transient ischemic attacks, reversible ischemic neurological deficits, or strokes) in the morning (and winter months) (57). The mechanisms responsible for the circadian pattern of stroke onset may include variation of the blood pressure, instability of the atherosclerotic plaque, a relatively prothrombotic state, and increased arrhythmogenesis.

It is known that blood pressure presents a circadian variation (58–62), and in hypertensive patients, it has been suggested that the early morning onset of cerebral hemorrhage (as well as subarachnoid hemorrhage) is the result of a rapidly increasing arterial blood pressure in the morning (43,58). The association between intracerebral hemorrhage and the diurnal variation of blood pressure seems to be very strong in untreated hypertensives (48). The nondipping or dipping pattern of the 24 h monitoring of blood pressure appears to be associated with the cerebrovascular disease.

Nondippers (hypertensives whose 24 h blood pressure does not follow the normal circadian pattern) have a higher risk of stroke (63). The nondipping status conferred risk for stroke even after adjustment for traditional stroke risk factors (64). Sometimes, the change from a "dipper" to a "nondipper" status may be attributed to a small lacunar infarct (65). The absence of "dipping" or the lower nocturnal blood pressure fall in elderly hypertensives might be associated with silent cerebrovascular disease (66). The diminished nocturnal blood pressure decline in cerebrovascular disease is thought to be caused by specific injury to the central autonomic nervous system (such as the striatum, midbrain, pontine tegmentum, or insular cortex) (67,68).

The preserved circadian "dip" in hypertensives (mostly in the early morning) might induce a "critical" local hypotension that can be responsible for the stroke (especially when superimposed on a critical stenosis of the cerebral vessels) (39, 69,70). Silent cerebrovascular lesions are more severe in elderly women with an extreme dipper pattern of circadian blood pressure variation (71).

Factors that may predispose to increased coagulation or vasoconstriction also demonstrate circadian variation are as follows:

- Peak hematocrit and blood viscosity (as important factors influencing cerebral flow) have been described to occur at 8 AM *(72)*.
- The highest fibrinolytic inhibition (and barely detectable tissue plasminogen activity in the blood) occurs between 3 and 8 AM *(73,74)*.
- Spontaneous increase in platelet sensitivity to epinephrine and the binding affinity of the α_2- adrenoreceptors were maximum at 8 AM *(75)*.
- Platelet aggregability increases between 9:30 and 11 AM (after assumption of the upright posture) *(76)*.
- Plasma renin activity of recumbent normal subjects presents the highest values between 2 and 8 AM (with a further increase when assuming the upright posture) *(77)*.
- Minimum vascular resistance is higher in the morning and night compared to noon and evening *(78)*.

FINAL CONSIDERATIONS

Several observations have shown the existence of a certain temporal (seasonal, weekly, and daily) variability in the onset of acute stroke. Further studies are necessary to better characterize and prevent the potential triggers of cardiovascular events (vulnerable plaque, refractory hypertension, nondipping status, etc.) *(79)* as well as to provide a better understanding of the role played by certain hormones (like melatonin) in the regulation of various circadian rhythms and stroke onset *(80–83)*.

REFERENCES

1. Stern S, Tzivoni D. Early detection of silent ischemic heart disease by 24-hour electrocardiographic monitoring of active subjects. Br Heart J 1974;36:481–486.
2. Rocco MB, Barry J, Campbell S, Nabel E, Cook EF, Goldman L, et al. Circadian variation of transient myocardial ischemia in patients with coronary artery disease. Circulation 1987;75:395–400.
3. Muller JE, Stone PH, Turi ZG, Rutherford JD, Czeisler CA, Parker C, et al., and the MILLIS Study Group. Circadian variation in the frequency of onset of acute myocardial infarction. N Engl J Med 1985;313:1315–1322.
4. Dewar HA, Weightman D. A study of embolism in mitral valve disease and atrial fibrillation. Br Heart J 1983;49:133–140.
5. Willich SN, Levy D, Rocco MB, Tofler GH, Stone PH, Muller JE. Circadian variation in the incidence of sudden cardiac death in the framingham heart study population. Am J Cardiol 1987;60:801–806.
6. Mittler MM, Hajdukovic RM, Shafor R, Hahn PM, Kripke DF. When people die. Cause of death versus time of death. Am J Med 1987;82:266–274.
7. Gallerani M, Manfredini R, Ricci L, Cocurullo A, Goldoni C, Bigoni M, et al. Chronobiological aspects of acute cerebrovascular diseases. Acta Neurol Scand 1993;87:482–487.
8. Garrison FH. An Introduction to the History of Medicine, With Medical Chrononlogy, Suggestions for Study and Bibliographic Data, 4th ed. Saunders, Philadelphia, 1929, p. 67.
9. Gintrac E. Traite theorique et pratique de l'appareil nerveux, vol. 2. Germer-Bailliere, Paris, 1869, p. 467.
10. Gowers WR. Diseases of the Nervous System, vol. 2, 2nd ed. Churchill, London 1893, p. 388.
11. Aring CD, Merritt HH. Differential diagnosis between cerebral hemorrhage and cerebral thrombosis. Arch Intern Med 1935;56:435–456.

12. Bokonjic R, Zec N. Strokes and the weather. A quantitative statistical study. J Neurol Sci 1968;6:483–491.
13. McDowell FH, Louis S, Monahan K. Seasonal variation of non-embolic cerebral infarction. J Chronic Dis 1970;23:29–32.
14. Olivares L, Castaneda E, Grife A, Alter M. Risk factors in stroke: a clinical study in Mexican patients. Stroke 1973;4:773–781.
15. Christie D. Stroke in Melbourne, Australia: an epidemiologic study. Stroke 1981;12(4):467–469.
16. Ramirez- Lassepas M, Haus E, Lakatua DJ. Seasonal (circannual) periodicity of spontaneous intracerebral hemorrhage in Minnesota. Ann Neurol 1980;8:539–541.
17. Haberman S, Capildeo R, Clifford Rose F. The seasonal variation in mortality from cerebrovascular disease. J Neurol Sci 1981;52:25–36.
18. Suzuki K, Kutsuzawa T, Takita K, Ito M, Sakamoto T, Hirayama A, et al. Clinico-epidemiologic study of stroke in Akita, Japan. Stroke 1987;18:402–406.
19. Sobel E, Zhang Z, Alter M, Lai S, Davanipour Z, Friday G, et al. Stroke in Lehig Valley: seasonal variation in incidence rates. Stroke 1987;18:38–42.
20. Gill JS, Davies P, Gill SK, Beevers DG. Wind-chill and the seasonal variation of cerebrovascular disease. J Clin Epidemiol 1988;41(3):225–230.
21. Biller J, Jones MP, Bruno A, Adams HP Jr, Banwart K. Seasonal variation of stroke—does it exist? Neuroepidemiology 1988;7:89–98.
22. Pasqualetti P, Natali G, Casale R, Colantonio D. Epidemiological chronorisk of stroke. Acta Neurol Scand 1990;81:71–74.
23. Shinkawa A, Ueda K, Hasuo Y, Kiyohara Y, Fujishima M. Seasonal variation in stroke incidence in Hisayama, Japan. Stroke 1990;21:1262–1267.
24. Bull GM. Meteorological correlates with myocardial and cerebral infarction and respiratory disease. Brit J Prev Soc Med 1973;27:108–113.
25. Chyatte D, Chen T, Bronstein K, Brass L. Seasonal fluctuations in the incidence of intracranial aneurysm rupture and its relationship to changing climatic conditions. Stroke 1993;24:187 (abstract).
26. Woo J, Kay R, Nicholls MG. Environmental temperature and stroke in a subtropical climate. Neuroepidemiology 1991;10:260–265.
27. Berginer VM, Goldsmith J, Batz U, Vardi H, Shapiro Y. Clustering of strokes in association with meteorologic factors in the Negev Desert of Israel: 1981–1983. Stroke 1989;20:65–69.
28. Ricci S, Celani MG, Vitali R, La Rosa F, Righetti E, Duca E. Diurnal and seasonal variations in the occurance of stroke: a community-based study. Neuroepidemiology 1992;11:59–64.
29. Capon A, Demeurisse G, Zheng L. Seasonal variation of cerebral hemorrhage in 236 consecutive cases in Brussels. Stroke 1992;23:24–27.
30. Vinall PE, Maislin G, Michele JJ, Deitch C, Simeone FA. Seasonal and latitudinal occurrence of cerebral vasospasm and subarachnoid hemorrhage in the Northern Hemisphere. Epidemiology 1994;5:302–308.
31. Kelly-Hayes M, Wolf PA, Kase CS, Brand FN, McGuirk JM, D'Agostion RB. Temporal patterns of stroke onset. The Framingham Study. Stroke 1995;26:1343–1347.
32. Brennan PJ, Greenberg G, Miall WE, Thompson SG. Seasonal variation in arterial blood pressure. Br Med J 1982;285:919–923.
32a.Alter M, Christoferson L, Resch J, Myers G, Ford J. Cerebrovascular disease: frequency and population selectivity in an upper midwestern community. Stroke 1970;1:454–465.
33. Keatinge WR, Coleshaw SRK, Cotter F, Mattock M, Murphy M, Chelliah R. Increases in platelet and red cell counts, blood viscosity, and arterial pressure during mild surface cooling: factors in mortality from coronary and cerebral thrombosis in winter. Br Med J 1984;289: 1405–1408.
34. Bleiler RE, Yearick ES, Schnur SS , Singson IL, Ohlson MA. Seasonal variation of cholesterol in serum of men and women. Am J Clin Nutr 1963;12:12–16.

35. Doyle JT, Kinch SH, Brown DF. Seasonal variation in serum cholesterol concentration. J Chronic Dis 1965;18:657–664.
36. Gordon DJ, Hyde J, Trost DC, Whaley FS, Hannan PJ, Jacobs DR, et al. Cyclic seasonal variation in plasma lipid and lipoprotein levels: The Lipid Research Clinics Coronary Primary Prevention Trial Placebo Group. J Clin Epidemiol 1988;41:679–689.
37. Brackenridge CJ. Daily variation and other factors affecting the occurence of cerebrovascular accidents. J Gerontol 1981;36(2):176–179.
38. Johansson BB, Norrving B, Widner H, Wu J, Halberg F. Stroke incidence: circadian and circaseptan (about weekly) variations in onset. In: Hayes DK, Pauly JE, Deiter RJ (eds.), Chronobiology: Its Role in Clinical Medicine, General Biology and Agriculture. Wiley-Liss, New York, 1990, pp. 427–436.
39. Hossmann V. Circadian changes of blood pressure and stroke. In: Zulch KJ, ed. Cerebral Circulation and Stroke. Springer-Verlag, New York, 1971, pp. 203–208.
40. Marshall J. Diurnal variation in occurrence of strokes. Stroke 1977;8:230–231.
41. Arboix A, Marti-Vilalta JL. Acute stroke and circadian rhythm [Letter]. Stroke 1990;21:826.
42. Wroe SJ, Sandercock, Bamford J, Dennis M, Slattery J, Warlow C. Diurnal variation in the incidence of stroke: Oxfordshire Community Stroke Project. Br Med J 1992;304:155–157.
43. Sloan MA, Price TR, Foulkes MA, Marler JR, Mohr JP, Hier DB, et al. Circadian rhythmicity of stroke onset. Stroke 1992;23:1420–1426.
44. Marsh EE, Biller J, Adams HP, Marler JR, Hulbert JR, Love BB, et al. Circadian variation in onset of acute ischemic stroke. Arch Neurol 1990;47:1178–1180.
45. Argentiono C, Toni D, Rasura M, Violi F, Sacchetti ML, Allegretta A, et al. Circadian variation in the frequency of ischemic stroke. Stroke 1990;21:387–389.
46. Jovicic A. Bioritam i ishemicni cerebrovaskularni poremecaji. Vojnosanitetski Pregled 1983; 40:347–351.
47. Marler JR, Price TR, Clark GL, Muller JE, Robertson T, Mohr JP, et al. Morning increase in onset of ischemic stroke. Stroke 1989;20:473–476.
48. Tsementzis SA, Gill JS, Hitchcock ER, Gill SK, Beevers DG. Diurnal variation of and activity during the onset of stroke. Neurosurgery 1985;17:901–904.
49. Agnoli A, Manfredi M, Mossuto L, Piccinelli A. Rapport Entre les Rythmes Hemeronyctaux de la Tension Arterielle et sa Pathogenie de L'Insuffisance Vasculaire Cerebrale. Rev Neurol (Paris) 1975;131:597–606.
50. Lago A, Geffner D, Tembl J, Landete L, Valero C, Baquero M. Circadian variation in acute ischemic stroke. Stroke 1998;29:1873–1875.
51. Pardiwalla FK, Yeolekar ME, Bakshi SK. Circadian rhythms in acute stroke. JAPI 1993;41(4): 203–204.
52. Kaps M, Busse O, Hofmann O. Zur Circadianen Haufigkeitsverteilung Ischamischer Insulte. Nervenarzt 1983;54:655–657.
53. Van Der Windt C, Van Gijn J. Cerebral Infarction does not occur typically at night. J Neurol Neurosurg Psychiatry 1988;51:109–111.
54. Ince B. Circadian variation in stroke [Letter]. Arch Neurol 1992;49:900.
55. Alberts MJ. Circadian variation in stroke [Letter]. Arch Neurol 1991;48:790.
56. Marler J. Circadian variation in stroke onset. In: Deedwania PC, ed. Circadian Rhythms of Cardiovascular Disorders. Futura, Armonk, NY, 1997, pp. 163–172.
57. Butchart EG, De la Santa PM, Rooney SJ, Lewis PA. The Role of risk factors and trigger factors in cerebrovascular events after mitral valve replacement: implications for antithrombotic management. J Card Surg 1994;9(Suppl):228–236.
58. Millar-Craig MW, Bishop CN, Raftery EB. Circadian variation of blood-pressure. Lancet 1978;i:795–797.
59. Muller C. Die Messung des Blutdrucks am Schlafenden als klinische Methode. Acta Med Scand 1921;55:381–485.

60. Mueller SC, Brown GE. Hourly rhythms in blood pressure in persons with normal and elevated pressures. Ann Intern Med 1930;3:1190–1200.
61. Shaw DB, Knapp MS, Davies DH. Variations of blood pressure in hypertensives during sleep. Lancet 1963;i:797–799.
62. Richardson DW, Honour AJ, Fenton GW, Stott FH, Pickering GW. Variation in arterial pressure throughout the day and night. Clin Sci 1964;26:445–460.
63. O'Brien O, Sheridan J, O'Malley K. Dippers and non-dippers [Letter]. Lancet 1988;i:397.
64. Phillips RA, Sheinart K, Godbold JH, Tuhrim S. Absence of nocturnal dip in blood pressure increases stroke in a multi- ethnic population. Hypertension 1998;32:606A (abstract).
65. Kario K, Shimada K. Change in diurnal blood pressure rhythm due to small lacunar infarct [Letter]. Lancet 1994;344:200.
66. Shimada K, Kawamoto A, Matsubayashi K, Nishinaga M, Kimura S, Ozawa T. Diurnal blood pressure variations and silent cerebrovascular damage in elderly patients with hypertension. J Hypertens 1992;10:875–878.
67. Sander D, Klingelhofer J. Changes of circadian blood pressure patterns after hemodynamic and thromboembolic brain infarction. Stroke 1994;25:1730–1737.
68. Yamamoto Y, Akiguchi I, Oiwa K, Satoi H, Kimura J. Diminished nocturnal blood pressure decline and lesion site in cerebrovascular disease. Stroke 1995;26:829–833.
69. Pierach A. Local and relative hypotension as the cause of cerebrovascular accidents. In: Zulch KJ, ed. Cerebral Circulation and Stroke. Springer-Verlag, New York, 1971, pp. 198–202.
70. Zulch KJ. Clinical ischemia: brain infarcts. In: Zulch KJ, Kaufmann W, Hossmann KA, Hossmann V, eds. Brain and Heart Infarct. Springer-Verlag, New York, 1977, pp. 288–296.
71. Imai Y, Tsuji I, Nagai K, Watanabe N, Ohkubo T, Sakuma M, et al. Circadian blood pressure variation related to morbidity and mortality from cerebrovascular and cardiovascular diseases. Ann NY Acad Sci 1996;783:173–185.
72. Kubota K, Sakurai T, Tamura J, Shirakura T. Is the circadian change in hematocrit and blood viscosity a factor triggering cerebral and myocardial infarction? [Letter]. Stroke 1987;18:812–813.
73. Rosing DR, Brakman P, Redwood DR, Goldstein RE, Beiser GD, Astrup T, et al. Blood fibrinolytic activity in man. Circ Res 1970;27:171–184..
74. Andreotti F, Davies GJ, Hackett DR, Khan MI, De Bart ACW, Aber VR, et al. Major circadian fluctuations in fibrinolytic factors and possible relevance to time of onset of myocardial infarction, sudden cardiac death and stroke. Am J Cardiol 1988;62:635–637.
75. Mehta JL, Lawson D, Mehta P, Lopez L. Circadian variation in platelet aggregation and alpha 2 adrenoceptor binding affinity. Circulation 1987;76(Suppl IV):IV–364 (abstract).
76. Brezinski DA, Tofler GH, Muller JE, Pohjola- Sintonen S, Willich SN, Schafer AI, et al. Morning increase in platelet aggregability. association with assumption of the upright posture. Circulation 1988;78:35–40.
77. Gordon RD, Wolfe LK, Island DP, Liddle GW. A diurnal rhythm in plasma renin activity in man. J Clin Investig 1966;45 (10):1587–1592.
78. Quyyumi AA, Panza JA, Lakatos E, Epstein SE. Circadian variation in ischemic events: causal role of variation in ischemic threshold due to changes in vascular resistance. Circulation 1988;78(Suppl II):331 (abstract).
79. Kullo IJ, Edwards WD, Schwartz RS. Vulnerable plaque: pathobiology and clinical implications. Ann Intern Med 1998;129:1050–1060.
80. Cagnacci A. Melatonin in relation to physiology in adult humans. J Pineal Res 1996;21(4):200–213.
81. Murphy PJ, Campbell SS. Physiology of the circadian system in animals and humans. J Clin Neurophysiol 1996;13(1):2–16.
82. Portaluppi F, Vergnani L, Manfredini R, Fersini C. Endocrine mechanisms of blood pressure rhythms. Ann NY Acad Sci 1996;783:113–131.
83. Fiorina P, Lattuada G, Ponari O, Silvestrini C, Dall'Aglio P. Impaired nocturnal melatonin excretion and changes of immunological status in ischaemic stroke patients [Letter]. Lancet 1996;347:692–693.

III Twenty-Four-Hour Blood Pressure Monitoring and Therapy

12 Cardiovascular Chronobiology and Chronopharmacology
Importance of Timing of Dosing*

Björn Lemmer, MD

CONTENTS

INTRODUCTION
CHRONOBIOLOGY OF THE CARDIOVASCULAR SYSTEM
CLINICAL CHRONOPHARMACOLOGY OF HYPERTENSION
DURATION OF THE ANTIHYPERTENSIVE EFFECT
CONCLUSION
REFERENCES

INTRODUCTION

Heart rate was among the earliest physiological functions reported not to be constant throughout the 24 h of a day *(1)*. As early as at the beginning of the 17th century, daily variations in pulse rate, as well as a rapid increase on awakening, were described *(2)*. In the 18th and 19th centuries, general observations as well as detailed data on daily variations in pulse rate and pulse quality were reported *(3–11)*. The pulse of a healthy subject as determined in the late afternoon was even proposed as a easily available "metronom" to be used by musicians *(12)* (*see* Fig. 1). The metronom itself was not invented until 1816 by Mälzel.

The development of the pulse-watch by Floyer (1707–1710) and the introduction of a "third hand" into the clock to precisely measure the seconds allowed the determination of changes in the pulse rate *(4)*. It is of interest to note that the symptoms of "office hypertension or white coat hypertension"—nowadays of increasing medical importance *(13–18)*—has already been precisely described more than 300 years ago independently by several authors *(17–20)* (*see* Fig. 2).

*This chapter is dedicated to the memory of Jürgen Aschoff (1913–1998).

From: *Contemporary Cardiology:*
Blood Pressure Monitoring in Cardiovascular Medicine and Therapeutics
Edited by: W. B. White © Humana Press Inc., Totowa, NJ

255

"What I found to be an appropriate timegiver for the tempo .... is the pulse at the hand of a healthy man."

"One should take the pulse of a merry and good tempered man .... as it is after lunch until evening and the tempo will be fine."

Fig.1. From: Johann Joachim Quantz, "Versuch einer Anweisung die Flöte traversière zu spielen" *(12)*.

Joachim Targiri (1698)
"Most of all one has to have an experienced knowledge to study the pulse of the artery, the movement of which can be manifold increased, decreased, and disturbed by internal causes and external conditions. Even catching sight of the doctor and the doctor's stepping in may not be of minor importance,....because this, indeed, can induce changes in the movement of the pulse."

Christoph Hellwig (1738)
"It is important to note that the patient's puls may change remarkably...most commenly this is caused by the advent of the doctor."

Théophile de Bordeu (1756)
"In order to estimate the quality of the pulse it is neccessary to feel the pulse several times; it is an exception that the presence of the doctor does not lead occasionally to some changes which may *elevate* or *increase* it: the practitioners never forget to keep in mind the pulse which they call the *pulse of the doctor*."

Fig. 2. Early reports on the symptoms of "white coat hypertension" *(17–19)*.

Moreover, Hellwig proposed that the doctor should sit down and should talk to the patient for a while before examining the quality of the pulse once or several (sic!) times *(18)*, a recommendation reflecting our modern guidelines when measuring the blood pressure. Shortly thereafter Théophile de Bordeu, professor at the University of Montpellier, named the same observation "*le pouls du médicin*" *(19)*.

In the 17th century, when minute watches were not yet available, it was difficult to exactly commemorate the patient's pulse rate. In order to overcome this diagnostic deficiency, Sanctorius Sanctorius, professor of medicine at the University of Padua, in 1631 invented the "pulsilogium" by which he was able to record the pulse rate present at different days of the disease or at different times of the day *(21)* (*see* Fig. 3).

> "In order to get good and rapid information I have invented a pulse measuring device (pulsilogium) with which I can precisely measure, observe and commemorate the beats and the rest of the arteries in comparison to those of earlier days."
>
> "The pulsilogium tells us at what day and a what hour of the day the pulse of the patient varies from the natural state."

Fig. 3. Description of the "pulsilogium" *(21)* (translated by BL).

When plethysmographic devices became available *(22–24)*, it was also noted that the level in blood pressure in healthy and in diseased persons were not the same throughout 24 h *(23,25–34)*. Zadek *(23)* was the first to present detailed data on daily variations ("Tagesschwankungen") in blood pressure with an increase in the afternoon and a drop at night. At the beginning of the 20th century, even different types of hypertension were verified by their different blood pressure profiles *(32–34)*.

There are also very early reports describing the nightly occurrence of the symptoms and/or the onset of angina pectoris attacks and of myocardial infarction *(4,35)*. In the light of these observations, it is not surprising that more than 200 yr ago, Reil *(24)* recommended that "the time of day of drug application and the dose must be in harmony with each other."

CHRONOBIOLOGY
OF THE CARDIOVASCULAR SYSTEM

In recent years, numerous more sophisticated studies have provided convincing evidence for circadian rhythms in cardiovascular functions both in healthy subjects and in patients suffering from cardiovascular diseases *(36–42)*. Although the rhythms in heart rate and blood pressure are the best-known periodic functions in the cardiovascular system, other parameters have been shown to exhibit circadian variations as well, including stroke volume, cardiac output, blood flow, peripheral resistance, parameters of electrocardiogram (ECG) recordings, the plasma concentrations of pressor hormones such as noradrenaline, renin, angiotensin, aldosterone, atrial natriuretic hormone and plasma cAMP concentration, and blood viscosity, aggregability, and fibrinolytic activity. Figure 4 gives a simplified scheme of the physiological parameters involved in the regulation of the blood pressure.

In recent years, the development of easy-to-use devices to continuously monitor blood pressure and heart rate in man by ambulatory blood pressure monitoring (ABPM) devices not only demonstrated that the level of blood pressure in normotensive and in hypertensive patients are clearly dependent on the time of

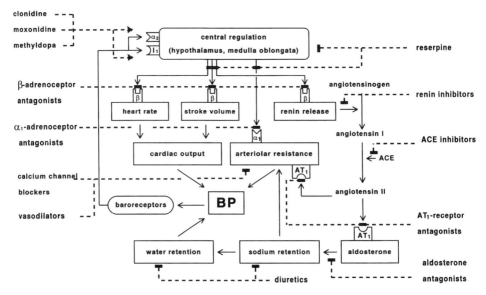

Fig. 4. Simplified scheme of the mechanisms involved in the regulation of blood pressure and the main target mechanisms by which drugs lower blood pressure.

day (Fig. 5) but also that drugs can differently affect the blood pressure rhythm depending on circadian time of drug dosing. There is no doubt about the usefulness of ABPM in assessing antihypertensive treatment and in testing for clinical relevance *(43,44)*.

Moreover, different forms of hypertension can exhibit different circadian patterns. In normotension as well as in primary hypertension, there is, in general, a nightly drop in blood pressure, those patients are termed "dippers" (Fig. 5), whereas in secondary hypertension resulting from renal disease, Cushing's disease, and diabetes mellitus, the rhythm in blood pressure is abolished or even reversed in 70% of patients with highest values at night, termed "nondippers" *(45–49)*. This is of particular interest because the loss in nocturnal blood pressure fall (nondipping) correlates with increased end-organ damage in cardiac, cerebral, vascular, and renal tissues; nocturnal hypertension is a risk factor *(50)*.

CLINICAL CHRONOPHARMACOLOGY OF HYPERTENSION

Chronopharmacodynamics

Drug treament of hypertension includes various types of drugs such as diuretics, β- and α-adrenoceptor blocking drugs, calcium channel blockers, converting enzyme inhibitors, AT$_1$-receptor blockers, and others, which differ in their sites of action as depicted in Fig. 4. Because the main steps in the mechanisms regulating the blood pressure (Fig. 4) are circadian phase dependent, it is not

Normotensives   **Primary Hypertensives**

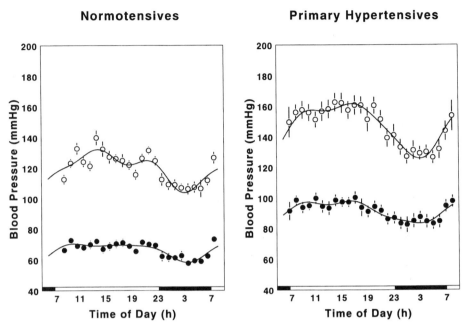

Fig. 5. 24-Hour blood pressure profiles in systolic and diastolic blood pressures in normotensives and primary hypertensive patients as determined by ambulatory blood pressure recording, shown are mean hourly data ± SEM of 12–17 subjects *(53)*. Solid lines represent nonlinear fitting of partial Fourier series to the ABPM data *(108)*.

surprising to note that antihypertensive drugs may display a circadian time dependency in their effects and/or their pharmacokinetics as well *(51–53)*.

Moreover, the different groups of antihypertensive drugs as well as the various compounds within one group of antihypertensives differ in pharmacokinetic half-life, galenic formulation, duration of drug effect, and, thus, in dosing interval. However, despite the great number of studies published in evaluating antihypertensive drug efficacy, the time of day of drug application has only rarely been a specific point of investigation.

β-ADRENOCEPTOR BLOCKING DRUGS

Unfortunately, in hypertensive patients, no crossover (morning vs evening) study with β-adrenoceptor antagonists has been published. From the studies performed without time-specified drug dosing, however, it is difficult to draw definite conclusions on the importance of the circadian time of drug dosing for antihypertensive drug efficacy. A resume of 20 "conventionally" performed studies *(54)* showed that β-adrenoceptor antagonists (either $β_1$-selective, nonselective, or with intrinsic sympathomimetic activity [ISA]) either have no effect or reduce the rhythmic pattern in blood pressure. In general, however, there is a tendency for β-adrenoceptor antagonists to predominately reduce daytime blood pressure levels and not

Table 1
Chronopharmacology of Propranolol
After Oral Dosing of 80 mg of (±)-Propranolol in Four Healthy Subjects
Applied in a Crossover Dosing at Four Different Circadian Times

	Time of (±)-propranolol (80 mg po) application			
	0800 h	1400 h	2000 h	0200 h
Pharmacokinetics				
C_{max} (ng/mL)	38.6 ± 11.2	20.0 ± 6.5	26.2 ± 5.3	18.4 ± 4.4*
T_{max} (h)	2.5 ± 0.5	3.5 ± 0.5	3.0 ± 0.6	3.5 ± 1.0
AUC (ng/mL/h)	169 ± 47	106 ± 30	140 ± 23	92 ± 22
$t_{1/2}$ β (h)	3.3 ± 0.4	4.2 ± 0.5	4.9 ± 0.2	4.4 ± 0.6**
C_{max} / T_{max} (ng/mL/h)	17.9 ± 6.4	7.5 ± 3.9	10.6 ± 3.7	7.1 ± 2.4*
Hemodynamics (heart rate)				
E_{max} (bpm)	16.0 ± 2.4	11.7 ± 1.8	16.3 ± 1.5	15.3 ± 4.6
T_{max} (h)	2.3 ± 0.6	4.5 ± 1.0	6.5 ± 1.5	7.0 ± 1.0*

Note: Shown are the pharmacokinetics of (–)-propranolol and the effects on heart rate (E_{max} = peak effect, T_{max} = time-to-peak effect) in comparison to the circadian control values. ANOVA: $*p < 0.05$; $**p < 0.01$.

Source: Data from ref. *55*.

to greatly affect nighttime values, being less effective or noneffective in reducing the early morning rise in blood pressure *(49,54,)*. Consistently, decreases in heart rate by β-adrenoceptor antagonists are more pronounced during daytime hours. Similarly, in healthy subjects, a crossover study with propranolol showed a more pronounced decrease in heart rate and blood pressure during daytime hours than at night *(55)*. Interestingly, the agent with partial agonist activity, pindolol, actually increased heart rate at night *(56)* (*see* Table 1).

Thus, clinical data indicate that β-adrenoceptor-mediated regulation of blood pressure dominates during daytime hours and is of less or minor importance during the night and the early morning hours. This correlates well with the circadian rhythm in sympathetic tone, as indicated by the rhythm in plasma noradrenaline and cAMP *(57,58)*.

CALCIUM CHANNEL BLOCKERS

The effects of calcium channel blockers were also analyzed mainly by visual inspection of the blood pressure profiles *(49)*. In primary hypertensives, dosing of immediate-release verapamil three times per day did not greatly change the blood pressure profile, but was less effective at night *(59)*. A single morning dose of a sustained-release verapamil showed good 24-h blood pressure control *(60)*, whereas a sustained-release formulation of diltiazem was less effective at night *(61)*. Dihydropyridine derivatives, differing in pharmacokinetics, seem to reduce blood pressure to a varying degree during the day and night; drug formulation and dosing interval may play an additional role *(59)*.

Table 2
Effects of Calcium Channel Blockers on the 24-h Pattern in Blood Pressure

Drug	Dose		Patients (n), diagnosis	Effect on 24-h blood pressure			Ref.
	mg/d	Duration dosing time		Day	Night	24-h profile	
Amlodipine	5	4 wk	20, EH				62
		AM		++	++	Preserved	
		PM		++	++	Preserved	
Amlodipine	5	3 wk	12, EH				69
		0800 h		+	+	Preserved	
		2000 h		+	+	Preserved	
Isradipine	5	4 wk	18, EH				63
		0700 h		++	++	Preserved	
		1900 h		++	++	Preserved	
Nifedipine GITS	30	1 or 2 wk	10, EH				65
		1000 h		++	++	Preserved	
		2200 h		++	++	Preserved	
Nitrendipine	20	4 wk	41, EH				67
		0700 h		+	+	Preserved	
		1900 h		+	+	Preserved	
Nitrendipine	10	3 d	6, EH				68
		0600 h		++	++	Preserved	
		1800 h		+	++	Changed	
Isradipine	5	4 wk	16, RH[a]				64
		0800 h		++	++	Not normalized	
		2000 h		+	+++	Normalized	
Nifedipine i.r.	10	Single dose	12, NT				66
		0800 h		+	++	Preserved	
		1900 h		+	+	Preserved	

Note: Table includes only data from crossover studies. EH = essential (primary) hypertensives, RH = renal (secondary) hypertensives, NT = normotensives.
[a] = Abolished 24-h blood pressure profile.

Eight studies using a crossover design to assess the pharmacodynamics of calcium channel blockers have been published (62–69) (Table 2). In essential hypertensives, amlodipine, sustained-release isradipine, and nifedipine Gastrointestinal Therapeutic System (GITS) and in normotensives, immediate-release nifedipine did not differentially affect the 24-h blood pressure profile after once-morning or once-evening dosing; with nitrendipine the profile remained either unaffected or slightly changed after evening dosing (Table 2). In primary hypertensive patients, twice-daily nifedipine also effectively lowered the blood pressure throughout a 24-h period (66). Most interestingly, the greatly disturbed blood pressure profile in secondary hypertensives as a result of renal failure was only normalized after evening but not after morning dosing of isradipine (64) (Table 2).

ACE INHIBITORS

Five crossover studies (morning vs evening dosing) with enzyme-converting inhibitors in essential hypertensive patients have been reported (Table 3). They

Table 3
Effects of ACE Inhibitors on the 24-h Pattern in Blood Pressure

Drug	Dose		Patients (n), diagnosis	Effect on 24-h blood pressure			Ref.
	mg/d	Duration dosing time		Day	Night	24-h profile	
Benazepril	10	Single dose	10, EH				99
		0900 h		+++	++	Preserved	
		2100 h		+	++	Changed	
Enalapril	10	Single dose	10, EH				76
		0700		++	+	Preserved	
		1900 h		++	+++	Changed	
		3 wk					
		0700 h		++	+	Preserved	
		1900 h		+	++	Changed	
Quinapril	20	4 wk	18, EH				99
		0800 h		++	+	Preserved	
		2200 h		++	++	Preserved	
Ramipril	2.5	4 wk	33, EH				100
		0800 h		+	(+)	Preserved	
		2000 h		(+)	+	Preserved	
Perindopril	2	4 wk	18, RH				101
		0900 h		++	+	Preserved	
		2100 h		+	++	Changed	

Note: Table includes only data from crossover studies. EH = essential (primary) hypertensives.

demonstrate that in contrast to morning dosing, evening dosing of benazepril and enalapril resulted in a more pronounced nightly drop, with a distortion of the 24-h blood pressure (BP) profile by evening dosing of enalapril. Evening dosing of quinapril also resulted in a more pronounced effect than morning dosing. The BP pattern, however, was not greatly modified. In light of a reduced cardiac reserve of patients with hypertension at risk, a too-pronounced nightly drop in BP after evening dosing might be a potential risk factor for the occurrence of ischemic events *(49)*.

OTHER ANTIHYPERTENSIVE DRUGS

Antihypertensives of other classes have rarely been studied in relation to possible circadian variation. Once-daily morning dosing of the diuretics xipamide *(70)* and indapamide *(71)* reduced the BP in essential hypertensives without changing the 24-h BP pattern. On twice-daily dosing the α-adrenoceptor antagonists indoramin *(72)* and prazosin *(73)* also did not change the BP profile. A single nighttime dose of the α-adrenoceptor antagonist doxazosin reduced both systolic and diastolic BP throughout day and night, but the greatest reduction occurred in the morning hours *(74)*. Because α-adrenoceptor blockade more effectively reduced the peripheral resistance during the early morning hours than at other times of

Table 4
Pharmacokinetic Parameters of Cardiovascular
Active Drugs Determined in Crossover Studies

Drug	Dose (mg), duration	C_{max} (ng/mL) Morning	Evening	T_{max} (h) Morning	Evening	Ref.
Digoxin	0.5, sd	3.6*	1.8	1.2	3.2	102
Enalaprilat						
After Enalapril	10, sd	33.8	41.9	4.4	4.5	76
After Enalapril	10, 3w	46.7	53.5	3.5*	5.6	
IS-5-MN i.r.	60, sd	1605.0	1588.0	0.9*	2.1	103
						40
IS-5-MN s.r.	60, sd	509.0	530.0	5.2	4.9	66
Molsidomine	8, sd	27.0	23.5	1.7	1.9	82
Nifedipine i.r.	10, sd	82.0*	45.7	0.4*	0.6	95,96
Nifedipine s.r.	2×20, 1w	48.5	50.1	2.3	2.8	95,96
Atenolol	50, sd	440.0	391.8	3.2	4.0	83
Oxprenolol[a]	80, sd	507.0	375.0	1.0	1.1	104
Propranolol[b]	80, sd	38.6*	26.2	2.5	3.0	55
Propranolol (±)	80, sd	68	60	2.3	2.7	105
Verapamil s.r.	360, 2w	389.0	386.0	7.2*	10.6	106
Verapamil	80, sd	59.4*	25.6	1.3	2.0	107

Note: At least two dosing times (around 0600–0800 h and 1800–2000 h) were studied. In some studies, up to six circadian times were included. Only the parameters C_{max} (peak drug concentration) and T_{max} (time to C_{max}) are given. sd = single dose, w = weeks, i.r. = immediate-release preparation, s.r. = sustained-release preparation. *p morning versus evening at least <0.05.
[a] Significant difference in half-life.
[b] (±)-Propranolol was given, kinetic data for (–)-propranolol.

the day (75), these findings point to the importance of α-adrenoceptor-mediated regulation of BP during the early morning hours. In addition, the peak treatment effect after nigthtime dosing of doxazosin occcured later than predicted from the drug's pharmacokinetics (74), an observation that supports nicely similar findings on a circadian phase dependency in the dose-response relationship of nifedipine (66), enalapril (76), and propranolol (55).

Chronopharmacokinetics

There is good evidence that the kinetics of cardiovascular active drugs may also be dependent on the time of day (77–81). Our own studies have shown that cardiovascular active compounds such as propranolol (see Table 1), oral nitrates, and the calcium channel blocker nifedipine showed higher peak drug concentrations (C_{max}) and/or a shorter time-to-peak concentration (T_{max}) after morning than evening oral drug dosing, at least when immediate release formulations were used (Table 4). In the case of the retard formulation of isorbide-5-mononitrate and nifedipine, however, no circadian phase dependency in their pharmacokinetics was found (Table 4). There was also no circadian time dependency in the kinetics of sustained-release molsidomine (82) nor in the kinetics of the hydrophilic β-blocker atenolol (83).

Concerning the underlying mechanisms responsible for this chronokinetic behavior of these lipophilic compounds, a faster gastric emptying time in the morning (84) and, more importantly, a higher gastrointestinal perfusion in the morning than in the evening are assumed to be involved (85).

DURATION OF THE ANTIHYPERTENSIVE EFFECT

As mentioned earlier, ABPM has been widely used to evaluate the duration of drug action. In general, ABPM is performed for a single 24-h span. However, the restriction of ABPM to 24 h may cause potential pitfalls, as can be demonstrated from several studies (86). A 4-wk treatment of hypertensive patients with the β_1-selective adrenoceptor blocking drug bisoprolol showed that the duration persisted up to 48 h after cessation of therapy (87). Similarly, after chronic morning dosing of the β-adrenoceptor blocking drug atenolol, the BP lowering effect was no longer observed 20–24 h after the last dose (Fig. 6). However, continuing ABPM for 48 h revealed that the reduction in BP was observed again on the next day off therapy (Fig. 6) (88).

Almost the same findings were reported after 3 wk of once-a-day morning or once-a-day evening administration of the ACE inhibitor enalapril when the BP profile was monitored for 48 h after the last dose (Fig. 7) (77). Conversely, the duration of the antihypertensive effect of short-term treatment with a sustained-release preparation of diltiazem was restricted to about 18 h when the BP was monitored by ABPM for 48 h after the last dose (61).

These data show that the conventional method for estimating the duration of an antihypertensive effect by the peak-to-trough ratio within 24 h can be misleading. The peak-to-trough ratio does not consider that regulatory mechanisms of the blood pressure rhythm predominate at certain times of day and are of minor importance at other times (52). β-Adrenergic tone, for example, is higher during the daytime activity phase than at night; β-adenoceptor blockers are therefore less active at night (see above). Panza et al. (75) showed that the vascular tone is higher in the morning and decreases thereafter, leading to a more pronounced reduction of the peripheral resistance by the α-adrenoceptor blocking drug phentolamine in the morning than at other times of the day. As a consequence, it may be worthwhile to not restrict the ABPM to a 24-h span in order to avoid misleading conclusions on the duration of action of an antihypertensive drug.

CONCLUSION

Various functions of the cardiovascular system, including the blood pressure and heart rate, are well organized in time (49). There is also good evidence that

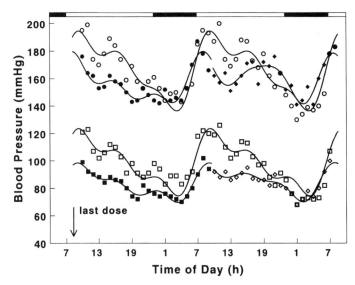

Fig. 6. Circadian blood pressure profile of hypertensive patients before (filled circles) and after once-a-day treatment with atenolol (100 mg/d) for 6 wk (open circles); 48-h ambulatory blood pressure data after last dose. Note the convergence of blood pressure data curves at night and separation again during d 2. Data from ref. *88* were submitted to a nonlinear rhythm analysis by ABPM-FIT *(108)* and redrawn accordingly *(86)*.

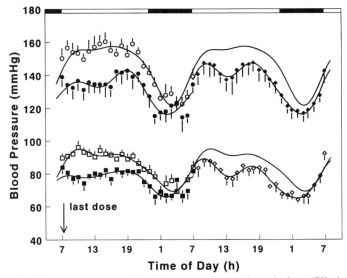

Fig. 7. Circadian blood pressure profile of hypertensive patients before (filled circles) and after once-a-day morning treatment with enalapril (10 mg/d) for 3 wk (open circles); 48-h ambulatory blood pressure data after last dose. Note that the antihypertensive effect reappears again on the second day off therapy. Solid lines represent nonlinear fitting of partial Fourier series to the ABPM data *(108)*; data from ref. *(76)*.

a disease is able to disturb, reverse, or even destroy a rhythmic pattern. At least in the rat, the rhythms in systolic and diastolic blood pressures are mainly endogenous in nature (i.e., driven by an internal pacemaker) *(89–91)*. In man, there are indirect data for the involvement of an endogenous pacemaker in the blood pressure rhythm and—even more evident—in heart rate rhythm as derived from transmeridian flights *(92,93)* and from studies performed under unmasking conditions under constant routine *(94)*.

Moreover, it has been shown that different cardiovascular active compounds such as propranolol, oral nitrates, and the calcium channel blockers nifedipine and verapamil can display higher peak drug concentrations (C_{max}) and/or a shorter time-to-peak concentration (T_{max}) after oral morning than evening drug dosing, at least when immediate-release formulations were used. In the case of sustained-release formulation of isorbide-5-mononitrate, nifedipine and molsidomine no circadian phase dependency in their pharmacokinetics were found (Table 4) *(95–97)*.

The cardiovascular active drugs mentioned are, in general, absorbed by passive diffusion; the underlying mechanisms responsible for their chronokinetics can be explained by a faster gastric emptying time in the morning *(84)* and, more importantly, by a higher gastrointestinal perfusion in the morning *(85)*, resulting in higher C_{max} and/or shorter T_{max} in the morning than in the evening.

There is evidence that in hypertensive dippers, antihypertensive drugs should be given in the early morning hours, whereas in nondippers it may be necessary to add an evening dose or to even apply a single evening dose in order not only to reduce high morning blood pressure but also to normalize a disturbed 24-h blood pressure profile. However, because the pharmacokinetics can be circadian phase dependent, the galenic formulation and/or the indigenous half-life of a drug has to be considered in order to come to a final recommendation concerning the most appropriate dosing time within 24 h.

In conclusion, recent studies clearly demonstrate that the effects as well as the kinetics of cardiovascular active drugs can be dependent on the circadian phase (i.e., time of day or circadian time) of drug dosing. However, possible daily variation in drug kinetics seem to be of some importance for the degree in the circadian-time-dependent effects of these compounds. Nevertheless, the data published with respect to time-of-day of dosing of cardiovascular agents clearly demonstrate that the dose-response relationship can be circadian phase dependent.

REFERENCES

1. Aschoff J. Day–night variations in the cardiovascular system. Historical and other notes by an outsider. In: Schmidt TFH, Engel BT, Blümchen G, eds. Temporal Variations of the Cardiovascular System. Springer-Verlag, Berlin, 1992, pp. 3–14.
2. Struthius J. Ars sphygmica. Königs, Basel, 1602, pp. 127ff.
3. Elsner ChF. Beyträge zur Fieber=Lehre. Wagner und Denzel, Königsberg 1782, pp. 28–29.

4. Zimmermann JG. Von der Erfahrung in der Arzneykunst. Neue Auflage, Edlen von Trattnern, Agram, 1793, pp. 233ff.

5. Reil JC. Von der Lebenskraft. Arch Physiol 1796;1:8–162.

6. Falconer W. Beobachtungen über den Pulse. Heinsius, Leipzig, 1797, pp. 24ff.

7. Hufeland CW. Die Kunst das menschliche Leben zu verlängern. Akademische Buchhandlung, Jena, 1797, pp. 552.

8. Autenrieth JHF. Handbuch der empirischen Physiologie, Teil 1. Heerbrandt, Tübingen, 1801, pp. 209.

9. Wilhelm GT. Unterhaltungen über den Menschen. Dritter Theil, Von dem Körper und seinen Theilen und Functionen insbesondere. Engelbrechtsche Kunsthandlung, Augsburg, 1806, pp. 352ff.

10. Barthez PJ. Nouveaux éléments de la science de l'homme, 2nd ed. Goujon et Brunot, Paris, 1806, part II, p. 147 and Note 1806, pp. 66 and 69.

11. Knox R. On the relation subsisting between the time of the day, and various functions of the human body; and on the manner in which the pulsation of the heart and arteries are affected by muscular exertion. Edinburgh Med Surg J 1815;11:52–65.

12. Quantz JJ. Versuch einer Anweisung die Flöte traversière zu spielen. Voß, Berlin, 1752, p. 261.

13. Pickering TG, Levenstein M, Walmsley P, for the Hypertension and Lipid Trial Study Group. Differential effects of doxazosin on clinic and ambulatory pressure according to age, gender, and presence of white coat hypertension. Results of the HALT study. Am J Hypertens 1994;7:848–852.

14. Krakoff LR. Doxazosin studies provide clearer picture of blood pressure profiles [Editorial]. Am J Hypertens 1994;7:853–854.

15. Middeke M, Schrader J. Nocturnal blood pressure in normotensive subjects and those with white coat, primary, and secondary hypertension. Br Med J 1994;308:630–632.

16. Middeke M, Lemmer B. Office hypertension: abnormal blood pressure regulation and increased sympathetic activity compared with normotension. Blood Pressure Monit 1996;1:403–407.

17. Targiri J. Medicina compendaria. Fredericum Haringius, Lyon, 1698, p. 662.

18. Hellwig Ch (pseudonym: Kräutermann V). Curieuser und vernünftiger Urin-Artzt, welcher eines Theils lehret und zeiget, wie man aus dem Urin nicht allein die meisten und vornehmsten Kranckheiten .. erkennen,. Anderen Theils, wie man auch aus dem Pulse den Zustand des Gebläts, die Stärcke und Schwäche der Lebens-Geister, Ab- und Zunahme der Kranckheit ersehen. Beumelburg JJ, 3rd ed. Arnstadt, Leipzig, 1738, pp. 134 and 140.

19. Bordeu T. de Recherches sur le pouls. de Bure l'ainé, Paris, 1756, p. 471.

20. Lemmer B. White coat hypertension: described more than 250 years ago. Am J Hypertens 1995;8:437–438.

21. Sanctorius S. Methodi vitandorum errorum omnium qui in arte medica contingunt. Aubertum, Geneva, 1631, p. 289.

22. von Basch S. Ueber die Messung des Blutdrucks am Menschen. Z Klin Med 1881;2:79–96.

23. Zadek J. Die Messung des Blutdrucks des Menschen mittels des Basch'schen Apparates. Z Klin Med 1881;2:509–551.

24. Riva-Rocci S. Un nuovo sfigmomanometro. Gazz Med Dir Torino 1896;47:981–969.

25. Howell WHA. Contribution to the physiology of sleep, based on plethysmographic experiments. J Exp Med 1897;2:313.

26. Hill L. On rest, sleep and work and the concomitant changes in the circulation of the blood. Lancet 1898;1:282–285.

27. Jellinek S. Über den Blutdruck des gesunden Menschen. Z Klin Med 1900;39:447–472.

28. Weiss H. Blutdruckmessung mit Gärtler's Tonometer. Münch Med Wschr 1900;47:69–71.

29. Hensen H. Beiträge zur Physiologie und Pathologie des Blutdruckes. Dtsch Arch Klin Med 1900;67:436–530.

30. Brush CE, Fayerweather R. Observations on the changes in blood pressure during normal sleep. Am J Physiol 1901;5:199–210.
31. Weysse AW, Lutz BR. Diurnal variations in arterial blood pressure. Am J Physiol 1915;37: 330–347.
32. Müller C. Die Messung des Blutdrucks am Schlafenden als klinische Methode—speciell bei der gutartigen (primären) Hypertonie und der Glomerulonephritis I. Acta Med Scand 1921; 55:381–442.
33. Müller C. Die Messung des Blutdrucks am Schlafenden als klinische Methode—speciell bei der gutartigen (primären) Hypertonie und der Glomerulonephritis II. Acta Med Scand 1921; 55:443–485.
34. Katsch G, Pansdorf H. Die Schlafbewegung des Blutdrucks. Münch Med Wschr 1922;69: 1715–1718.
35. Testa AJ. Über die Krankheiten des Herzens. German translation by K Sprengel. Gebauer, Halle, 1815, p. 323.
36. Reinberg A, Halberg F. Circadian chronopharmacology. Annu Rev Pharmacol 1971;11: 455–492.
37. Reinberg A, Smolensky MH. Biological Rhythms and Medicine. Springer-Verlag, Berlin,1983.
38. Smolensky MH, Tatar SE, Bergmann SA, Losman JG, Barnard CN, Dacso CC, Kraft IA. Circadian rhythmic aspects of human cardiovascular functions: a review by chronobiologic statistical methods. Chronobiologia 1976;3:337–371.
39. Lemmer B. Chronopharmakologie—Tagesrhythmen und Arzneimittelwirkung, 2nd ed. Wissenschaftliche Verlagsgesellschaft, Stuttgart 1984, pp. 71–87.
40. Lemmer B. Temporal aspects in the effects of cardiovascular active drugs in man. In: Lemmer B, ed. Chronopharmacology—Cellular and Biochemical Interactions. Marcel Dekker, New York, 1989, pp. 525–542.
41. Lemmer B. The cardiovascular system and daily variation in response to antihypertensive and antianginal drugs: recent advances. Pharmacol Ther 1991;51:269–274.
42. Willich SN, Muller JE. Triggering of Acute Coronary Syndromes. Kluwer, Dordrecht, 1996.
43. White WB. The usefulness of ambulatory blood pressure monitoring to assess antihypertensive therapy. Blood Pressure Monit 1996;1:149–150.
44. White WB. Circadian variation of blood pressure: clinical relevance and implications for cardiovascular chronotherapeutics. Blood Pressure Monit 1997;2:47–51.
45. Imai Y, Abe K, Sasaki S, Minami N, Munakata M, Nihei M, et al. Exogenous glucocorticoid eliminates or reverses circadian blood pressure variations. J Hypertens 1989;7:113–120.
46. Middeke M, Mika E, Schreiber MA, Beck B, Wachter B, Holzgreve H. Ambulante indirekte Blutdrucklangzeitmessung bei primärer und sekundärer Hypertonie. Klin Wochenschr 1989; 67:713–716.
47. Portaluppi F, Montanari L, Massari M, Di Chiara V, Capanna M. Loss of nocturnal decline of blood pressure in hypertension due to chronic renal failure. Am J Hypertens 1991;4:20–26.
48. Baumgart P, Walger P, Gemen S, von Eiff M, Raidt H, Rahn KH. Blood pressure elevation during the night in chronic renal failure, haemodialysis and after renal transplantation. Nephron 1991;57:293–298.
49. Lemmer B, Portaluppi F. Chronopharmacology of cardiovascular diseases. In: Redfern P, Lemmer B, eds. Handbook of Experimental Pharmacology, Vol. 125, Physiology and Pharmacology of Biological Rhythms. Springer-Verlag, Heidelberg, 1997, pp. 251–297.
50. Middeke MRF. Risk factor nocturnal hypertension. Causes and consequences. Cardiovasc Risk Factors 1998;7:214–221.
51. Lemmer B. Timing of cardiovascular medications—pitfalls and challenges. Br J Cardiol 1995;2:303–309.
52. Lemmer B. Differential effects of antihypertensive drugs on circadian rhythm in blood pressure from the chronobiological point of view. Blood Pressure Monit 1996;1:161–169.

53. Lemmer B. Circadian rhythm in blood pressure: signal transduction, regulatory mechanisms and cardiovascular medication. In: Lemmer B, ed. From the Biological Clock to Chrono-pharmacology. Medpharm Publ., Stuttgart, 1996, pp. 91–117.
54. Stanton A, O'Brien E. Auswirkungen der Therapie auf das zirkadiane Blutdruckprofil. Kar-dio 1994;3:1–8.
55. Langner B, Lemmer B. Circadian changes in the pharmacokinetics and cardiovascular effects of oral propranolol in healthy subjects. Eur J Clin Pharmacol 1988;33:619–624.
56. Quyyumi AA, Wright C, Mockus L, Fox KM. Effect of partial agonist activity in β blockers in severe angina pectoris: a double blind comparison of pindolol and atenolol. Br Med J 1984;289:951–953.
57. de Leeuw PW, Falke HE, Kho TL, Vandongen R, Wester A, Birkenhager WH. Effects of beta-adrenergic blockade on diurnal variability of blood pressure and plasma noradrenaline levels. Acta Med Scand 1977;202:389–392.
58. Brühl T, Pflug B, Köhler W, Touitou Y. Effects of bright light on circadian patterns of cAMP, melatonin and cortisol in healthy subjets. Eur J Endocrinol 1994;130:472–477.
59. Gould BA, Mann S, Kieso H, Balasubramanian V, Raftery EB. The 24-hour ambulatory blood pressure profile with verapamil. Circulation 1982;65:22–27.
60. Caruana M, Heber M, Bridgen G, Raftery EB. Assessment of "once daily" verapamil for the treatment of hypertension using ambulatory, intra-arterial pressure recording. Eur J Clin Pharmacol 1987;32:549–553.
61. Lemmer B, Sasse U, Witte K, Hopf R. Pharmacokinetics and cardiovascular effects of a new sustained-release formulation of diltiazem. Naunyn-Schmiedeberg's Arch Pharmacol 1994; 349:R141.
62. Mengden T, Binswanger B, Gruene S. Dynamics of drug compliance and 24-hour blood pressure control of once daily morning vs evening amlodipine. J Hypertens 1992;10(Suppl 4): S136.
63. Fogari R, Malocco E, Tettamanti F, Tettamanti F, Gnemmi AE, Milani M. Evening vs morning isradipine sustained release in essential hypertension: a double-blind study with 24 h ambulatory monitoring. Br J Clin Pharmacol 1993;35:51–54.
64. Portaluppi F, Vergnani L, Manfredini R, degli Uberti EC, Fersini C. Time-dependent effect of isradipine on the nocturnal hypertension of chronic renal failure. Am J Hypertens 1995;8: 719–726.
65. Greminger P, Suter PM, Holm D, Kobelt R, Vetter W. Morning versus evening administra-tion of nifedipine gastrointestinal therapeutic system in the management of essential hyper-tension. Clin Invest 1994;72:864–869.
66. Lemmer B, Nold G, Behne S, Kaiser R. Chronopharmacokinetics and cardiovascular effects of nifedipine. Chronobiol Int 1991;8:485–494.
67. Meilhac B, Mallion JM, Carre A, Chanudet X, Poggi L, Gosse P, et al. Étude de l'influence de l'horaire de la prise sur l'effet antihypertenseur et la tolérance de la nitrendipine chez des patients hypertendus essentiels légers à modérés. Therapie 1992;47:205–210.
68. Umeda T, Naomi S, Iwaoka T, Inoue J, Sasaki M, Ideguchi Y, et al. Timing for administra-tion of an antihypertensive drug in the treatment of essential hypertension. Hypertension 1994;23(Suppl I):I211–I214.
69. Nold G, Strobel G, Lemmer B. Morning versus evening amlodipine treatment: effect on circadian blood pressure profile in essential hypertensive patients. Blood Pressure Monit 1998;3:17–25.
70. Raftery EB, Melville DI, Gould BA, Mann S, Whittington JR. A study of the antihyperten-sive action of xipamide using ambulatory intra-arterial monitoring. Br J Clin Pharmacol 1981;12:381–385.
71. Ocon J, Mora J. Twenty-four-hour blood pressure monitoring and effects of indapamide. Am J Cardiol 1990;65:58H–61H.

72. Gould BA, Mann S, Davies A, Altman DG, Raftery EB. Indoramin: 24-hour profile of intra-arterial ambulatory blood pressure, a double-blind placebo controlled crossover study. Br J Clin Pharmacol 1981;12(Suppl):67s–73s.

73. Weber MA, Tonkon MJ, Klein RC. Effect of antihypertensive therapy on the circadian blood pressure pattern. Am J Med 1987;82(Suppl 1A):50–52.

74. Pickering TG, Levenstein M, Walmsley P, for the Hypertension and Lipid Trial Study Group. Night-time dosing of doxazosin has peak effect on morning ambulatory blood pressure. Results of the HALT study. Am J Hypertens 1994;7:844–847.

75. Panza JA, Epstein SE, Quyyumi AA. Circadian variation in vascular tone and its relation to alpha-sympathetic vasoconstrictor activity. N Engl J Med 1991;325:986–990.

76. Witte K, Weisser K, Neubeck M, Mutschler E, Lehmann K, Hopf R, et al. Cardiovascular effects, pharmacokinetics and converting enzyme inhibition of enalapril after morning versus evening administration. Clin Pharmacol Ther 1993;54:177–186.

77. Reinberg A, Smolensky MH. Circadian changes of drug disposition in man. Clin Pharmacokinet 1982;7:401–420.

78. Bruguerolle B, Lemmer B. Recent advances in chronopharmacokinetics: methodological problems. Life Sci 1993;52:1809–1824.

79. Lemmer B, Bruguerolle B. Chronopharmacokinetics—are they clinically relevant? Clin Pharmacokinet 1994;26:419–427.

80. Bélanger PM, Bruguerolle B, Labrecque G. Rhythms in pharmacokinetics: absorption, distribution, metabolism, and excretion. Chronopharmacology of cardiovascular diseases. In: Redfern P, Lemmer B, eds. Handbook of Experimental Pharmacology, Vol. 125, Physiology and Pharmacology of Biological Rhythms. Springer-Verlag, New York, 1997, pp. 177–204.

81. Lemmer B. Chronopharmacokinetics—implications for drug treatment. J Pharm Pharmacol 1999;51:887–890.

82. Nold G, Lemmer B. Pharmacokinetics of sustained-release molsidomine after morning versus evening application in healthy subjects. Naunyn-Schmiedeberg's Arch Pharmacol 1998; 357:R173.

83. Shiga T, Fujimura A, Tateishi T, Ohashi K, Ebihara A. Differences of chronopharmacokinetic profiles between propranolol and atenolol in hypertensive subjects. J Clin Pharmacol 1993;33:756–761.

84. Goo RH, Moore JG, Greenberg E, Alazraki NP. Circadian variation in gastric emptying of meals in humans. Gastroenterology 1987;93:515–518.

85. Lemmer B, Nold G. Circadian changes in estimated hepatic blood flow in healthy subjects. Br J Clin Pharmacol 1991;32:627–629.

86. Lemmer B. Chronopharmacological aspects of PK/PD-modelling. Int J Clin Pharmacol Ther 1997;35:458–464.

87. Asmar R, Hughes Ch, Pannier B, Daou J, Safar ME. Duration of action of bisoprolol after cessation of a 4 weeks treatment and its influence on pulse wave velocity and aortic diameter: a pilot study in hypertensive patients. Eur Heart J 1987;8(Suppl):115–120.

88. Gould BA, Raftery EB. Twenty-four-hour blood pressure control: an intraarterial review. Chronobiol Int 1991;8:495–505.

89. Lemmer B, Mattes A, Böhm M, Ganten D. Circadian blood pressure variation in transgenic hypertensive rats. Hypertension 1993;22:97–101.

90. Witte K, Lemmer B. Free-running rhythms in blood pressure and heart rate in normotensive and transgenic hypertensive rats. Chronobiol Int 1995;12:237–247.

91. Witte K, Schnecko A, Buijs RM, Vliet J van der, Scalbert E, Delagrange Ph, et al. Effects of SCN-lesions on circadian blood pressure rhythm in normotensive and transgenic hypertensive rats. Chronobiol Int 1998;15:135–145.

92. Nold G, Kern R, Lohrer H, Lemmer B. Effects of jet-lag on circadian blood pressure and heart rate rhythms in top athletes. Chronobiol Int 1996;13(Suppl 1):97.

93. Lemmer B, Nold G, Kern R, Lohrer H. Jet lag at the Olympics: 24-hour blood pressure profile and synchronisation by light. Photodermatol Photoimmunol Photomed 1998;14:195.

94. Kräuchi K, Wirz-Justice A. Circadian rhythm of heat production, heart rate, and skin and core temperature under unmasking conditions in men. Am J Physiol 1994;267:R819–R829.

95. Lemmer B, Scheidel B, Blume H, Becker HJ. Clinical chronopharmacology of oral sustained-release isosorbide-5-mononitrate in healthy subjects. Eur J Clin Pharmacol 1991;40: 71–75.

96. Lemmer B, Scheidel B, Behne S. Chronopharmacokinetics and chronophar-macodynamics of cardiovascular active drugs: propranolol, organic nitrates, nifedipine. Ann NY Acad Sci 1991;618:166–181.

97. Lemmer B, Scheidel B, Stenzhorn G, Blume H, Lenhard G, Grether D, et al. Clinical chronopharmacology of oral nitrates. Z Kardiol 1889;87(Suppl 2):61–63.

98. Palatini P, Mos L, Motolese M, Mormino P, DelTorre M, Varotto L, Pavan E, et al. Effect of evening versus morning benazepril on 24-hour blood pressure: a comparative study with continuous intraarterial monitoring. Int J Clin Pharmacol Ther Toxicol 1993;31:295–300.

99. Palatini P, Racioppa A, Raule G, Zaninotti M, Penzo M, Pessina AC. Effect of timing of administration on the plasma ACE inhibitory activity and the antihypertensive effect of quinapril. Clin Pharmacol Ther 1992;52:378–383.

100. Myburgh DP, Verho M, Botes JH, Erasmus ThP, Luus HG. 24-Hour pressure control with ramipril: comparison of once-daily morning and evening administration. Curr Ther Res 1995;56:1298–1306.

101. Morgan T, Anderson A, Jones E. The effect on 24 h blood pressure control of an angiotensin converting enzyme inhibitor (perindopril) administered in the morning or at night. J Hypertens 1997;15:205–211.

102. Bruguerolle B, Bouvenot G, Bartolin R, Manolis J. Chronopharmacocinétique de la digoxine chez le sujet de plus de soixante-dix ans. Therapie 1988;43, 251–253.

103. Scheidel B, Lemmer B. Chronopharmacology of oral nitrates in healthy subjects. Chronobiol Int 1991;8:409–419.

104. Koopmans R, Oosterhuis B, Karemaker JM, Weiner J, van Boxtel CJ. The effect of oxprenolol dosage time on its pharmacokinetics and haemodynamic effects during exercise in man. Eur J Clin Pharmacol 1993;44:171–176.

105. Semenowicz-Siuda K, Markiewicz A, Korczynska-Wardecka J. Circadian bioavailability and some effects of propranolol in healthy subjects and liver cirrhosis. Int J Clin Pharmacol Ther Toxicol 1984;22:653–658.

106. Jespersen CM, Frederiksen M, Hansen JF, Klitgaard NA, Sorum C. Circadian variation in the pharmacokinetics of verapamil. Eur J Clin Pharmacol 1989;37:613–615.

107. Hla KK, Latham AN, Henry JA. Influence of time of administration on verapamil pharmacokinetics. Clin Pharmacol Ther 1992;51:366–370.

108. Zuther P, Witte K, Lemmer B. ABPM and CV-SORT: an easy-to-use software package for detailed analysis of data from ambulatory blood pressure monitoring. Blood Pressure Monit 1996;1:347–354.

13

Advances in Ambulatory Blood Pressure Monitoring for the Evaluation of Antihypertensive Therapy in Research and Practice

William B. White, MD

CONTENTS

From: *Contemporary Cardiology:*
Blood Pressure Monitoring in Cardiovascular Medicine and Therapeutics
Edited by: W. B. White © Humana Press Inc., Totowa, NJ

INTRODUCTION

Over the past decade, there has been a marked increase in the utilization of 24-h ambulatory blood pressure (BP) monitoring to assess new drugs for hypertension beginning with the first and second phases of drug development (studies that establish the range of doses in patients with hypertension) to the fourth phase, in which the drugs are tested in comparison to other registered drugs in a particular patient population, such as the elderly or diabetic patient with hypertension.

Several specific attributes have made ambulatory monitoring of the BP important in clinical trials involving the assessment of antihypertensive drug therapy *(1-4)*. Some of these benefits include removal of observer bias or error *(5)*, better short-term and long-term BP reproducibility *(6,7)*, elimination of the "white coat" effect during patient selection *(8,9)*, and the ability to assess the effects of therapy on diurnal and nocturnal BP variability *(10)*. Furthermore, recent data have demonstrated that ambulatory BP is a superior predictor of hemodynamic abnormalities in the hypertensive patient *(11)*, hypertensive target organ involvement *(12,13)*, and prognostic outcomes, including myocardial infarction, stroke, and other types of cardiovascular morbidity *(14–18)*.

In this chapter, an overview of the utility of ambulatory BP monitoring in clinical pharmacology research will be provided, with several examples using data from randomized, controlled, or comparator trials. Furthermore, examples that show the utility of ambulatory monitoring for the assessment of patients in clinical practice will also be discussed.

IMPORTANCE OF BLOOD PRESSURE VARIABILITY ON THE REPRODUCIBILITY OF OFFICE VERSUS AMBULATORY BLOOD PRESSURE AS IT RELATES TO DRUG DEVELOPMENT

The typical reduction in systolic or diastolic BP observed in a clinical trial of an antihypertensive drug (generally in the range of 5–20%) must be viewed against the magnitude of the relatively large variability of the office BP from one visit to the next (12–18%). Studies that have examined the repeatability of office and ambulatory BP in patients with hypertension consistently have demonstrated much less variance with the ambulatory BP *(7,19)*. For example, Conway et al. *(19)* recorded the diastolic BP of 75 hypertensive subjects on 2 occasions, 1 mo apart, while they were being administered a placebo. With clinic measurements, the mean difference in diastolic BP was 1.7 mmHg and the standard deviation of this difference was 12.3 mmHg. In contrast, the daytime ambulatory BP fell by 0.9 mmHg and the standard deviation of the difference was halved to 6.3 mmHg. The implications of this marked reduction in BP variability with ambulatory BP recordings compared to the clinic pressure is that it will double the precision of a

Table 1
Reproducibility of Clinic and Ambulatory Blood Pressure
Studies Separated by up to 2 Years in Patients with Hypertension

Blood pressure measure	Diastolic			Systolic		
	R value	SDD	CV	R value	SDD	CV
Office	0.48	17.0	11.0	0.31	10.0	10.0
24-h mean	0.87[a]	9.8[a]	7.0	0.90[a]	4.7[a]	5.6
Awake	0.86[a]	10.7[a]	7.4	0.88[a]	5.8[a]	6.5
Sleep	0.92[a]	7.7	6.3	0.88[a]	5.2	7.1

Note: R value = correlation coefficient; SDD = standard deviation of the differences; CV = coefficient of variation.

[a] Significantly different from the office blood pressure correlation coefficients, SDD, and CV.

Source: Modified from Mansoor GA, McCabe EJ, White WB. Long-term reproducibility of ambulatory blood pressure. J Hypertens 1994;12:703–707 (with permission).

short-term trial and allow as much as a fourfold reduction in the number of patients required to achieve an accurate result.

Similarly, the long-term reproducibility of ambulatory BP is also superior to the office BP *(7)*. In patients for whom there was nearly 2 yr between visits (hypertensives studied under the same therapeutic and environmental conditions on two different occasions), the standard deviation of the differences were significantly lower and the correlation coefficients significantly higher for ambulatory BP than for the office BP (Table 1). The improved reproducibility of ambulatory over office BP continued to be present when the data were divided into awake and sleep periods. These data suggest that clinical trials involving ambulatory BP over long periods would also require smaller sample sizes than similarly designed trials in which the statistical power is based on the ability to show changes in a more highly variable clinic BP.

In contrast, there may be little advantage of ambulatory BP over the clinic pressure in clinical trials when the measure of interest is a small block of time, such as 1 or 2 h. In an evaluation of a group of hypertensives using both noninvasive and intra-arterial BP over 24 h, Mancia and colleagues *(20)* showed that the standard deviation of the differences for 24-h mean BP values were similar for the two methodologies. However, despite the much larger number of BP values obtained in an intra-arterial study, the hourly BP reproducibility was no different for the direct measurements than it was for noninvasive BP monitoring. Thus, unlike the larger blocks of time (e.g., 24 h, the awake period, or the sleep period), the reproducibility of hourly ambulatory BP data has not been shown to be superior to that of office BP measurements *(20)*. Hence, ambulatory BP recordings will not allow a reduction in sample sizes if the end point is for short periods of time. This increased variability in the hourly BP levels is probably secondary to differences in the activities of patients who are monitored on two different days. As controlling for hourly physical and mental activities is nearly impossible in free-ranging subjects, longer periods of time (e.g., ≥4 h) will remain the time periods that are statistically and practically appropriate for clinical trials involving ambulatory BP monitoring.

Benefits of ambulatory monitoring of the BP over clinic BP with regard to sample size requirements in clinical trials of the elderly may be substantially reduced, however. One report in elderly hypertensive patients with isolated systolic hypertension suggests that there would not be improvement in reproducibility for ambulatory BP over clinic BP measurements, as the between-subject variance was not much different for the two methods (21). Staessen et al. reported that 60 subjects with isolated systolic hypertension would be required to detect a 10 mmHg difference in systolic BP between 2 treatments in a parallel design using clinic readings, whereas if ambulatory BP monitoring was used, the number would only fall to 54. In contrast, if a crossover design was used, the number of subjects needed to show the same systolic BP difference would be just 18 and 14, respectively, for clinic versus ambulatory BP measurements.

USEFULNESS OF AMBULATORY BP IN EVALUATING PATIENTS FOR ENTRY INTO A CLINICAL TRIAL OF AN ANTIHYPERTENSIVE DRUG

At the recruitment and enrollment phases of a clinical hypertension trial, current antihypertensive medication is discontinued, and "baseline" BPs and heart rates are obtained during a single-blind placebo period that generally lasts for 2–5 wk. Conventional inclusion criteria for these trials have been based on the supine or seated clinic systolic or diastolic BPs at the end of the single-blind placebo period. In recent years though, many protocols have also included ambulatory BP values as primary or secondary criteria for inclusion into the study. For example, it is not uncommon to require that the seated diastolic BP in the clinic exceed 90 or 95 mmHg and that the awake (or daytime) ambulatory BP exceed 85 or 90 mmHg. (1). The impact of various awake ambulatory BP values for exclusion of patients during the screening process can be fairly dramatic when the requirement for the office diastolic BP is 90 mmHg or greater. An example of this is shown in an analysis from a multicenter U.S. clinical trial (Fig. 1). In this study, a seated clinic diastolic BP of > 95 and < 115 mmHg was used as the criterion for entering and remaining in the single-blind portion of the trial. To progress into the double-blind randomized portion of the study, ambulatory BP values at certain thresholds were used. However, when using an ambulatory awake BP cut-off value of 85 mmHg, nearly 30% of the study group was excluded from randomization into the double-blind part of the trial. When 90 mmHg was the cutoff value for ambulatory diastolic pressure, over 50% of the group was excluded from randomization.

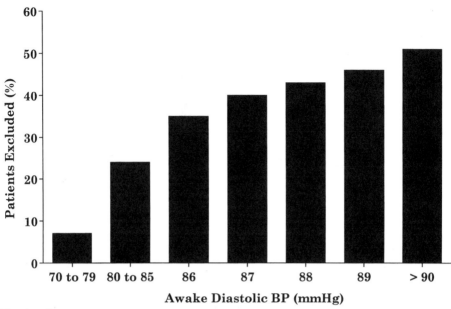

Fig. 1. Effects of patient recruitment using an office diastolic blood pressure > 90 mmHg and various awake ambulatory diastolic blood pressures as the selection criteria in antihypertensive drug trials. (Modified from Mansoor GA, White WB. J Cardiovasc Risk 1994;1: 136–142 with permission.)

The major reason for the high exclusion rate based on the ambulatory BP values compared to the office pressure is that a relatively high percentage of patients entering these trials have a "white coat" effect *(4,8,22)*. There has always been substantial ontroversy as to whether patients with "white coat" hypertension should be included or excluded from participation in clinical trials of antihypertensive drugs. The viewpoint of those favoring inclusion of the white coat hypertensive patients is that it is relevant to study their hemodynamic response to the new drug because it is likely that many patients with the white coat syndrome will have therapy prescribed by physicians who base treatment decisions solely on office BP measurements. Although not an unreasonable concern, there are a number of studies that have demonstrated that patients with white coat hypertension have minimal–to–no ambulatory BP responses by antihypertensive drugs *(23,24)* The typical compromise in recent years has been to include an intermediate cutoff BP entry value for ambulatory BP that is lower than the office BP entry criteria. By using the ambulatory BP criteria, less patients will be required in the randomized portion of the study, but the number of individuals screened in the single-blind period is typically increased *(1,10,19)*. Even in 2000, it remains commonplace to recruit about 130–140% of the required final number of evaluable patients to assure that the statistical power required to show the desired changes from baseline will be achieved.

MULTICENTER TRIALS
TO EVALUATE ANTIHYPERTENSIVE THERAPY

A multicenter trial is a clinical trial conducted simultaneously by several investigators working in different institutions but using the same protocol and identical methods in order to pool the data collected and analyze them together (25,26). Two key reasons for conducting multicenter hypertension studies over single-center studies is to enhance patient recruitment and to make the study group more "representative" of the entire patient population, as there may be unique or homogeneous local population characteristics from a single center.

In North America and Europe, sponsors of antihypertensive drug trials often select centers based on personal experience with the center, reputation for recruitment, and good study conduct, and, in some instances, the ability to analyze and report the results of the multicenter study. Often at issue is whether it is best to use a large number of centers with a small number of patients per center or a smaller number of centers with a larger number of patients per center. For a common disease such as hypertension it has generally been easier to standardize, to follow, and to motivate a small number of centers (i.e., 15–30) with a moderate number of patients (i.e., 10–20) per center. When the criteria for study entry become more complex (e.g., severe hypertension with left ventricular hypertrophy or certain ambulatory BP selection criteria), the general trend has been to use more centers and less patients per center. This may lead to problems with final analyses however, as the extreme situation of one to two patients in a center does not enable differentiating between a center-related effect and one related to the treatments.

Analyses of Multicenter Hypertension Trials:
Relevant Problems for Ambulatory Blood Pressure Recordings

There are several problems specific to multicenter hypertension trials, including those utilizing ambulatory BP measurements. First, there is the "center" factor: Incorporation of the center factor into the analysis improves the power of comparison of treatments. One can assess the variability among centers from the residual variability in order to improve the sensitivity in detecting differences between treatments. As mentioned earlier, if the sample size in some centers are very small, then these centers may be pooled into a large center. Second, it is important to evaluate whether the differences between treatment modalities vary outside of random fluctuations across all centers. If a major difference does exist, it may be proven statistically by performing a test of treatment-by-center interaction.

It is important to evaluate the causes of treatment by center interactions, as they may invalidate the principal findings of a study (27), including those using ambulatory BP monitoring. Some of the causes of treatment-by-center interactions are listed in Table 2. Differences in patient features from one center to another

Table 2

Causes of Treatment-by-Center Interactions in Multicenter Clinical Trials

Differences in patient features from one center to another

Abnormal frequency of protocol violations, losses to follow-up, or
noncompliancy in one or more centers

Outlier center (small number of "doubtful" cases)

Real variations of differences between treatments according to centers

Source: White WB, Walsh SJ. Blood Pressure Monit 1996;1:227–229.

may result in confounding of the results. An abnormal or unusual frequency of protocol violations, losses to follow-up, or noncompliant patients may occur in one or more centers. When this occurs, it may reflect poor adherence to the protocol or insufficient motivation of the investigators or study coordinators at these centers. For example, when a center has inexperienced or apathetic personnel involved in an ambulatory BP monitoring protocol, there may be excessive data loss during the recording period, poor correlation between cuff and device measurements, or inaccuracy with regard to drug dosing and recorder hookup times *(4,8,28)*.

Outlier centers, possibly because of a small number of doubtful cases, may decrease credibility concerning these data and also may cause a center effect. However, tests for outliers may be misleading in a large clinical trial. For example, if three or four centers are identified as outliers, it is possible that these are the clinics that are doing a good job while the others are not. Thus, statistical tests for outliers (which are essentially tests of homogeneity) must be used carefully and intelligently by the statisticians in charge of the final analyses. Finally, real variations of differences between treatments according to centers may occur and restrict the general applicability of the results.

Bias in a Multicenter Trial
Using Ambulatory Blood Pressure Monitoring

Bias enters into a multicenter trial through two primary mechanisms: selection bias and misclassification bias. An example of selection bias in an antihypertensive drug trial involving ambulatory BP monitoring might be recruiting a more severely hypertensive population to avoid inclusion of white coat hypertensives. Many investigators have learned to avoid screen failures (Fig. 1) (which has a possible financial impact on the center), so they will enroll either a patient with higher clinic pressures or one who has a "known" ambulatory BP from a previous trial. Misclassification bias in the multicenter trial is exemplified by clinic BP measurement error (e.g., using improper methodology for measurement) and may induce a center effect if untrained or inexperienced personnel are used. Whereas misclassification bias is probably uncommon in studies using experienced investigators and coordinators, many of the newer and ongoing large outcome trials are using centers inexperienced in performing clinical research in general and measurement error may end up being more prevalent.

Practical Concerns in the Conduct of Multicenter Trials That Use Ambulatory Blood Pressure Recorders

The use of ambulatory BP monitors in a clinical trial requires the availabilty of skilled, trained technicians. Multiple devices are necessary in order to complete a clinical trial in a timely fashion, to facilitate the scheduling of large numbers of participants, and to minimize the impact of mechanical problems when they occur. These requirements may increase study costs. An additional concern is the possibility that the data of some individuals may be excluded from analyses because of the poor quality of an ambulatory BP recording or to mechanical difficulties (29). Infrequently, the use of ambulatory BP monitoring may potentially hinder recruitment efforts because certain individuals may decline participation in a trial as a result of the perceived burden of wearing and returning a recorder. Appel et al. (29) have reported that patient recruitment efforts will improve when the technique is presented as a standard part of the study. Then, the expectation is that the ambulatory BP data collection is a primary part of the study as opposed to an optional or ancillary procedure.

IMPORTANCE OF THE PLACEBO EFFECT ON CLINIC VERSUS AMBULATORY BLOOD PRESSURE

It is standard practice to include a placebo group in clinical trials involving antihypertensive therapy, especially those studies that are considered dose ranging or "pivotal" ones during the earlier phases of drug development. Because of the substantial variability of office BP, most investigators have found it necessary to distinguish true drug effect from placebo effect in blood pressure trials. Several factors might create the placebo effect, including regression to the mean (30), the presence of a pressor response in the doctor's office (the white coat effect) (31,32), and expectations of the patient and the clinical observer (5).

In contrast to studies that employ the clinic pressure as the primary means to obtain the primary study end point, the placebo effect is either minimal or absent when ambulatory BP monitoring is used in antihypertensive drug trials (33–35). The lack of observed placebo effect on ambulatory BP is probably secondary to both the lack of observer bias and the increased number of BP values obtained over a 24-h study period. In contrast, ambulatory BP monitoring probably would not remove regression to the mean or other potential patient factors that contribute to the placebo effect. In fact, it is somewhat difficult to separate the regression to the mean effect from the placebo effect and the decrease in a white coat effect over time.

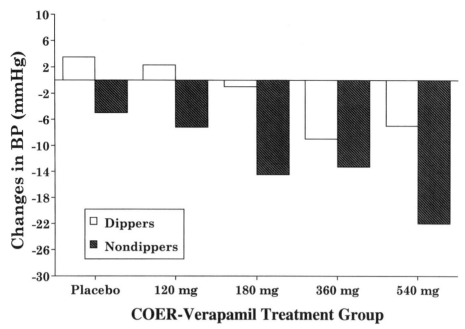

COER-Verapamil Treatment Group

Fig. 2. Changes in nocturnal (10 PM to 5 AM) BP from baseline measured by ambulatory BP monitoring in dippers (decline in mean BP from the daytime period to the nocturnal period was >10%) contrasted with changes in nocturnal BP in nondippers (<10% decline in nocturnal BP) on placebo and four doses of controlled-onset extended-release (COER) verapamil. (Modified from White WB, Mehrotra DV, Black HR, Fakouhi TD. Am J Cardiol 1997;80:469–474 with permission.)

This phenomenon of regression to the mean in an ambulatory BP monitoring study has been shown quite clearly in a recent study by White and colleagues *(36)*. In this trial, patients with hypertension were randomized to receive either placebo or controlled-onset extended-release (COER) verapamil for 8 wk after a 3- to 4-wk single-blind placebo baseline period. The patients were then divided into those patients whose BP fell by >10% during sleep compared to their awake values (dippers) and those whose BP fell by <10% during sleep (nondippers). In the nondipper patients randomized to receive placebo, nocturnal systolic BP fell by 4 mmHg compared to the first baseline study (also on placebo but during the single-blind period). In the dipper patients randomized to receive placebo, nocturnal systolic BP increased by about 4 mmHg compared to the baseline BP. Thus, the spread between the two types of patients in the placebo group for nocturnal pressure was nearly 8 mmHg (Fig. 2). The changes in nocturnal BP on active drug were also consistently greater across all doses and greater in nondippers compared to dippers. Thus, if this remarkable regression to the mean on placebo had not been accounted for, then the response to active treatment with COER verapamil in the dippers would have been substantially underestimated and the response in the nondippers would have been overestimated.

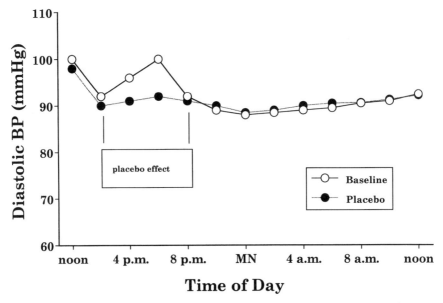

Fig. 3. Ambulatory diastolic blood pressures before and after 4 wk of placebo. The overall means were not significantly different; however, an effect of placebo was observed during the first 8 h after dosing. (Modified from Mutti E, Trazzi S, Omboni S, et al. J Hypertens 1991;9:361–366 with permission.)

In a study by Mutti and co-workers *(35)*, the office BP fell signficantly by 10/3 ± 3/2 mmHg following 4 wk of placebo administration, whereas the overall 24-h BP was unchanged. However, the ambulatory BP did fall slightly during the first 8 h of placebo administration (Fig. 3), which the authors attributed to the white coat effect. Of note is that this initial fall did not have a statistically effect on the overall mean BP.

In a much longer-term study by Staessen et al. *(37)* in older patients with isolated systolic hypertension, one treatment arm was randomized to placebo for 1 yr. Compared to the baseline period, the clinic systolic BP fell by 7 ± 16 mmHg on placebo and the 24-h systolic BP fell by just 2 ± 11 mmHg. Because the ambulatory BP has a superior repeatability index compared to the clinic pressure, the changes in 24-h systolic BP met statistical significance, whereas the larger mean reduction in clinic BP showed only a trend ($p = 0.06$). As this was a patient population with normal diastolic BP, there were no statistically significant changes in clinic or ambulatory diastolic BP on placebo therapy during this study. The authors also noted that the 24-h systolic BP was more likely to decrease on placebo if it was higher at baseline and if the follow-up was longer. The authors discounted regression to the mean or the white coat effect as having an impact on these placebo effects and recommended that long-term studies in older patients

Table 3
Methods for Evaluating Ambulatory Blood Pressure Data in Clinical Trials

24-Hour means (and standard deviation as a measure of variability)
Awake and sleep means based on patient diaries or activity recorders
Hourly means
Blood pressure load (proportion method)
Area under the blood pressure curve
Placebo-subtracted curves showing hourly means
Various data smoothing techniques (including cosinor analyses or fast Fourier
    transformation)
Modeling of 24-h curves

using noninvasive ambulatory BP monitoring should require a placebo-controlled design.

ANALYSES OF AMBULATORY BP DATA IN ANTIHYPERTENSIVE DRUG TRIALS

Data from ambulatory BP studies in hypertension trials may be analyzed in a number of ways (Table 3). A consensus regarding a superior, single method of analysis has never been reached despite numerous attempts by many committees in several countries. The use of 24-h means, daytime and nighttime means (or preferably awake and sleep values), blood pressure loads (the proportion of values above a cutoff value during wakefulness [>140/90 mmHg] or sleep [>120/80 mmHg] divided by the total number of BP readings), area under the 24-h BP curve, and smoothing techniques designed to remove some of the variability from the raw BP data analysis are among the most popularly utilized methods of analysis *(1–4,10,11)*.

Features of any method of analysis for ambulatory BP data should include the statistical ease of calculation, clinical relevance of the measure, and relationship of the parameter to the hypertensive disease process. Many of these analytic methods meet all of these criteria. For example, the 24-h mean BP remains an important parameter for evaluation in antihypertensive drug trials because it appears to be a strong predictor of hypertensive target organ disease *(2)*, is easy to calculate, utilizes all of the ambulatory BP data, and, as previously mentioned, is remarkably reproducible in both short-term *(6)* and long-term *(7)* studies.

The blood pressure load has been used as a simple method of analysis in evaluating the effects of antihypertensive drugs. Blood pressure load has been defined in our laboratory as the percentage of BPs exceeding 140/90 mmHg while the patient is awake plus the percentage of BPs exceeding 120/80 mmHg during sleep *(38)*. A number of years ago, we evaluated the relationship between this BP load and cardiac target organ indexes in previously untreated hypertensives. At a 40%

Table 4
Relationship Among Blood Pressure, Blood Pressure Load
(AUC Method), and Hemodynamic Indices in Untreated Hypertensive Patients

| | *Correlation coefficients* | |
BP measure	*TPRI* (*resting*)	*Stroke index* (*exercise*)
Clinic systolic BP	0.25	0.11
Clinic diastolic BP	0.31*	0.06
24-h systolic BP	0.53**	−0.27
24-h diastolic BP	0.48**	−0.25
140/120 mmHg systolic BP load	0.48**	−0.36**
90/80 mmHg diastolic BP load	0.56^	−0.56^

Note: TPRI = total peripheral resistance index. $*p < 0.05$; $**p < 0.01$; $^p < 0.001$.
Source: White WB, Lund-Johansen P, Weiss S, et al. J Hypertens 1994;12:1075–1081.

diastolic BP load, the incidence of left ventricular hypertrophy (LVH) was nearly 80%, but below a 40% diastolic BP load, the prevalence of LVH fell to about 8%. In contrast, the office BP and even the 24-h average BP were not as discriminating in predicting LVH in this group of previously untreated patients. Thus, in mild to moderately hypertensive patients, one would desire a low (conservatively, <30%) BP load while being treated with antihypertensive drug therapy.

In studies in which the patient population has a greater range in BP, the proportional (or percentage) BP load may become less useful. As the upper limit of the BP load is 100%, this value may represent a substantial number of individuals with broad ranges of moderate to severe hypertension. To overcome this problem, we devised a method to integrate the area under the ambulatory BP curve and relate its values to predicting hemodynamic indices in untreated essential hypertensives *(11)*. Areas under the BP curve were computed separately for periods of wakefulness and sleep and combined to form the 24-h area under the BP curve (AUC). Threshold values were used to calculate AUC such as 135 or 140 mmHg systolic while awake and 85 or 90 mmHg diastolic while awake. Values during sleep were reduced to 115 and 120 mmHg systolic and 75 and 80 mmHg diastolic.

The results of univariate regression studies of the casual, 24-h mean, and AUCs with the two most important hemodynamic indices, peripheral resistance and exercise stroke volume, are shown in Table 4. Both hemodynamic indices were significantly predicted by the AUC; hence, the data imply that these integrated AUCs could also be used to assess the extent of the hypertensive burden in antihypertensive therapeutic trials.

Smoothing of ambulatory BP data may be used to aid in the identification of the peak and trough effects of an antihypertensive drug. The extent of variability in an individual's BP curve may be large as a result of both mental and physical activity; thus, evaluating the peak antihypertensive effect of a short-acting or intermediate-acting drug may be difficult. Other than the benefits associated with examining pharmacodynamic effects of new antihypertensive drugs, data and curve smoothing for 24-h BP monitoring appear to have little clinical relevance. Furthermore, editing protocols are not uniform in the literature and missing data may alter the balance of mean values for shorter periods of time. To avoid excessive data reduction in a clinical trial, one statistical expert suggested that data smoothing should be performed on individual BP profiles rather than on group means *(39)*.

SITUATIONS IN WHICH AMBULATORY BP MONITORING HAS BEEN USEFUL IN ANTIHYPERTENSIVE DRUG TRIALS

Treating the White Coat Hypertensive Patient

The inclusion of white coat hypertensive patients in an antihypertensive drug trial that uses only office BP criteria for study entry will have a potentially confounding effect on efficacy, as these patients are not hypertensive outside of the medical care environment *(8,9,13,14)*. Furthermore, patients may develop excessive drug-induced side effects without much change in BP, especially if titration of the dose is based on office pressures.

In a study by Weber and colleagues *(24)*, a sustained fall in BP was found across a study group taking a long-acting form of diltiazem. In a subset of six patients who had hypertensive office BP readings but whose ambulatory BPs were normotensive (i.e,, a white coat hypertensive group), no significant ambulatory BP changes from placebo baseline (0/1 mmHg) were observed. In contrast, the diltiazem therapy decreased 24-h BPs by 18/13 mmHg in the subgroup of nine patients who were hypertensive by both office and ambulatory BP. Thus, treating white coat hypertensive patients may be of little to no benefit if the only place where BP reduction is observed is in the medical care environment.

Utility of Ambulatory Blood Pressure Monitoring in Dose-Finding Studies

Since the early 1990s, numerous studies have been performed with ambulatory BP monitoring to fully assess the efficacy of a wide range of doses of new antihypertensive agents. The advantage of ambulatory BP monitoring in dose-finding studies is related in part to the improved statistical power to show differences among the treatment groups compared to clinic pressures. Examples are shown below.

EPROSARTAN

To determine the dose responsiveness of a new angiotensin II receptor antagonist eprosartan during phase II of development, we studied the drug at doses of

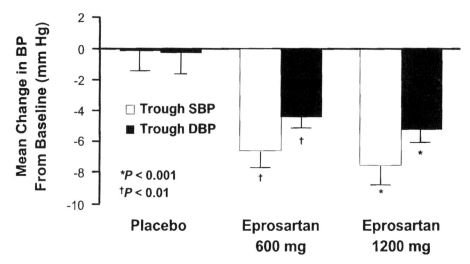

Fig. 4. Changes in trough ambulatory blood pressure (last 4 h of the 24-h dosing period) following 4 wk treatment with once-daily dosing of the angiotensin II receptor blocking agent eprosartan. *p*-Values contrast drug effects versus placebo effects. (Data derived from White WB, Anwar YA, Sica DA, Dubb J. Am J Hypertens 1999;12:27A.)

100, 200, 300, and 400 mg daily (in twice-daily divided doses) using ambulatory BP monitoring *(40)*. Compared to placebo, only the 400-mg daily dose showed consistently significant reductions in ambulatory systolic and diastolic BP. These findings led to the use of higher doses in the phase III clinical development program and a larger once-daily trial using 600 and 1200 mg once daily versus placebo *(41)*. As shown in Fig. 4, the trough BP (last 4 h of the dosing period) changes from baseline were significantly greater than placebo for both doses of the drug with a trend for greater reductions on 1200 mg versus 600 mg once daily. When assessing the changes from baseline using the *clinic* BPs, the differences for 1200 mg versus 600 mg once daily against placebo were not significant.

EPLERENONE

The efficacy of a novel selective aldosterone receptor antagonist, eplerenone, was studied in 417 patients with essential hypertension using a multicenter, randomized, placebo-controlled design *(42)*. In this trial, the drug was assessed using either a once-daily dosing regimen of 50, 100, or 400 mg or a twice-daily dosing regimen of 25 mg, 50 mg, or 200 mg. Clinic and ambulatory BPs were compared to both baseline values and to the effects of placebo. As shown in Fig. 5, there was a dose-related reduction in systolic BP at the trough for both clinic and ambulatory BP (similar results were seen for the changes in diastolic BP). Twice-daily dosing of eplerenone led to greater reductions in BP compared to the once-daily dosing regimen, but these differences were not statistically significant.

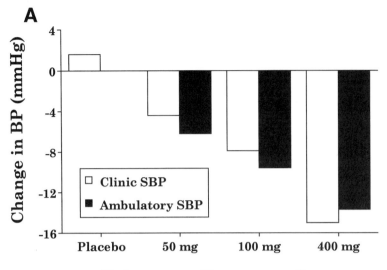

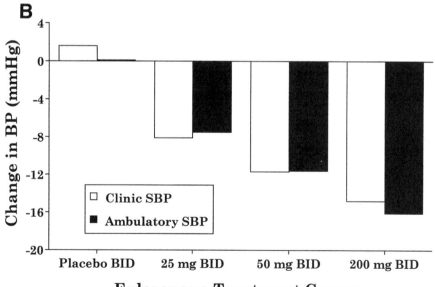

Fig. 5. Changes from baseline in ambulatory versus clinic systolic blood pressure in a dose-ranging trial with a selective aldosterone antagonist, eplerenone. Panel A shows the effects of once-daily dosing; panel B shows the effects of twice-daily dosing. (Data derived from Epstein M, Menard J, Alexander J, Roniker B. Circulation 1998;98(17):I98–I99.)

Utility of Ambulatory Blood Pressure Monitoring in Comparator Trials

Ambulatory BP monitoring has been very helpful in comparing antihypertensive drugs, especially when assessing duration of action. There are numerous examples in the literature that now illustrate this benefit, including the superiority of ambulatory BP over clinic BP in assessing the trough-to-peak ratio of various agents *(43)*.

COMPARISONS WITHIN THE SAME CLASS

In a recent multicenter study, Neutel et al. *(44)* compared the β-blockers bisoprolol and atenolol in 606 patients using both clinic and ambulatory BP. Following therapy, trough BP in the clinic was reduced 12/12 mmHg by bisoprolol and 11/12 mmHg by atenolol. Although these changes were significantly different from baseline therapy, there were no differences when comparing the effects of each drug. In contrast, daytime systolic and diastolic BPs (6 AM to 10 PM) and the last 4 h of the dosing interval (6 AM to 10 AM) were lowered significantly greater by bisoprolol than by atenolol. This finding was present whether the assessment was made by examination of the overall means, area under the curve, or BP loads. These data demonstrated that despite there being no difference in office BP, bisoprolol had significant differences in efficacy and duration of action compared with atenolol when assessed by 24-h BP monitoring.

The antihypertensive efficacy of the selective angiotensin II receptor antagonists telmisartan and losartan were compared with placebo in randomized, parallel group, double-blind trial of 223 patients with stage II and III hypertension *(45)*. After 4 wk of single-blind placebo baseline treatment, patients were randomized to receive 40 mg telmisartan, 80 mg telmisartan, 50 mg losartan, or placebo once daily. Based on clinic BP measurements, the reductions in trough BP were 14/9 mmHg on the lower dose of telmisartan and 16/10 mmHg on the higher dose of telmisartan, whereas on losartan, BP fell by 10/6 mmHg. Changes in BP induced by the 80-mg dose of telmisartan were significantly greater than the reductions in BP observed with losartan. Ambulatory BP monitoring after 6 wk showed that both telmisartan and losartan produced significant reductions from baseline in 24-h mean BP compared to placebo. As shown in Fig. 6, during the 18- to 24-h period after dosing, the reductions in systolic BP with telmisartan (−10.7 mmHg) and 80 mg (−12.2 mmHg) were each significantly greater than the changes observed for losartan (−6 mmHg). Thus, ambulatory BP monitoring was able to discern differences in the low dose of telmisartan and losartan, whereas the clinic BP was not able to consistently show these changes. The ability of ambulatory BP monitoring to statistically reveal these smaller changes between treatment groups compared to clinic BP is most likely related to the lower variance that occurs with repeated ambulatory BP studies compared to repeated clinic BP *(1,6,19)*.

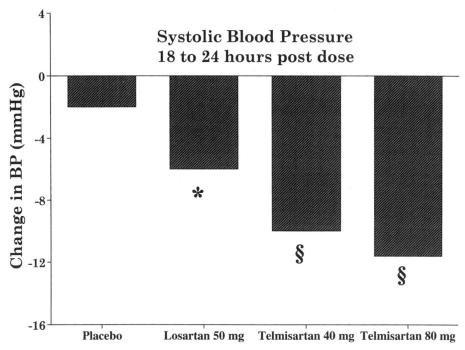

Fig. 6. Adjusted changes from baseline in mean blood pressure for the 18- to 24-h postdose period as measured by ambulatory BP monitoring on two doses (40 and 80 mg) of the angiotensin II receptor blockers telmisartan and 50 mg of losartan. *$p < 0.05$ versus placebo; §$p < 0.05$ compared with losartan and placebo. (Modified from Mallion JM, Siche JP, Lacourciere Y. J Hum Hypertens 1999;13:657–664 with permission.)

COMPARISONS OF DRUGS IN DIFFERENT CLASSES

In a study performed by LaCourciere and co-workers in Canada *(46)*, the angiotensin II receptor blocker telmisartan (doses of 40–120 mg once daily) was compared to the long-acting calcium antagonist amlodipine (5–10 mg once daily) in a clinical trial that used 24-h ambulatory BP monitoring at baseline and following 12 wk of double-blind treatment. Although both of these agents have similar plasma half-lives close to 24 h, they have entirely different mechanisms of action. This bears relevance because it is known that as BP and heart rate fall during sleep, plasma renin activity gradually increases. In the morning upon awakening, the sympathethic nervous system is activated, which enhances renin secretion from the juxtaglomerular apparatus in the kidney. Thus, the renin–angiotensin–aldosterone system is further activated in the early morning upon awakening, increasing the contribution of angiotensin to the postawakening surge in BP.

Both amlodipine and telmisartan lowered *clinic* BP to similar extents at the end of the dosing period. However, reductions in ambulatory diastolic BP with

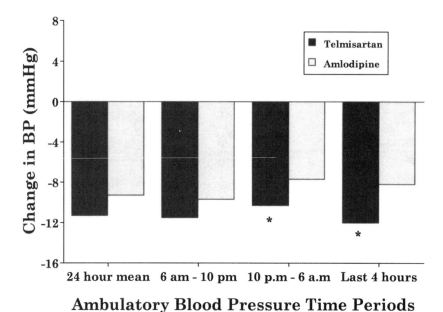

Ambulatory Blood Pressure Time Periods

Fig. 7. Mean changes from baseline in 24-h ambulatory diastolic blood pressure on the angiotensin II receptor blocker telmisartan (doses of 40–120 mg once daily) and the calcium antagonist amlodipine (doses of 5–10 mg once daily). *$p < 0.05$ versus amlodipine. (Modified from Lacourciere Y, Lenis J, Orchard R, et al. Blood Pressure Monit 1998;3:295–302 with permission.)

telmisartan were greater than those with amlodipine during the nighttime as well as during the last 4 h of the dosing interval (Fig. 7). In addition, the ambulatory BP control rates (24-h diastolic BP < 85 mmHg) were higher following telmisartan treatment (71%) than following amlodipine (55%). Thus, these findings serve as additional data that demonstrate the improved ability of ambulatory monitoring of the BP to discern pharmacodynamic changes between two drugs with relatively similar pharmacokinetic profiles.

USE OF AMBULATORY MONITORING TO ASSESS THE EFFECTS OF CHRONOTHERAPEUTIC AGENTS

Chronotherapeutics is a term that was infrequently used in the clinical hypertension and cardiovascular literature until recently. In general, chronotherapeutics attempts to match the effects of a drug to the timing of the disease being treated or prevented *(47–49)*. In the case of hypertension and coronary artery disease, this imparts a great deal of clinical relevance because BP and heart rate have distinct, reproducible circadian rhythms. In most patients, the BP and heart rate are lowest during sleep and highest during the day. As noted previously by

Table 5
Daytime and Nighttime Blood Pressure and Heart Rate
After Placebo Administration and at the End of Two Regimens
of 20 mg of Quinapril (8 AM vs 10 PM Dosing Times)

Parameter	Placebo	Morning quinapril	Evening quinapril
Daytime SBP (mmHg)	154 ± 16	138 ± 16	137 ± 14
Daytime DBP (mmHg)	101 ± 7	89 ± 9	90 ± 9
Nighttime SBP (mmHg)	140 ± 15	132 ± 20	127 ± 18**
Nighttime DBP (mmHg)	90 ± 7	83 ± 10	81 ± 9*
24-h heart rate (beats/min)	73 ± 9	71 ± 10	72 ± 8

Note: SBP = systolic BP; DBP = diastolic BP.

$*p < 0.05$ versus morning administration; $**p < 0.01$ versus morning administration.

Source: Modified from Palatini et al. *(56)*, with permission.

several authors in this volume, most cardiovascular diseases, including myocardial infarction *(50)*, angina and myocardial ischemia *(51)*, and stroke *(52)* have circadian patterns that are all characterized by the highest incidences in the early morning hours.

Timing of Drug Administration

The approach for the chronotherapy of hypertension and angina pectoris differs from conventional "homeostatic" treatments that deliver medication to achieve a constant effect, regardless of the circadian rhythm of BP *(53–55)*. Several authors have made attempts to alter the effects of conventional drugs by dosing them prior to sleep versus upon arising *(56–59)*. In one of these studies *(56)*, the angiotensin-converting enzyme inhibitor quinapril was dosed in the early morning versus at bedtime in 18 moderately hypertensive patients. The study was conducted in a double-blind crossover design with quinapril dosed at either 8 AM or 10 PM for 4 wk in each period. Ambulatory BP monitoring was carried out before and at the end of each 4-wk double-blind period. As shown in Table 5, daytime BP was reduced similarly by both dosing regimens. In contrast, nighttime systolic and diastolic BP was decreased to a significantly greater extent with the evening administration of quinapril. Measurement of ACE activity showed that evening administration of quinapril induced a more sustained decline in plasma ACE but not a more pronounced change. The findings in this study are of substantial interest because nocturnal BP has largely been ignored in the past *(60)*, and in many types of hypertensive patients, the BP during sleep may remain unknowingly elevated despite "normal" BP in the doctor's office.

Other studies *(57–59)* show that little change in BP or heart rate occurs by altering the dosing time of these long-acting agents to nighttime. However, most of the studies have small sample sizes and had low statistical power to show changes less than 5–10 mmHg in ambulatory BP. Thus, whether or not altering the dosing time of a long-acting antihypertensive agent truly changes the level of ambulatory BP has not been shown with any great degree of confidence.

Specific Chronotherapeutic Delivery Systems

There are two delivery systems specifically developed for the chronotherapeutic delivery of antihypertensive therapy; these are the controlled-onset extended-release (COER) delivery system *(53–55)* and the chronotherapeutic oral drug absorption system (CODAS) delivery system *(61)* and both use verapamil HCl as the active agent. In the first case, the COER verapamil system has been extensively studied and approved for the treatment of hypertension and angina pectoris; in the latter case, the CODAS verapamil system has been studied and approved for hypertension.

In a large multicenter ($n = 51$ centers and 557 patients), randomized, double-blind clinical trial, the effects of COER verapamil administered at bedtime were compared with a conventional homeostatic therapy [nifedipine gastrointestinal therapeutic GITS)] taken in the morning, on early morning BP, heart rate, and the heart rate–systolic BP product *(54)*. Changes in the early morning BP were similar for the two treatment arms. However, changes in the rate–pressure product were significantly greater following COER verapamil therapy versus nifedipine GITs (Fig. 8) (−1437 beats/min-mmHg vs −703 beats/min-mmHg, respectively; $p < 0.001$). These findings may be of clinical importance in hypertensive patients, especially those who have increased risk of coronary disease, as epidemiologic analyses show that heart rate is an independent predictor of cardiovascular risk in patients with hypertension *(62)*. Furthermore, the reduction in the rate–pressure product, an index of myocardial oxygen demand, may benefit patients whose increased rate–pressure product increases their risk for myocardial ischemia, as shown by Deedwania and Nelson *(63)*.

In patients with chronic stable angina pectoris, the effects of COER verapamil on silent myocardial ischemia compared to the dihydropyridine calcium antagonist amlodipine alone and in combination with the β-blocker, atenolol was assessed using 48-h Holter monitoring studies *(55)*. During the 6-h time interval of 6 AM to noon, the average total duration of ischemia was found to be significantly greater in the amlodipine monotherapy and placebo-treatment groups compared to COER verapamil and the combination of amlodipine and atenolol (Fig. 9).

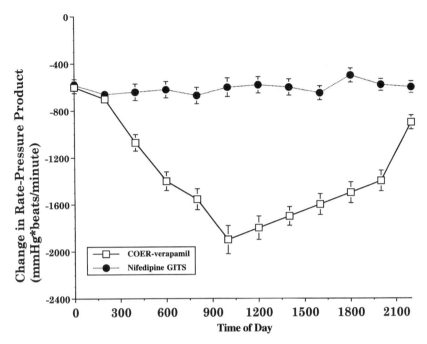

Fig. 8. Changes from baseline in the 24-h rate–pressure product after administration of the calcium antagonists nifedipine GITS given in the morning or COER verapamil given at bedtime. Treatment studies were performed after 4 wk of stable therapy. (Modified from White WB, Black HR, Weber MA, et al. Am J Cardiol 1998;81:424–431 with permission.)

Analyses of heart rate data from the Holter monitoring studies showed that amlodipine patients clearly had higher early morning heart rates than patients in the placebo group. Furthermore, COER verapamil and atenolol induced significant reductions in ambulatory heart rate compared to both placebo and amlodipine throughout the dosing period.

These two large clinical trials with chronotherapeutic delivery of a calcium antagonist suggest pharmacologic benefit beyond what is typically observed for this class of drugs in hypertension and angina pectoris. However, to further evaluate the long-term effect of this type of chronotherapy, a large, randomized, prospective parallel-group international trial involving over 16,000 older patients with hypertension has been initiated *(64)*. The Controlled Onset Verapamil Investigation of Cardiovascular Endpoints (CONVINCE) Trial will compare the incidence of fatal or nonfatal myocardial infarction, fatal or nonfatal stroke, or cardiovascular disease related death in two antihypertensive treatment regimens: (1) the bedtime dosing of COER verapamil versus (2) morning dosing of either the diuretic hydrochlorothiazide or the β-blocker atenolol. This study is expected to determine whether there is equivalence between these two treatment strategies for the primary prevention of cardiovascular morbidity and mortality

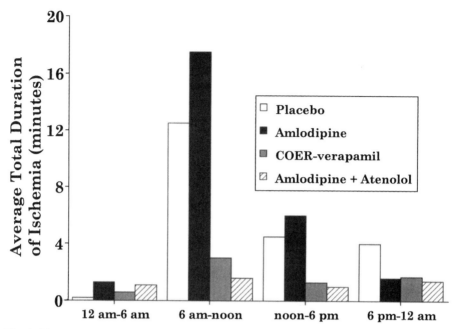

Fig. 9. The average total duration of myocardial ischemia (in minutes) during 48-h Holter monitoring of patients with chronic stable angina pectoris. Studies were performed after 4 wk of placebo versus the calcium antagonists amlodipine and COER verapamil, and the combination of amlodipine and the β-blocker atenolol. (Modified from Frishman W, Glasser S, Stone P. Am J Cardiol 1999;83(4):507–514 with permission.)

in patients with hypertension. Furthermore, we hope to determine whether the timing of events can be altered and whether the incidence of early morning myocardial infarctions and stroke may be reduced.

CONCLUSIONS

The data from the past 15–20 yr of clinical trials now overwhelmingly support the usefulness of ambulatory BP monitoring in the assessment and development of new antihypertensive drugs. First, there are numerous reports that show that ambulatory BP is a powerful, independent predictor of cardiovascular morbidity (13–18). Additionally, several studies also show that ambulatory BP monitoring has excellent potential as a tool to aid in the management of hypertension (65,66), including determining whether the initation, adjustment, and withdrawal of antihypertensive treatment should be considered (67). Finally, based on most analyses (67,68), ambulatory monitoring of the BP is, at worst, cost-neutral and should become cost-effective in most countries when used for the appropriate clinical diagnoses and if charged at reasonable costs.

REFERENCES

1. Mansoor GA, White WB. Contribution of ambulatory blood pressure monitoring to the design and analysis of antihypertensive therapy trials. J Cardiovasc Risk 1994;1:136–142.
2. Mansoor GA, White WB. Ambulatory blood pressure and cardiovascular risk stratification. J Vasc Med Biol 1994;5:61–68.
3. White WB. The role of ambulatory monitoring of the blood pressure for assessment of antihypertensive agents. J Clin Pharmacol 1992;32:524–528.
4. White WB, Morganroth J. Usefulness of ambulatory monitoring of the blood pressure in assessing antihypertensive therapy. Am J Cardiol 1989;63:94–98.
5. Bruce NG, Shaper A, Walker M, Wannamethee G. Observer bias in blood pressure studies. J Hypertens 1988;6:375–378.
6. James GD, Pickering TG, Yee LS, et al. The reproducibility of average, ambulatory, home, and clinic pressures. Hypertension 1988;11:545–549.
7. Mansoor GA, McCabe EJ, White WB. Long-term reproducibility of ambulatory blood pressure. J Hypertens 1994;12:703–708.
8. Pickering TG, James GD, Boddie C, et al. How common is white-coat hypertension? JAMA 1988;259:225–228.
9. White WB. Assessment of patients with office hypertension by 24-hour noninvasive ambulatory blood pressure monitoring. Arch Intern Med 1986;146:2196–2199.
10. White WB. Methods of blood pressure determination to assess antihypertensive agents: are casual measurements enough? Clin Pharmacol Ther 1989;45:581–586.
11. White WB, Lund-Johansen P, Weiss S, et al. The relationships between casual and ambulatory blood pressure measurements and central hemodynamics in essential human hypertension. J Hypertens 1994;12:1075–1081.
12. Shimada K, Kawamoto A, Matsubayashi K, et al. Silent cerebrovascular disease in the elderly: correlation with ambulatory blood pressure. Hypertension 1990;16:692–697.
13. White WB, Schulman P, McCabe EJ, et al. Average daily blood pressure, not office blood pressure, determines cardiac function in patients with hypertension. JAMA 1989;261:873–877.
14. Perloff D, Sokolow M, Cowan RM. Prognostic value of ambulatory blood pressures. JAMA 1983;249:2792–2798.
15. Verdecchia P, Porcellati C, Schillaci G, et al. Ambulatory blood pressure: an independent predictor of prognosis in essential hypertension. Hypertension 1994;24:793–801.
16. Redon J, Campos C, Narciso ML, Rodicio JL, Pascual JM, Ruilope LM. Prognostic value of ambulatory blood pressure monitoring in refractory hypertension: a prospective study. Hypertension 1998;31:712–718.
17. Khattar RS, Senior R, Lahiri A. Cardiovascular outcome in white-coat versus sustained mild hypertension: a 10-year followup study. Circulation 1998;98:1892–1897.
18. Staessen JA, Fagard R, Thijs L, O'Brien ET, Clement D, de Leeuw PW, et al. Predicting cardiovascular risk using conventional vs ambulatory blood pressure in older patients with systolic hypertension. JAMA 1999;282:539–546.
19. Conway J, Johnston J, Coats A, Somers V, Sleight P. The use of ambulatory blood pressure monitoring to improve the accuracy and to reduce the number of subjects in clinical trials of antihypertensive agents. J Hypertens 1988;6:111–116.
20. Mancia G, Omboni S, Parati G, et al. Limited reproducibility of hourly blood pressure values obtained by ambulatory blood pressure monitoring: implications for studies of antihypertensive drugs. J Hypertens 1992;10:1531.
21. Staessen JA, Thijs L, Clement D, et al. Ambulatory blood pressure decreases on long-term placebo treatment in older patients with isolated systolic hypertension. J Hypertens 1994;12:1035–1041.

22. Gradman AH, Pangan P, Germain M. Lack of correlation between clinic and 24-hour ambulatory blood pressure in subjects participating in a therapeutic drug trial. J Clin Epidemiol 1989; 42:1049–1054.

23. Myers MG, Reeves RA. White coat phenomenon in patients receiving antihypertensive therapy. Am J Hypertens 1991;4:844–848.

24. Weber MA, Cheung DG, Graettinger WF, et al. Characterization of antihypertensive therapy by whole-day blood pressure monitoring. JAMA 1988;259:3281–3285.

25. Sylvester RJ, Pinedo HM, De Pauw M, et al. Quality of institutional participation in multicenter clinical trials. N Engl J Med 1981;305:852–855.

26. Meinert CL. Toward more definitive clinical trials. Control Clin Trials 1980;1:249–261.

27. Spriet A, Dupin-Spriet T, Simon P. Methodology of Clinical Drug Trials, 2nd ed. Karger, Basel, 1994, pp. 140–147.

28. White WB, Walsh SJ. Ambulatory monitoring of the blood pressure in multicenter clinical trials. Blood Pressure Monitor 1996;1:227–229.

29. Appel LJ, Marwaha S, Whelton PK, Patel M. The impact of automated blood pressure devices on the efficiency of clinical trials. Control Clin Trials 1992;13:240–247.

30. McDonald CJ, Mazzuca SA, McCabe GP. How much of the placebo effect is really statistical regression? Stat Med 1983;2:417–424.

31. Mancia G, Grassi G, Pomidossi G, et al. Effects of blood pressure measurement by the doctor on the patient's blood pressure and heart rate. Lancet 1983;2:196–199.

32. Mansoor GA, McCabe EJ, White WB. Determinants of the white-coat effect in hypertensive patients. J Human Hypertens 1996;10:87–92.

33. Bottini PB, Carr AA, Rhoades RB, et al. Variability of indirect methods used to determine blood pressure. Arch Intern Med 1992;152:139–145.

34. Dupont AG, van der Niepen P, Six RO. Placebo does not lower ambulatory blood pressure. Br J Clin Pharmacol 1987;24:106–110.

35. Mutti E, Trazzi S, Omboni S, et al. Effect of placebo on 24-h noninvasive ambulatory blood pressure. J Hypertens 1991;9:361–366.

36. White WB, Mehrotra DV, Black HR, Fakouhi TD. Effects of controlled-onset extended release verapamil on nocturnal blood pressure (dippers versus nondipper). Am J Cardiol 1997; 80:469–474.

37. Staessen JA, Thijs L, Mancia G, Parati G, O'Brien ET. Clinical trials with ambulatory blood pressure monitoring: fewer patients needed? Lancet 1994;344:1552–1554.

38. White WB, Dey HM, Schulman P. Assessment of the daily blood pressure load as a determinant of cardiac function in patients with mild to moderate hypertension. Am Heart J 1989;118: 782–795.

39. Dickson D, Hasford J. Twenty-four hour blood pressure measurement in antihypertensive drug trials: data requirements and methods of analysis. Stat Med 1992;11:2147–2157.

40. White WB, McCabe EJ, Mansoor GA. Comparison of office and ambulatory blood pressure measurements to assess the angiotensin II receptor antagonist eprosartan. Blood Pressure Monit 1996;1:45–50.

41. White WB, Anwar YA, Sica DA, Dubb J. Once-daily effects of the angiotensin receptor blocker, eprosartan on 24-hour blood pressure in patients with systemic hypertension. Am J Hypertens 1999;12:27A (abstract).

42. Epstein M, Menard J, Alexander J, Roniker B. Eplerenone, a novel and selective aldosterone receptor antagonist: efficacy in patients with mild to moderate hypertension. Circulation 1998; 98(17):I98–I99 (abstract).

43. White WB. Relevance of the trough-to-peak ratio to 24 hour blood pressure load. Am J Hypertens 1996;9:91s–96s.

44. Neutel JM, Smith DHG, Ram CVS, et al. Application of ambulatory blood pressure monitoring in differentiating between antihypertensive agents. Am J Med 1993;94, 181–186.

45. Mallion JM, Siche JP, Lacourciere Y. ABPM comparison of the antihypertensive profiles of the selective angiotensin II receptor antagonists telmisartan and losartan in patients with mild-to-moderate hypertension. J Hum Hypertens 1999;13:657–664.
46. Lacourciere Y, Lenis J, Orchard R, Lewanczuk R, Houde M, Pesant Y, et al. A comparison of the efficacies and duration of action of the angiotensin II receptor blocker telmisartan and amlodipine. Blood Pressure Monit 1998;2:295–302.
47. Smolensky MH, D'Alonzo GD. Medical chronobiology: concepts and applications. Am Rev Resp Dis 1993;147:S2–S19.
48. Straka RJ, Benson SR. Chronopharmacologic considerations when treating the patient with hypertension: a review. J Clin Pharmacol 1996;36:771–782.
49. White WB. A chronotherapeutic approach to the management of hypertension. Am J Hypertens 1996;10:29s–33s.
50. Muller JE, Tofler GH, Stone PH. Circadian variation and triggers of onset of acute cardiovascular disease. Circulation 1989;79:733–743.
51. Waters DD, Miller DD, Bouchard A, Bosch X, Theroux P. Circadian variation in variant angina. Am J Cardiol 1984;54:61–64.
52. Marler JR, Price TR, Clark GL, Muller JE, Robertson T, Mohr JP, et al. Morning increase in the onset of ischemic stroke. Stroke 1989;20:473–476.
53. White WB, Anders RJ, MacIntyre JM, Black HR, Sica DA. Nocturnal dosing of a novel delivery system of verapamil for systemic hypertension. Am J Cardiol 1995;76:375–380.
54. White WB, Black HR, Weber MA, Elliott WJ, Bryzinski B, Fakouhi TD. Comparison of effects of controlled onset extended release verapamil at bedtime and nifedipine gastrointestinal therapeutic system on arising on early morning blood pressure, heart rate, and the heart rate–blood pressure product. Am J Cardiol 1998;81:424–431.
55. Frishman WH, Glasser S, Stone P, Deedwania PC, Johnson M, Fakouhi TD. Comparison of controlled-onset extended release verapamil to amlodipine and amlodipine plus atenolol on exercise performance and ambulatory ischemia in patients with chronic stable angina pectoris. Am J Cardiol 1999;83(4):507–514.
56. Palatini P, Racioppa A, Raule G, et al. Effect of timing of administration on the plasma ACE inhibitor activity and the antihypertensive effect of quinapril. Clin Pharmacol Ther 1992;52: 378–383.
57. Lemmer B. Differential effects of antihypertensive drugs on circadian rhythm in blood pressure from a chronobiologic point of view. Blood Pressure Monit 1996;1:161–169.
58. Mengden T, Binswanger B, Gruene S. Dynamics of drug compliance and 24 hour blood pressure control of once daily morning versus evening amlodipine. J Hypertens 1992;10(Suppl 4): S136–S142.
59. White WB, Mansoor GA, Pickering TG, Vidt DG, Hutchinson HG, Johnson RB, et al. Differential effects of morning versus evening dosing of nisoldipine ER on circadian blood pressure and heart rate. Am J Hypertens 1999;12:806–814.
60. White WB, Mansoor GA, Tendler BE, Anwar YA. Nocturnal blood pressure: epidemiology, determinants, and effects of antihypertensive therapy. Blood Pressure Monit 1998;3:43–52.
61. Neutel JM, Smith DHG, Weber MA. The use of chronotherapeutics to achieve maximal blood pressure reduction during the early morning blood pressure surge, pending.
62. Gillman MW, Kannel WB, Belanger A, D'Agostino RB. Influence of heart rate on mortality among persons with hypertension: the Framingham study. Am Heart J 1993;125:1148–1154.
63. Deedwania PC, Nelson JR. Pathophysiology of silent myocardial ischemia during daily life: hemodynamic evaluation by simultaneously electrocardiographic and blood pressure monitoring. Circulation 1990;82:1296–1304.
64. Black HR, Elliott WJ, Neaton JD, Grandits G, Grambsch P, Grimm RH, et al. Rationale and design for the controlled onset verapamil investigation of cardiovascular endpoints (CONVINCE) Trial. Control Clin Trials 1998;19:370–390.

65. Grin JM, McCabe EJ, White WB. Management of hypertension after ambulatory blood pressure monitoring. Ann Intern Med 1993;118:833–837.
66. Pickering TG, Kaplan NM, Krakoff L, Prisant LM, Sheps SG, Weber MA, et al. American Society of Hypertension Expert Panel: conclusions and recommendations on the clinical use of home (self) and ambulatory blood pressure monitoring. Am J Hypertens 1995;9:1–11.
67. Staessen JA, Byttebier G, Buntinx F, Celis H, O'Brien ET, Fagard R. Antihypertensive treatment based on conventional or ambulatory blood pressure measurement. JAMA 1997;278:1065–1072.
68. Khoury S, Yarows SA, O'Brien TK. Ambulatory BP monitoring in a nonacademic setting: effects of age and sex. Am J Hypertens 1992;5:616–620.

INDEX

About the Editor

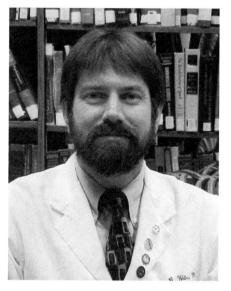

Dr. William White has been a Professor in the Department of Medicine and Chief of the Section of Hypertension and Clinical Pharmacology at the University of Connecticut School of Medicine for nearly 20 years. In addition, he is an attending physician at the John Dempsey Hospital in Farmington, Connecticut and a consulting physician in hypertension and vascular diseases at the Newington V. A. Medical Center (Newington, CT) and the Connecticut Children's Medical Center (Hartford).

After receiving his medical degree from the Medical College of Georgia, Dr. White completed his residency and chief residency at the University of Connecticut Consortium Hospitals in the greater Hartford area. Dr. White also completed a research fellowship in cardiovascular pharmacology at the University of Bergen in Norway under the leadership of Professor Per Lund-Johansen. Dr. White is U.S. board certified in both internal medicine and clinical pharmacology.

Dr. White is a Fellow of the American College of Physicians, the Council for High Blood Pressure Research of the American Heart Association, and the International Society for Hypertension in Blacks and a charter member of the American Society of Hypertension.

Dr. White has a long-standing interest in clinical hypertension, ambulatory blood pressure monitoring, and clinical trials of antihypertensive drugs. In 1981, he founded a hypertension unit at the University of Connecticut Health Center that included a faculty consultant practice as well as a clinical trials unit. He is the author or coauthor of over 230 articles and book chapters in the field of hypertension and clinical pharmacology.

In 1996, Dr. White developed the peer-reviewed, international journal *Blood Pressure Monitoring,* which is devoted to original research in the area of blood pressure measurement and variability. The journal is entering its 4th year of publication and has recently been indexed on EMBASE/Excerpta Medica and MEDLINE. He also serves on numerous editorial boards including the *American Journal of Hypertension, American Journal of Cardiology, American Journal of Medicine, Clinical Pharmacology and Therapeutics, Journal of Human Hypertension,* and the *American Journal of Clinical Hypertension.*